The NEW ENGLAND
JOURNAL of MEDICINE

Clinical Problem-Solving

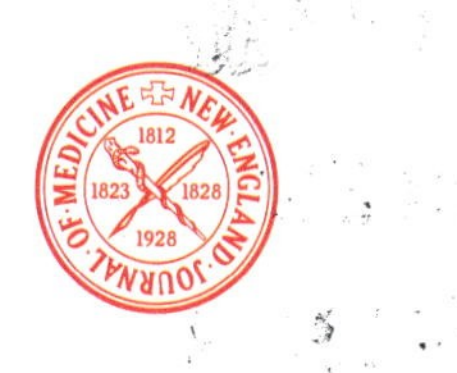

EDITED BY
SANJAY SAINT, M.D., M.P.H., JEFFREY M. DRAZEN, M.D.,
& CAREN G. SOLOMON, M.D., M.P.H.

McGraw-Hill
Medical Publishing Division

New York Chicago San Francisco Lisbon London Madrid
Mexico City Milan New Delhi San Juan Seoul Singapore Sydney Toronto

The McGraw-Hill Companies

Clinical Problem-Solving

1 2 3 4 5 6 7 8 9 0 DOC/DOC 0 9 8 7 6

ISBN 0-07-147162-6

NOTICE

Medicine is an ever-changing science. As new research and clinical experience broaden our knowledge, changes in treatment and drug therapy are required. The authors and the publisher of this work have checked with sources believed to be reliable in their efforts to provide information that is complete and generally in accord with the standards accepted at the time of publication. However, in view of the possibility of human error or changes in medical sciences, neither the authors nor the publisher nor any other party who has been involved in the preparation or publication of this work warrants that the information contained herein is in every respect accurate or complete, and they disclaim all responsibility for any errors or omissions or for the results obtained from use of the information contained in this work. Readers are encouraged to confirm the information contained herein with other sources. For example and in particular, readers are advised to check the product information sheet included in the package of each drug they plan to administer to be certain that the information contained in this work is accurate and that changes have not been made in the recommended dose or in the contraindications for administration. This recommendation is of particular importance in connection with new or infrequently used drugs.

This book is printed on acid-free paper.

The editors wish to thank the editorial, production and publishing staffs of the Journal *for their cheerful diligence in producing this volume. Their work was accomplished in the face of the unrelenting demands of a weekly publication.*

CLINICAL PROBLEM-SOLVING

Contents

CONTRIBUTORS

Thomas Bashore, MD
Duke University Medical Center
Durham, NC

Stephen Bent, MD
University of California, San Francisco
San Francisco, CA

Sandra Bliss, MD
Johns Hopkins University School of Medicine
Baltimore, MD

Peter Clarke, MD
John H. Stroger Hospital of Cook County
and Rush University
Chicago, IL

Michael D. Christian, MD
McMaster University
Hamilton, Ontario, Canada

Harold R. Collard, MD
University of California, San Francisco
San Francisco, CA

Paul B. Cornia, MD
VA Puget Sound Health Care System
and University of Washington
Seattle, WA

David A. DeGuzman, MD
University of Michigan
Ann Arbor, MI

Allan S. Detsky, MD, PhD
University of Toronto
Toronto, Ontario, Canada

Gurpreet Dhaliwal, MD
University of California, San Francisco
San Francisco, CA

Robert S. Dittus, MD, MPH
Vanderbilt University
Nashville, TN

Kim A. Eagle, MD
University of Michigan
Ann Arbor, MI

Mark W. Feinberg, MD
Harvard Medical School
Boston, MA

Scott A. Flanders, MD
University of Michigan
Ann Arbor, MI

Daniel Gilden, MD
Legacy Emanuel Hospital
Portland, OR

Susan Glick, MD
John H. Stroger Hospital of Cook County
and Rush University
Chicago, IL

Christopher J. Goulet, MD
Digestive Health Clinic
Boise, ID

Michael P. Gruber, MD
University of Colorado Health Sciences Center
Denver, CO

Jessica Haberer, MD
Stanford University
Stanford, CA

Anthony A. Hilliard, MD
Mayo Clinic and Foundation
Rochester, MN

Robert J. Hoffman, MD
University of Wisconsin
Madison, WI

Harry Hollander, MD
University of California, San Francisco
San Francisco, CA

William J. Janssen, MD
University of Colorado Health Sciences Center
Denver, CO

Ashish K. Jha, MD, MPH
Harvard Medical School
Harvard School of Public Health
Boston, MA

Asha R. Kallianpur, MD, MPH
Vanderbilt University
Nashville, TN

Kevin C. Katz, MD
University of Toronto
Toronto, Ontario, Canada

Jay S. Keystone, MD
University of Toronto
Toronto, Ontario, Canada

Jeffrey Kohlwes, MD, MPH
University of California, San Francisco
San Francisco, CA

Theodore J. Kolias, MD
University of Michigan
Ann Arbor, MI

Howard E. LeWine, MD
Harvard Medical School
Boston, MA

Benjamin A. Lipsky, MD, FACP, FIDSA
VA Puget Sound Health Care System
and University of Washington
Seattle, WA

Michael Lukela, MD
University of Michigan
Ann Arbor, MI

Anne G. McLeod, MD
Mount Sinai Hospital
Toronto, Ontario, Canada

Mark Meier, MD
University of Michigan
Ann Arbor, MI

David E. Midthun, MD
Mayo Clinic College of Medicine
Rochester, MN

Richard H. Moseley, MD
University of Michigan
Ann Arbor, MI

Brahmajee K. Nallamothu, MD, MPH
University of Michigan
Ann Arbor, MI

Lori S. Newman, MD, PhD
Harvard Medical School
Boston, MA

Petros Nikolinakos, MD
Morrill County Community Hospital
Bridgeport, NE

Uptal D. Patel, MD
Duke University Medical Center
Durham, NC

Katherine A. Poehling, MD, MPH
Vanderbilt University Medical Center
Nashville, TN

Brendan M. Reilly, MD
John H. Stroger Hospital of Cook County
Chicago, IL

Iqbal S. Sandhu, MD
University of Utah
Salt Lake City, UT

Kaveh G. Shojania, MD
University of Ottawa
Ottawa, Ontario, Canada

Andrew M. Tager, MD
Harvard Medical School
Boston, MA

Carey C. Thomson, MD, MPH
Harvard Medical School
Boston, MA

Lawrence M. Tierney, Jr., MD
University of California, San Francisco
San Francisco, CA

Claude Tonnerre, MD
Hôpital de Pourtalès
Neuchâtel, Switzerland

Neil Trivedi, MD
University of California, San Francisco
San Francisco, CA

Sharon Walmsley, MD
University of Toronto
Toronto, Ontario, Canada

Andrew Wang, MD
Duke University Medical Center
Durham, NC

Steven Weinberger, MD, FACP
American College of Physicians
and University of Pennsylvania
School of Medicine
Philadelphia, PA

Peter F. Weller, MD
Harvard Medical School
Boston, MA

Preface

One of the joys of medicine is learning how to think through challenging clinical problems. Our book is aimed at those who want to become better diagnosticians as well as those who simply enjoy working through a diagnostic problem to eventually arrive at the answer. These challenges include generating an appropriate initial list of differential diagnoses based on a patient's presenting signs and symptoms; modifying this initial list to reflect the information gleaned from the history, physical examination, and standard laboratory tests; identifying appropriate additional tests or historical information needed to reach the diagnosis; and determining when the information obtained is sufficient to make a provisional or a final diagnosis and to justify beginning therapy.

Students and resident physicians have traditionally acquired these skills by working alongside and under the supervision of experienced clinicians, who provide guidance as a patient's presenting symptoms and signs are addressed. When patients remained in the hospital for long periods, students and residents had the opportunity to follow them from presentation through diagnosis and beyond. As a result of dramatic changes in health care delivery and medical education – with patients being discharged more quickly and with students and residents having mandatory days off – there are fewer opportunities for students and residents to engage in the full process of problem-solving that eventually yields the correct diagnosis.

Yet students and residents need as much as ever to understand how seasoned and expert clinicians confront clinical problems. For example, we have observed that skilled clinicians often keep two lists of potential diagnoses active in their mind as they consider a patient's problems. The first list contains, usually in rank order, the most likely diagnoses that can account for the patient's complaint. This list is initially generated from the history of the present illness, the past medical and social history, the physical examination, and the initial data obtained. As new data are obtained, the rank order is modified. Some who have just begun their clinical training may, unfortunately, not go beyond this point. Knowledgeable clinicians, on the other hand, realize that considering only the most likely disorders may lead to missed diagnoses and ultimately to patient harm. For this reason, master clinicians compile a second list that contains those diagnoses – however unlikely – that could cause the patient to die or to decompensate quickly. Although usually not all of the diagnoses on this additional list are pursued by advanced diagnostic testing, the clinician searches carefully for any clues in the history, physical examination, or initial diagnostic evaluation that require further pursuit.

Our book is divided into two sections. In the first, we provide an overview of the decision science underlying the art of clinical decision-making. "Quantitative Medical Decision-Making," provides a quantitative approach to making clinical decisions, including an overview of Bayesian decision-making, thresholds for taking action (diagnostic and therapeutic), and test characteristics such as sensitivity, specificity, and likelihood ratios. Complementing the quantitative approach to solving clinical problems, the next chapter, "Clinical Decision-Making: Understanding How Clinicians Make a Diagnosis," provides the reader with an overview of important concepts in cognitive psychology that to a large extent explain how clinicians make diagnoses. Various types of heuristics (or "mental shortcuts") and biases are defined, discussed, and illustrated with examples.

Clinicians learn best from patients. Thus, the rest of the book is devoted to clinical examples. The remaining chapters describe real cases previously peer-reviewed and published in the "Clinical Problem-Solving" series of the *New England Journal of Medicine.* Consistent with the format of the series, information about an actual patient is presented in small increments (shown in boldface type) to an experienced clinician (or clinicians), who responds to the information by sharing his or her reasoning with the learner (shown in regular type). A commentary following each case includes a discussion of the clinical issues raised in the case, and for many cases also reviews the decision-making process or processes employed, drawing on many of the concepts described in the first two chapters. Clinically relevant figures (such as chest radiographs, computed tomographic scans, and microscopical images) are incorporated into each of these chapters in order to make the case as real as possible.

Teachers may use the cases in this book as educational exercises (for example, for discussion on rounds). In such a situation, we suggest using the case material without the expert commentary. We suspect that not only physicians and physicians-in-training will find this book useful; those in other fields – such as nurse practitioners and physician assistants – will also find the information invaluable for learning several of the nuances of problem-solving. Finally, reviewing the cases in this book may be useful for persons preparing for national board–type examinations, given the emphasis such tests place on clinical vignettes and problem-solving ability.

We hope this book captures some of the enjoyment of real-life patient care. Our explicit goal is to help you become a better problem solver. The ability to logically work through and solve clinical problems is one of the most important and exciting aspects of being a physician.

SANJAY SAINT, M.D., M.P.H.
Associate Professor, Internal Medicine
Ann Arbor VA Medical Center
University of Michigan Medical School

JEFFREY M. DRAZEN, M.D.
Editor-in-Chief
The New England Journal of Medicine
Distinguished Parker B. Francis Professor of Medicine
Harvard Medical School

CAREN G. SOLOMON, M.D., M.P.H.
Deputy Editor
The New England Journal of Medicine
Assistant Professor of Medicine
Harvard Medical School

Quantitative Medical Decision-Making

STEPHEN BENT, M.D.

OVERVIEW

Quantitative medical decision-making provides both a visual and a mathematical model that examines each step of a medical decision. Although the process is quantitative, the main goal of the technique (for individual clinicians) is to improve their understanding of clinical reasoning. Quantitative medical decision-making is the mathematics behind the practice of evidence-based medicine, which is the process of identifying, evaluating, and applying the highest-quality medical evidence. This chapter discusses the application of medical evidence to three specific decisions:

1) Does this patient have a given disease? (applying a diagnostic test);

2) Should I treat this patient? (treatment thresholds); and

3) Should I order another test? (testing thresholds).

Deciding Whether a Particular Patient Has a Given Disease

When a patient presents with a new symptom or complaint, the clinician seeks to determine the correct diagnosis, which will guide treatment. The first step is to generate a differential diagnosis and to use clinical information (e.g., history, physical examination, laboratory tests, and radiographic studies) to estimate the probability of the disease for each item on the differential diagnosis. Each piece of clinical information (such as an answer to a question during the taking of the medical history) can be thought of as a diagnostic test that changes the probability that a patient has a given disorder. Therefore, the gathering of clinical information is a process of refining probability by using the following model:

What we thought before	+	Clinical information	→	What we think afterwards
Pretest probability	+	Diagnostic test	→	Post-test probability

Table 1. A Hypothetical Differential Diagnosis for a Woman Presenting with Dysuria.	
Diagnosis	**Probability**
Urinary tract infection	50 percent
Sexually transmitted disease	20 percent
Vaginal yeast infection	20 percent
Bacterial vaginosis	10 percent
Other (e.g., Reiter's syndrome)	<1 percent

This process of refining probability to solve problems of logic was first described by the Reverend Thomas Bayes, an 18th-century mathematician, and is therefore often referred to as Bayesian analysis.[1]

Example: A 29-year-old woman leaves a phone message at your office stating that she has felt some burning during urination, and she would like to know what to do.

The first step is to generate a differential diagnosis. Since the only information you have at this point is that the patient has dysuria, the initial differential diagnosis might include urinary tract infection, sexually transmitted disease, vaginal yeast infection, and bacterial vaginosis. There are other, less common, causes of dysuria (e.g., Reiter's syndrome), but the goal of the initial evaluation is to focus on the most likely causes of the presenting sign or symptom (Table 1) . The probabilities of all diseases in the differential diagnosis must add up to 100 percent.

As the probability of one item in the differential diagnosis increases, the probability of the other items must decrease. The goal is for the probability of one disease to move close to 100 percent while the sum of the probabilities of the other diseases moves close to 0 percent. For simplicity in this example, we will focus on the first item (urinary tract infection), using a three-step process.

Step 1: Determine the pretest probability of a disease

The pretest probability is the probability, chance, or likelihood (these three terms are synonymous) that a patient has a given disease before a test is applied. Pretest probabilities are best determined from studies that carefully examine a large group of patients with the same presenting symptom (such as dysuria) to determine the cause of the disease for each patient. A recent systematic review examining the value of the history and physical examination in women with suspected urinary tract infection found that the pretest probability of urinary tract infection in a woman who presented with dysuria was approximately 50

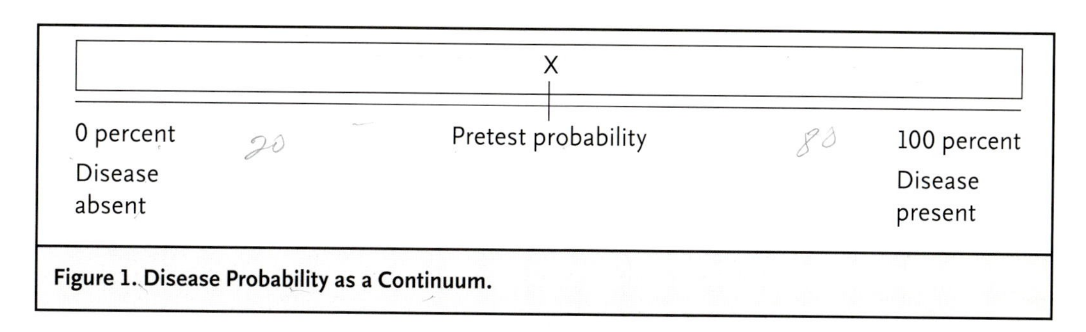

Figure 1. Disease Probability as a Continuum.

percent.[2] Since published pretest probabilities are most applicable to the population that was included in the study, clinicians should refine these pretest probabilities when performing quantitative medical decision-making in their own practice environments. For example, a clinician practicing in an inner-city free clinic where a large number of patients with sexually transmitted diseases are seen might correctly surmise that the pretest probability of urinary tract infection in a woman presenting with dysuria was only 20 percent, whereas the pretest probability of sexually transmitted disease might be 50 percent or even higher.

The probability of a disease can be thought of as a continuum, expressed in Figure 1. At initial presentation, the probability of many diseases falls somewhere in the middle of this continuum (between 20 and 80 percent). The goal of clinical reasoning is to use information from the history, physical examination, laboratory tests, and other sources to move the probability of a disease close to 0 percent (ruling out the disease) or 100 percent (ruling in the disease). In the current example, the pretest probability of urinary tract infection is 50 percent; additional information will serve to increase or decrease this probability.

Step 2: Apply a diagnostic test with the use of likelihood ratios

The information about the value of a diagnostic test may come in several forms, including sensitivity, specificity, positive and negative predictive values, and likelihood ratios. All of this information can be calculated from a standard 2×2 table describing a diagnostic test (Table 2).

Table 2. Two-by-Two Table Describing Test Result Relative to Presence of Disease.

		Disease	
		Present	Absent
Diagnostic test result	+	*a*	*b*
	–	*c*	*d*

The sensitivity is the proportion of patients with a disease who have a positive test for that disease, calculated by the formula a/(a+c). The specificity is the proportion of patients without a disease who have a negative test for that disease, calculated by the formula d/(b+d). The positive predictive value is the proportion of patients with a positive test who have the disease, calculated by the formula a/(a+b). The negative predictive value is the proportion of patients with a negative test who do not have the disease, calculated by the formula d/(c+d). This information tells us more about the test (sensitivity and specificity) or the population of patients tested (positive and negative predictive values) than about a particular clinical scenario.

Likelihood ratios allow the test results to be applied to a specific patient with a specific pretest probability of a disease. A likelihood ratio (LR) is calculated as one likelihood divided by another. LR+ denotes a positive likelihood ratio, and LR– a negative likelihood ratio.

$$\text{LR+} = \frac{\text{likelihood of a positive test in a patient with a disease}}{\text{likelihood of a positive test in a patient without the disease}} = \frac{a/(a+c)}{b/(b+d)} = \frac{\text{sensitivity}}{(1-\text{specificity})}$$

As the likelihood of a positive test in a patient with a disease increases and the likelihood of a positive test in a patient without the disease decreases, the positive likelihood ratio increases and becomes a more powerful test for ruling in the disease. A positive likelihood ratio greater than 1 increases the probability of the disease in a patient with a positive test. The larger the positive likelihood ratio, the more that a positive test result will increase the post-test probability of the disease.

$$\text{LR–} = \frac{\text{likelihood of a negative test in a patient with a disease}}{\text{likelihood of a negative test in a patient without the disease}} = \frac{c/(a+c)}{d/(b+d)} = \frac{(1-\text{sensitivity})}{\text{specificity}}$$

As the likelihood of a negative test in a patient with a disease decreases and the likelihood of a negative test in a patient without the disease increases, the negative likelihood ratio gets smaller and becomes more powerful for ruling out the disease. A negative likelihood ratio less than 1 decreases the probability of the disease in a patient with a negative test. The smaller the negative likelihood ratio, the more that a negative test result will decrease the post-test probability of the disease. Likelihood ratios range from 0 to infinity.

In most cases, positive likelihood ratios are greater than 1 and negative likelihood ratios are less than 1. However, there are certain clinical scenarios in which the finding of a positive likelihood ratio actually decreases the probability of a disease. For example, in a woman who presents with dysuria, an accompanying history of vaginal discharge has a positive likelihood ratio of 0.3, which decreases the probability of urinary tract infection. Intuitively, this makes sense, since the presence of vaginal discharge increases the likelihood of the other diagnoses on the list (yeast infection, bacterial vaginosis, and sexually transmitted disease) and therefore decreases the likelihood of urinary tract infection. However, it is sometimes difficult to remember that a positive likelihood ratio (and the presence of a positive finding) can decrease the probability of a disease.

Some rules about likelihood ratios can help guide their application in practice[3]:

> A relatively high likelihood ratio (5 to 10) will significantly increase the probability of a disease, given a positive test.
>
> A relatively low likelihood ratio (0.1 to 0.5) will significantly decrease the probability of a disease, given a negative test.
>
> Likelihood ratios of 2, 5, and 10 are associated with an increase in the probability of disease in the presence of a positive test, as follows:
>
> LR+ = 2 increases the probability of the disease by ~15 percent
> LR+ = 5 increases the probability of the disease by ~30 percent
> LR+ = 10 increases the probability of the disease by ~45 percent
>
> Likelihood ratios of 0.5, 0.2, and 0.1 are associated with a decrease in the probability of a disease in the presence of a negative test, as follows:
>
> LR– = 0.5 decreases the probability of the disease by ~15 percent
> LR– = 0.2 decreases the probability of the disease by ~30 percent
> LR– = 0.1 decreases the probability of the disease by ~45 percent

Returning to the example of the woman with dysuria, we can use the systematic review[2] described above to find the positive and negative likelihood ratios for relevant aspects of the history and physical examination. For example, if the patient with dysuria also reports frequent urination, the positive likelihood ratio for this "diagnostic test" is 1.8. Since 1.8 is close to 2.0, and we know from the approximations above that a positive likelihood ratio of 2.0 increases the post-test probability of urinary tract infection by about 15 percent, then this additional symptom (frequent urination) increases the probability of urinary

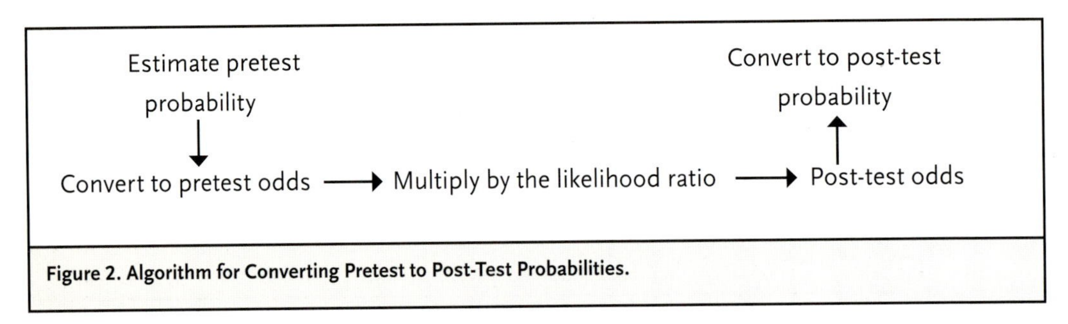

Figure 2. Algorithm for Converting Pretest to Post-Test Probabilities.

tract infection from a pretest value of 50 percent to a post-test value of 65 percent. If a urine dipstick test was performed and was positive (defined as a positive result for either leukocyte esterase or nitrate), the positive likelihood ratio for this result would be 4.2. We can estimate the change in probability by noting that a positive likelihood ratio of 4.2 is close to 5.0, which would increase the probability of the disease by about 30 percent. Therefore, a positive dipstick test would increase the post-test probability of the disease from 50 percent to 80 percent. These approximations suffice for most bedside decisions, but there are more precise ways to calculate the change in probability that occurs during the application of a diagnostic test, as shown in the following section.

Step 3: Generate precise post-test probabilities

It would be simple if we could just multiply the pretest probability by the likelihood ratio to generate a post-test probability. Unfortunately, because of the underlying mathematics, probabilities cannot be multiplied by likelihood ratios to generate post-test probabilities; they must first be converted to odds. The general format for converting pretest probabilities to post-test probabilities is shown in Figure 2.

Odds and probabilities

Odds and probabilities use the same numerator but different denominators:

$$\text{Odds} = \frac{\text{the number of people with a condition or exposure}}{\text{the number of people without the condition or exposure}}$$

$$\text{Probability} = \frac{\text{the number of people with a condition or exposure}}{\text{the total number of people}}$$

Most people are more comfortable thinking in terms of probabilities. For example, in a theoretical study of 100 women presenting to a clinic with dysuria, 50 are found to have

$$\text{Odds} = \frac{\text{probability}}{1-\text{probability}} \qquad \text{Probability} = \frac{\text{odds}}{\text{odds} + 1}$$

Figure 3. Converting Probabilities to Odds and Vice Versa.

urinary tract infections with positive urine cultures. On the basis of this study, the probability of a urinary tract infection in a woman presenting to a clinic with dysuria is 50/100 or 0.5 (50 percent). In contrast, the odds of a urinary tract infection are 50/50 or 1. For the purpose of diagnostic testing, you only need to know how to convert from probabilities to odds and from odds to probabilities (see Figure 3).

Continuing example

In the preceding example, the woman with dysuria has a 50 percent pretest probability of having a urinary tract infection. When asked if she also has been urinating more frequently, she answers "Yes," which corresponds to a positive likelihood ratio of 1.8. Her post-test probability of having a urinary tract infection on the basis of the presence of frequent urination is calculated as shown in Figure 4.

As you can see, the probability of urinary tract infection is increased, but not substantially. A test result with a positive likelihood ratio of 1.8 is not very powerful. However, if the woman came to your office for a urine dipstick test and that test was positive (LR+ = 4.2), her post-test probability of having a urinary tract infection would be 4.2/5.2 = 81 per-

Pretest probability = 50 percent

↓

$$\text{Pretest odds} = \frac{0.5}{0.5} = 1.0 \longrightarrow \times 1.8 \longrightarrow = 1.8 \text{ (post-test odds)}$$

↑

$$\text{Post-test probability} = \frac{1.8}{2.8} = 64 \text{ percent}$$

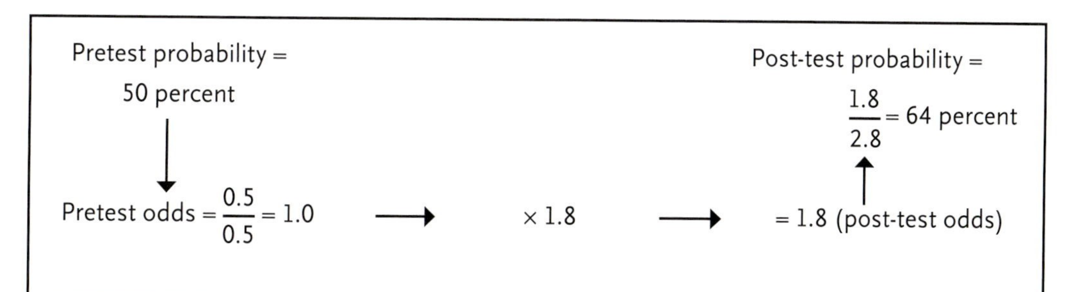

Figure 4. Calculating the Post-Test Probability.

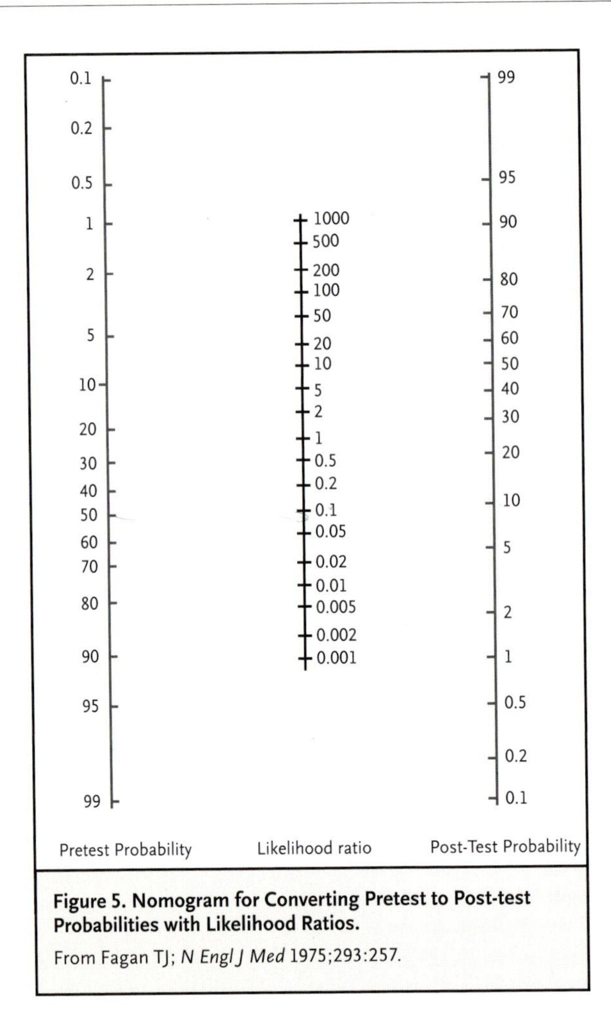

Figure 5. Nomogram for Converting Pretest to Post-test Probabilities with Likelihood Ratios.

From Fagan TJ; *N Engl J Med* 1975;293:257.

cent. This test is clearly much more powerful. It is also useful to note that this precise method resulted in post-test probabilities that were very similar to those generated by using the approximations described previously.

Using nomograms or handheld computers

If you prefer to avoid the calculations required to convert probabilities to odds and odds to probabilities, you can use a nomogram (Figure 5). The pretest probability is located on the left axis of the nomogram. A straightedge is then used to connect the pretest probability to the likelihood ratio, and the intersection of the straightedge with the right axis will give the post-test probability. Many programs that can perform these simple calculations for diagnostic tests are available for handheld computers.

Table 3. Initial Differential Diagnosis of a Man with Dyspnea.	
Diagnosis	**Probability**
Pulmonary embolism	30 percent
Viral upper respiratory infection	30 percent
Chronic obstructive pulmonary disease exacerbation	30 percent
Congestive heart failure	10 percent

Clinical utility of quantitative diagnostic testing

Quantitative medical decision-making derives most of its value not from generating precise post-test probabilities, but from helping the clinician understand what is taking place during the application of a diagnostic test. A patient presents with some probability of having a disease, information is gathered to modify that probability, and the final post-test probability helps determine whether any further action should be taken (should we treat, not treat, or perform another test?).

Deciding Whether to Treat

A 56-year-old man with a 50-pack-year history of smoking presents to the emergency department at midnight with unilateral left calf swelling and a three-day history of mild dyspnea. The chest radiograph and electrocardiogram, which were obtained before you arrived, were both normal. Again, your first step is to generate a differential diagnosis for dyspnea in this patient (Table 3).

You are worried that this patient might have a pulmonary embolism, and you have estimated that his pretest probability of having this disease is 30 percent (on the basis of his age, history of smoking, unilateral calf swelling, and normal radiograph and electrocardiogram). Although most estimates in practice are derived from clinical experience, published algorithms are available that use clinical and laboratory data to estimate the pretest probability of pulmonary embolism; according to one such algorithm, this patient's history places him at moderate risk, with a pretest probability of 28 percent.[4]

The emergency department happens to be in a small rural hospital, and it is not possible to obtain additional diagnostic tests tonight (e.g., ventilation–perfusion scan or spiral computed tomography). Therefore, you must decide whether to treat this patient with an anticoagulant agent now, before further diagnostic testing is performed. How will you decide whether to treat him?

Treatment threshold

The treatment threshold defines a probability of disease above which treatment is more likely to result in the desired outcome, and below which withholding treatment is more likely to result in the desired outcome. It can be thought of as the switching point: treat above the treatment threshold and do not treat below the treatment threshold.

The treatment threshold depends on both the risks (or costs) of treatment and its benefits. The treatment threshold is often abbreviated as Rx, and the formula for calculating the treatment threshold is

$$\text{Treatment threshold (Rx)} = \frac{\text{cost}}{\text{cost} + \text{benefit}}$$

In this equation, note that "cost" refers to the cost of treating nondiseased patients and "benefit" refers to the benefit of treating diseased patients. If the cost of treatment is low and the benefit of treatment is high, the treatment threshold is low. An example of a treatment with a low threshold is the administration of antibiotic drugs to a patient who may have pneumonia. The cost of treatment is low (the risk of a side effect of antibiotics in a nondiseased patient), and the benefit of treatment is great (prevention of complications of pneumonia, including death in a patient with disease); therefore, the treatment threshold is low. In other words, you would be willing to treat a patient with a relatively low pretest probability of pneumonia (say, 10 percent) if you were uncertain about the diagnosis and additional testing was not available.

It is important to note that treatment thresholds can be calculated from many different perspectives. In this case, we are only taking the patient's perspective, and we are assuming that the patient incurs no financial costs. If we were taking the perspective of a health care plan, we might consider the cost of the antibiotics (which would raise the cost in the equation and therefore raise the treatment threshold). If we were taking the perspective of society, we would probably consider the cost of the increased resistance to antibiotics that results when antibiotics are given to large numbers of patients (which would also increase the cost in the equation and raise the treatment threshold). A more complex calculation of treatment thresholds would involve decision analysis, which is beyond the scope of this chapter but is discussed in several textbooks.[5-7]

If the costs of treatment are high (e.g., chemotherapy for small-cell lung cancer) and the benefits are low (a few months of additional survival), the treatment threshold is high. In these situations, the probability of disease must be very high (such as in cases in which a diagnosis can be made by histologic examination) to raise the treatment threshold high enough to justify administering chemotherapy.

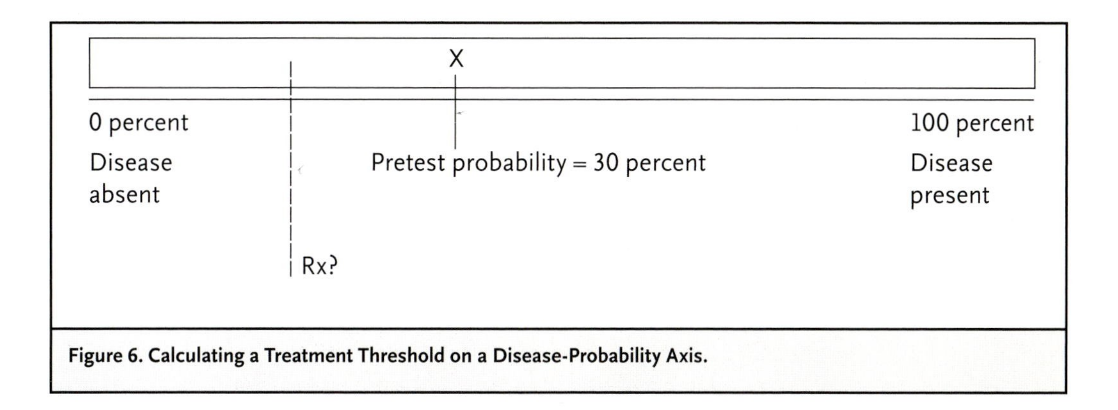

Figure 6. Calculating a Treatment Threshold on a Disease-Probability Axis.

Returning to our original example of the patient with suspected pulmonary embolism, we could represent his pretest probability of disease as shown in Figure 6.

If we are to decide whether this patient should be treated for pulmonary embolism with anticoagulant agents (intravenous heparin or intramuscular low-molecular-weight heparin), we must calculate the treatment threshold to determine whether the patient is above or below this threshold.

The main cost (or risk) of treating a patient with anticoagulant agents is the possibility of a major bleeding event (lethal or serious central nervous system bleeding or major gastrointestinal bleeding). Using low-molecular-weight heparin as an example, previous studies have suggested a risk of serious bleeding of 1.2 percent during the initial treatment period (typically less than 2 weeks).[8]

The benefit of anticoagulant therapy in a patient with pulmonary embolism is a major decrease in the risk of death (generally from recurrent embolism) from approximately 30 percent (in an untreated patient) to approximately 9 percent (in a treated patient), which is equivalent to a reduction of the risk of death by 21 percentage points.[9]

Therefore, the simple cost/(cost + benefit) equation yields a treatment threshold of:

$$\text{Rx} = \frac{\text{cost}}{\text{cost+benefit}} = \frac{\text{1.2 percent}}{\text{(1.2 percent + 21 percent)}} = \text{5.4 percent}$$

Since the patient's current probability of having a pulmonary embolism is 30 percent, he is above the treatment threshold, and treatment is indicated.

Caveats

The example described uses a simplified version of a more detailed analysis that might be conducted to estimate a treatment threshold precisely. For example, the risk of bleeding in a patient receiving low-molecular-weight heparin was estimated at 1.2 percent during the initial treatment period (typically less than 2 weeks), but estimates of this risk vary substantially depending on the patient's age and coexisting illnesses. For example, elderly patients, those at risk of falling, and those with known previous major bleeding events are likely to be at much higher risk of bleeding and therefore have higher individual treatment thresholds. Furthermore, the benefit of low-molecular-weight heparin in terms of reducing the risk of death depends on the severity of disease at presentation; patients with more severe disease are likely to receive more benefit. More complex determinations of treatment thresholds would require a formal decision analysis; these techniques are described in detail elsewhere.[5-7] The main use of the simple cost/(cost + benefit) equation is to enable the clinician to make a reasonable estimate of whether the treatment threshold is high, medium, or low. These estimates can then provide general guidelines about whether or not to treat patients. Some medical centers have decision-analysis teams that use complex computer modeling to assist in complicated medical decisions at the bedside.

Deciding Whether to Order Another Test

One of the basic principles of diagnostic testing is that tests should be ordered only if they are likely to affect the treatment of a patient. One could argue that there are other reasons to order diagnostic tests (e.g., for patient reassurance, even when a diagnosis has been almost certainly ruled in or out); but from the standpoint of quantitative medical decision-making, the primary reason to order diagnostic tests is to change the estimated probability of disease sufficiently to affect a treatment decision.

Recall that the decision whether or not to treat a patient changes at the treatment threshold. Therefore, for a diagnostic test to be useful (i.e., to be able to affect a treatment decision) it must have enough power to cause the pretest probability of disease to cross the treatment threshold. Let's use the example of suspected pulmonary embolism to determine whether a ventilation–perfusion scan would be a useful diagnostic test for this patient, whom we estimated to have a 30 percent pretest probability of having pulmonary embolism (Figure 7).

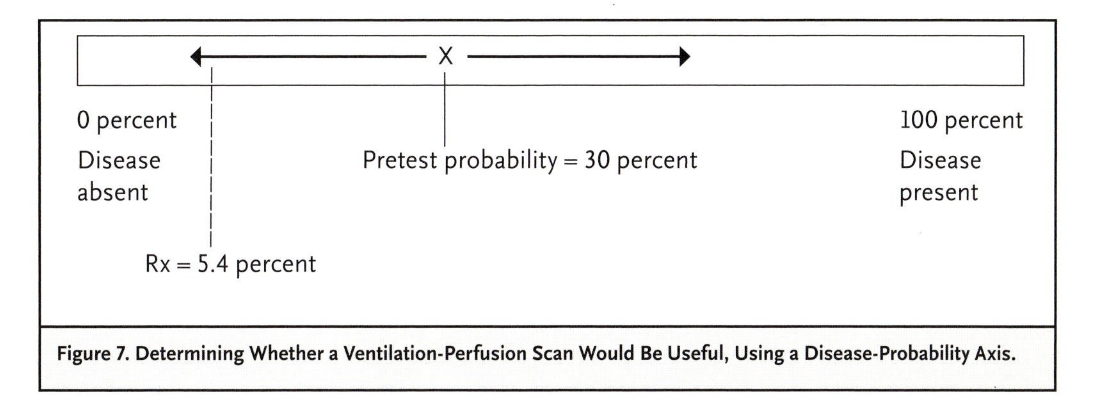

Figure 7. Determining Whether a Ventilation-Perfusion Scan Would Be Useful, Using a Disease-Probability Axis.

The arrows in the figure show how a positive test will result in a post-test probability of pulmonary embolism that is higher, and how a negative test will result in a post-test probability of the disease that is lower. In terms of medical decision-making, a positive test will not change the treatment of this patient (the probability of the disease is above the treatment threshold, so we would treat the patient whether or not the test was positive). Therefore, the test is only useful (i.e., will only cause us to change a treatment decision) if it is able to lower the post-test probability of the disease below the treatment threshold (or cross the treatment threshold).

Let's take a look at the likelihood ratios for various results from a ventilation–perfusion scan, based on results from the 1990 PIOPED study[10] (Table 4).

In this case, the question is whether a normal test result, with a likelihood ratio of 0.1, would lower the probability of pulmonary embolism below the treatment threshold of 5.4 percent, in which case we would change our decision to treat the patient to a decision not to treat him. First, we convert the pretest probability of the disease to the odds of the disease; we next multiply by the likelihood ratio of 0.1 and then convert the post-test odds back to probability (Figure 8).

Table 4. Likelihood Ratios of Pulmonary Embolism According to the 1990 PIOPED Study.

Ventilation–perfusion scan result	Likelihood ratio
High probability of disease	18.3
Intermediate probability of disease	1.2
Low probability of disease	0.4
Normal result	0.1

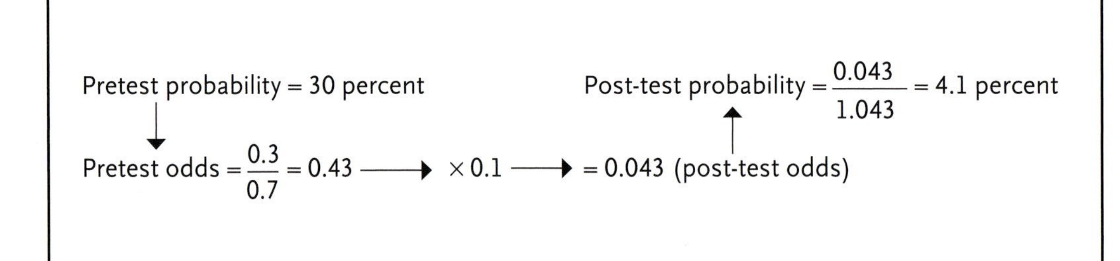

Figure 8. Pretest and Post-Test Probabilities in the Patient.

Thus, the test does have the power to lower the post-test probability of the disease below the treatment threshold, and a negative test would prompt us to withhold treatment. However, note that the post-test probability of the disease (4.1 percent) is very close to the treatment threshold (5.4 percent), and given the uncertainty of the exact treatment threshold, we might choose to estimate the risks and benefits of treatment in this particular patient more carefully, or we might want to consider a different diagnostic test (such as a spiral computed tomographic scan or a D-dimer test) to attempt to lower the probability of the disease even further.

The upper and lower testing thresholds (T_U and T_L) define the range of probabilities over which a diagnostic test can change the decision whether or not to treat the patient.

Figure 9 shows the testing thresholds in relation to the treatment threshold and defines three medical decisions: do not test or treat, test, and treat without testing.

Each diagnostic test will have its own unique upper and lower testing thresholds. The lower testing T_L threshold is the probability value at which a positive test will result in a post-test probability of the disease equal to the treatment threshold. Conversely, the upper testing threshold T_U is the probability value at which a negative test will result in a post-test

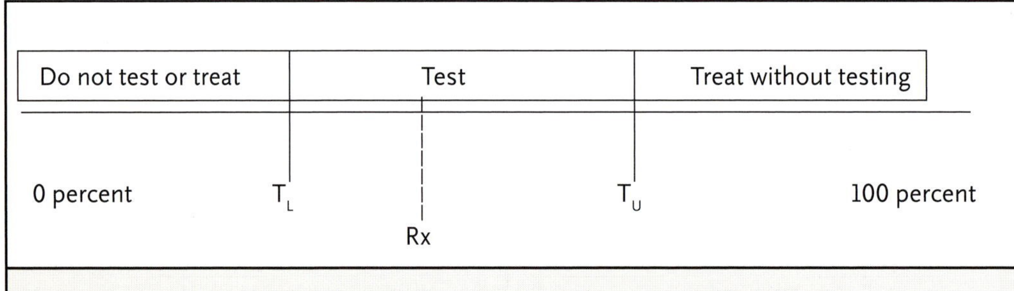

Figure 9. Testing Thresholds in Relation to the Treatment Threshold on a Disease-Probability Axis.

T_L denotes lower testing threshold, T_U upper testing threshold, and Rx treatment threshold. Adapted from Friedland.[5]

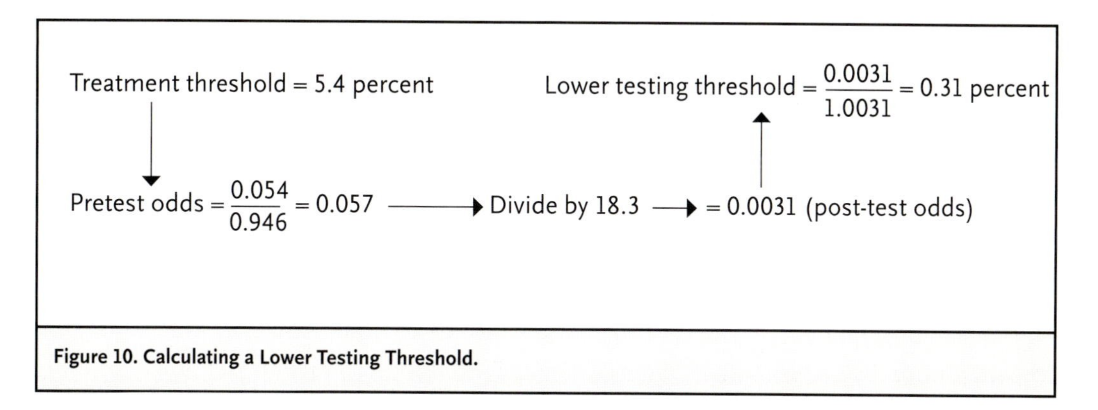

Figure 10. Calculating a Lower Testing Threshold.

probability of the disease equal to the treatment threshold. These probabilities of disease are calculated by taking the treatment threshold, converting it to odds, dividing it by the largest and smallest likelihood ratios to calculate T_L and T_U, respectively, and converting back to probability.

In the case of ventilation–perfusion scans, the lower testing threshold is calculated as shown in Figure 10.

Similar calculations show that the upper testing threshold is 36 percent. Therefore, the ventilation–perfusion scan has the potential to change a treatment decision over a wide range of pretest probabilities that encompasses the pretest probabilities of disease for most patients (from 0.31 percent to 36 percent). Unfortunately, the value of this testing is limited by the fact that intermediate results (intermediate or low probability), which are unlikely to influence decision-making, are common.

Caveats

Testing thresholds provide a model for how to think about the use of diagnostic tests, and the resulting threshold probabilities are based on estimates of the treatment threshold and the likelihood ratios of the diagnostic test. The testing thresholds should not be interpreted as exact values, but rather as rough measures of the usefulness of a given test in a particular patient. Testing thresholds evaluate only one test at a time. However, there are many diagnostic tests that can be performed to evaluate a given patient for a specific disease. If the tests are performed in series, it is almost always possible to raise or lower the probability of the disease sufficiently to cross the treatment threshold (if all tests have either positive or negative results). Clinical judgment must be used to determine when enough tests have been ordered.

Conclusions

This chapter focuses on estimating the probability that a given patient has a specific disease, using diagnostic tests to modify that probability, and judging whether the probability is sufficiently high or low to recommend treatment or additional testing. Physicians seldom know with certainty whether a patient has or does not have a specific disease, and it is often difficult to access data on the precise test characteristics or treatment thresholds relevant to a clinical decision. However, the process of modeling clinical decision-making with quantitative tools may improve a clinician's ability to understand the process of clinical reasoning. By systematically considering the likelihood of various diagnoses and the implications of the diagnoses, methods using probability theory help physicians and patients to make reasonable decisions in the face of uncertainty.

REFERENCES

1.
Bayes T. An essay toward solving a problem in the doctrine of chances. Philos Trans R Soc Lond 1763;53:370-418.

2.
Bent S, Nallamothu BK, Simel DL, Fihn SD, Saint S. Does this woman have an acute uncomplicated urinary tract infection? JAMA 2002;287:2701-10.

3.
McGee S. Simplifying likelihood ratios. J Gen Intern Med 2002;17:646-9.

4.
Wells PS, Ginsberg JS, Anderson DR, et al. Use of a clinical model for safe management of patients with suspected pulmonary embolism. Ann Intern Med 1998;129:997-1005.

5.
Friedland DJ, Go AS, Davoren JB, et al. Evidence-based medicine: a framework for clinical practice. Stamford, Conn.: Appleton & Lange, 1998.

6.
Petitti DB. Meta-analysis, decision analysis, and cost-effective analysis: methods for quantitative synthesis in medicine. Vol. 31 of Monographs in epidemiology and biostatistics. 2nd ed. New York: Oxford University Press, 2000.

7.
Sox HC Jr, Blatt MA, Higgins MC, Marton KI. Medical decision making. Boston: Butterworths, 1988.

8.
van Dongen CJ, van den Belt AG, Prins MH, Lensing AW. Fixed dose subcutaneous low molecular weight heparins versus adjusted dose unfractionated heparin for venous thromboembolism. Cochrane Database Syst Rev 2004: CD001100.

9.
Quinn RJ, Butler SP. A decision analysis approach to the treatment of patients with suspected pulmonary emboli and an intermediate probability lung scan. J Nucl Med 1991;32:2050-6.

10.
The PIOPED Investigators. Value of the ventilation/perfusion scan in acute pulmonary embolism: results of the Prospective Investigation of Pulmonary Embolism Diagnosis (PIOPED). JAMA 1990;263:2753-9.

Clinical Decision-Making: Understanding How Clinicians Make a Diagnosis

Gurpreet Dhaliwal, M.D.

The typical encounter between a patient and a health professional begins with a "problem" — the patient's chief presenting symptom, a particular vital sign, an abnormal laboratory value — which the physician is asked to "solve." Problem-solving is a skill all physicians must learn and that some clearly perform better than others, yet few can articulate how they do it. If pressed, physicians are apt to explain to students that diagnoses are made by taking a complete history and performing a complete physical examination, followed by a search of their memory for a disease that explains the findings. Unfortunately, this response does not capture the essence of how physicians think. This chapter addresses the mental functions that underlie the diagnostic process, the cognitive structures and characteristics of skilled diagnosticians, and the cognitive errors that all physicians — experienced or not — are likely to make. It is intended to summarize a selected group of theories and models — largely developed by educators and psychologists — and make them relevant and accessible to practicing clinicians and students.

Pattern Recognition versus Analytic Reasoning

The majority of clinical encounters involve common illnesses that physicians see frequently and recognize with little diagnostic quandary when they present in their typical forms.[1] Examples include allergic rhinitis, urinary tract infection, and cellulitis. From experience, the clinician recognizes the characteristic symptoms and signs and makes a diagnosis without needing to seriously consider alternative diagnoses. At the simplest level, this form of reasoning (*pattern recognition*) involves comparing the current case with previous cases (which are stored in memory either individually or in an abstract form) and making a judgment about the probability of a match. Pattern recognition occurs automatically and is rapid, efficient, and easy. Although it is usually an accurate method of making a diagnosis, these same features make it seductive in the setting of complex problems and can lead to mistakes. As Leape wrote, "Humans prefer pattern recognition to calculation, so they are strongly biased to search for a prepackaged solution, i.e., a 'rule,' before resorting to more strenuous knowledge-based functioning."[2]

When physicians are confronted with a more challenging patient who does not fit a previously recognized pattern, they are forced to employ a more time-consuming and deliberate assessment (*analytic reasoning*). This requires searching memory and knowledge stores, invoking pathophysiological mechanisms, and deriving new solutions to clinical problems.[2-4] A patient with right arm weakness, right facial droop, and aphasia will promptly receive a diagnosis of left middle cerebral artery stroke (pattern recognition); in contrast, a patient with right arm weakness and a T4 sensory level, which does not immediately invoke an obvious neuroanatomic correlate, will compel the physician to review memory and knowledge stores for a possible explanation.

The predominant form of reasoning in any given case is determined by the physician's unique clinical experience and knowledge base.[4,5] For example, a physician working at a university hospital with a major organ-transplantation unit will use pattern recognition to rapidly recognize a commonly encountered problem, such as cyclosporine nephrotoxicity, whereas an equally skilled clinician in a rural hospital may search his or her memory (and available resources) to arrive at the same diagnosis. Conversely, in the case of a common rural toxidrome, such as organophosphate poisoning, it is the community physician who will use pattern recognition, whereas the university physician will employ an intensive analytic process.

Even in cases of rapid pattern recognition and diagnosis, there is a role for analytic reasoning to verify the diagnosis and to safeguard against diagnostic errors.[6] When an elderly patient with a history of coronary heart disease presents with dyspnea and lower-extremity edema, the clinician will expect to diagnose congestive heart failure (pattern recognition) but should also seek information to rule out other possible causes, such as venous thromboembolism (analytic reasoning).

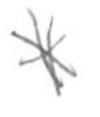

Problem-Solving Strategies and Methods

One of the most widely cited models of the diagnostic process and analytic reasoning is the hypothetico-deductive method,[7,8] an adaptation of the general scientific method, whereby hypotheses are proposed, tested, and verified or rejected.

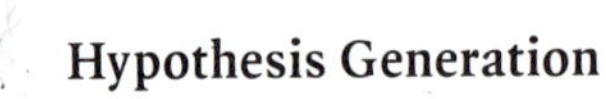

Hypothesis Generation

Very early in the encounter with the patient (within 30 seconds to 2 minutes), the physician forms a limited number (generally, two to five) of diagnostic hypotheses on the basis of the chief presenting symptom, the patient's demographic characteristics, and a few additional historical details.[7,9-11] Physicians sometimes form these tentative diagnoses before the first word is uttered in the interview, using nonverbal cues such as the patient's appearance, dress, gait, and mannerisms[10] or information previously available (e.g., the triage nurse's notation of the chief presenting symptom).[12]

Tentative diagnoses are generated on the basis of limited information and with little effort by the use of pattern recognition.[6] If the patient's initial history and nonverbal cues match a physician's mental image of a disease, that illness will be an early consideration. For example, the otherwise well-appearing young patient who walks into the examination room with an obvious facial droop most likely has Bell's palsy. The triage nurse's report of fever, sore throat, and myalgia will lead the clinician to suspect an upper respiratory tract infection before the patient is ever seen.

The initial hypothesis can be broad (e.g., rheumatologic disorder) or specific (e.g., Henoch–Schönlein purpura). In either case, these hypotheses — or tentative diagnoses — serve an important function for the human mind, which is limited in its ability to consider large amounts of information.[13] A hypothesis transforms an open medical problem (e.g., "What is this patient's illness?") into a set of well-circumscribed questions that are much easier for the human mind to address and solve (e.g., "Is this illness influenza, malaria, or urosepsis?").[14] The hypotheses collectively form a "filing system" to organize the new information as it is collected.[10]

Gathering and Analysis of Information

Much of the first encounter between the patient and the health professional is spent sorting out the initial two to five tentative diagnoses. The physician usually collects information (from the history, physical examination, laboratory tests, and imaging studies) within the confines of the initial hypotheses, searching for information that supports or refutes the possible diagnoses.[3,7,9,11,15,16] Some initial hypotheses are rejected, new hypotheses are activated, and general hypotheses are replaced by more specific ones.

Along with pattern recognition, physicians employ specific forms of reasoning as they invoke tentative diagnoses: probability (What are the most common causes of abdominal pain in a 26-year-old woman?); prognostic implications, including potential lethality (What is the most worrisome cause of abdominal pain in this patient?); cause-and-effect relationships (What could cause abdominal pain in this patient one week after she had unprotected sex?); or precompiled rules ("*Always* rule out pregnancy in a young woman with abdominal pain").[9,17]

As the clinician accumulates a complete data set about the patient, he or she also employs a number of strategies to narrow down the list of possible diagnoses. Findings that separate one disease state from another (e.g., the gradual onset of appendicitis vs. the abrupt onset of a perforated ulcer), support the leading diagnosis (e.g., cervical motion tenderness in a woman with suspected pelvic inflammatory disease), and help exclude competing diagnoses (e.g., negative urine pregnancy test when ectopic pregnancy is a possible diagnosis) are particularly emphasized.[9,18] In selected cases, for example, when the chief presenting symptom lends itself to an algorithmic approach (e.g., jaundice, anemia, or renal failure), physicians may alternatively seek clinical data directed at the branch points on an algorithm that helps distinguish between diagnostic possibilities (scheme-inductive reasoning), rather than information that allows them to accept or reject diagnostic hypotheses.[19,20]

Verification

When the clinician has arrived at one or two suspected diagnoses, these hypotheses are subjected to a process of verification.[9,18] The physician re-examines the available information, confirming that most normal and abnormal findings are explained by a given diagnosis; that the patient's risk factors, presentation, and natural history are consistent with the diagnosis; and that competing diagnoses — which generally do not meet the above criteria — have been eliminated with confidence by seeking contradictory evidence. The single simplest explanation for the presentation should be sought (according to the principle of Occam's razor), although such parsimony is not always applicable in complex clinical situations in which multiple illnesses may coexist. After the physician accumulates a certain amount of data (which varies from clinician to clinician), the probability of a given disease is judged as sufficiently high (treatment threshold) that no further testing is indicated, and specific treatment is instituted.[21,22] Since absolute diagnostic certainty is often not possible, management plans are often predicated on treating patients for the most likely diagnosis on the basis of the imperfect information at hand.

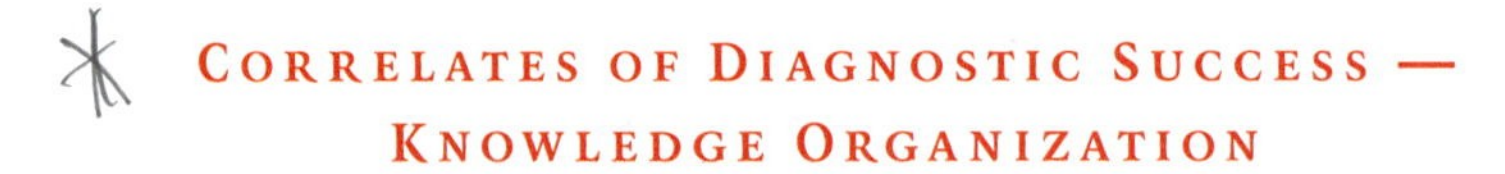

Correlates of Diagnostic Success — Knowledge Organization

A number of studies comparing the problem-solving strategies used by students and physicians,[15] residents and attending physicians,[23] specialists and nonspecialists,[9] and expert and average physicians[7] have failed to demonstrate any differences in the qualitative methods used to arrive at diagnoses. In each comparison, both groups generated a limited number of early hypotheses and used these hypotheses to direct further lines of inquiry. However, these studies and others — along with everyday observations — demonstrate that more successful diagnosticians (experts, specialists, or attending physicians) proceed through the process with greater accuracy and efficiency at each step. They ask fewer questions, consider fewer diagnoses, entertain the correct diagnosis earlier, and spend a larger amount of time confirming their "hunch" (rather than conducting a nonfocused generalized review of systems that generates more hypotheses and thus more investigation).[7,15,24,25]

This efficient and accurate diagnostic process is not explained simply by the accumulation of medical facts (students who memorize the most information are not always the best diagnosticians), by experience with many patients (more years of practice do not guarantee diagnostic skill), or by enhanced memory skills (studies demonstrate that more years of experience in clinical practice are not associated with enhanced memory skills[26,27]). Rather, diagnostic skill is highly dependent on how physicians' knowledge and experience are structured and organized in memory.

A study in which a case of endocarditis was presented in an organized and familiar format (the standard history and physical sequence) found that attending physicians were able to recall more case details than students. However, when the same case was presented in a random and unorganized fashion, the experts' recall deteriorated to that of the students.[27] In another study, the attending physicians' recall of laboratory data for a hypothetical patient exceeded that of the students only when the patient was assigned a diagnosis; when the laboratory data were simply memorized in the absence of a diagnosis, the students' ability to recall values equaled that of the practitioners.[28] These studies suggest that experienced physicians utilize a mental structure in which they store and organize information about diseases, but that they do not possess enhanced memory skills.[29] Clinicians compare patient information they collect with the information stored in their mental picture of a disease. When this information is unorganized, the framework within which they "file" the case details becomes disrupted.

Proposed mental models of how physicians store and organize knowledge of disease states include *prototypes* (e.g., recall of a typical case of pneumonia),[30] *instances* (recall of an uncommon disease or of a particularly memorable case, such as one of pneumococcal meningitis),[31] and *illness scripts*.[29,32] An illness script describes the way in which clinicians catalogue their own comprehensive pictures of disease states on the basis of previous experience. It combines a knowledge of predisposing conditions (demographic and risk factors) and a basic understanding of pathophysiological mechanisms with a detailed representation of a disease process and its manifestations. For example, a typical illness

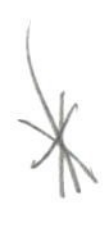

script for myocardial infarction encompasses risk factors such as smoking and diabetes, a mismatch of supply and demand at the myocardial level, and clinical findings of chest pain, dyspnea, and electrocardiographic changes. Illness scripts are fluid and adapted to real-world variations, since few disease presentations are textbook examples or are exactly in line with the clinician's previous experience. Because they reflect previous experience, the illness scripts of individual physicians often differ substantially from those in textbooks or from those of other physicians.

Clinicians use illness scripts as templates against which they compare the clinical information from the patient. If the clinical data are immediately concordant with the physician's illness script, then the easy and efficient process of pattern recognition unfolds. For example, an elderly diabetic smoker with substernal chest pain for two hours and ST-segment elevations on the electrocardiogram is likely to immediately trigger an illness script for myocardial infarction (pattern recognition). If, however, any of the acquired information is atypical of myocardial infarction (e.g., a report of pleuritic chest pain), more cognitive effort (analytic reasoning) is required to assess whether the findings are within the expected variation of disease presentation, or whether activation of a new script — invoking a new hypothesis — is required.

For precise and efficient diagnosis to occur, illness scripts must be accurate and accessible to the physician in real time.[33] This critical step is facilitated by *problem representation*, whereby the patient's signs and symptoms are transformed into a series of salient or distinguishing descriptive features (e.g., unilateral vs. bilateral, slowly progressive vs. rapid, acute vs. chronic). This limits the number of diagnostic possibilities and allows the case to be swiftly compared and contrasted with a focused number of illness scripts, allowing for the rapid exclusion of inappropriate diagnoses and the activation of appropriate scripts.[25,34-36]

For example, a 68-year-old man reports a "bad stomachache." On further inquiry, he points to the area under his right rib cage and reports that the pain "happens after meals," "has occurred for the past two weeks," "comes on quickly," "is very severe," and "goes away after 15 to 30 minutes." Whereas a novice physician may form differential diagnoses for each of these components of the history and then search for an overlap, an experienced clinician will mentally transform this narrative into a summary statement that is rich in distinguishing details: "an elderly man with recurrent, acute, postprandial, right upper quadrant pain." In this case, the physician scans his or her illness scripts for the subset of diseases that fit this well-defined scenario (e.g., biliary colic or peptic ulcer disease).[37,38] Relatively few additional historical features, examination maneuvers, laboratory tests, or imaging studies are needed at this point to choose among the limited number of diagnoses. Years of study and clinical experience — along with continued and deliberate practice (see conclusion) — allow for this rapid search among detailed, nuanced, and accurate illness scripts that leads to successful and sometimes effortless clinical problem-solving by skilled diagnosticians.

COGNITIVE ERRORS IN THE DIAGNOSTIC PROCESS

The study of clinical decision-making can be divided into two distinct areas: a normative component, which outlines how decisions *should* be made (e.g., the use of Bayes's theorem or decision trees), and a descriptive component, which describes how decisions are *actually* made.[39] Because physicians are imperfect quantitative reasoners, there are notable differences between human cognition and Bayesian reasoning. This discrepancy often underlies mistakes in the diagnostic process. (Other determinants of diagnostic errors, such as systems issues, are not discussed here.)

Bayesian or normative reasoning is predicated on having accurate data and subjecting it to accurate calculations. However, a physician's mental concept of a given disease (illness script) does not usually include detailed knowledge of the prevalence of the disease or of the sensitivities and specificities of particular symptoms, signs, and tests for diagnosing the disease.[40,41] Physicians — and all other human decision makers — routinely use imperfect numerical estimates made by inference from small samples, perceive patterns or associations when no such connections exist,[41-43] and liberally employ heuristics.

Heuristics are mental shortcuts ("rules of thumb") that usually lead to efficient and correct decisions and thus are used extensively by experienced clinicians.[44] Unfortunately, the use of heuristics also leads to predictable and recurrent errors.[45-47] Heuristics are necessary because thinking carefully, analyzing information, and deriving conclusions at each encounter is too difficult and inefficient; heuristics greatly simplify the task of judging probability and frequency.[45]

The *representative heuristic* leads the clinician to judge the probability of a disease by the extent to which the case matches expectations (the physician's illness script) rather than by taking into account the specificity and sensitivity of individual features for a given diagnosis and considering the overall prevalence of the illness. For example, a hypertensive patient with headache, sweating, and palpitations may be assessed as likely to have a pheochromocytoma, since the clinical features are a perfect match with the textbook description; this reasoning ignores the facts that each of these individual features is common in the absence of pheochromocytoma and that the prevalence of pheochromocytoma is extremely low.

The *availability heuristic* leads the clinician to judge the probability of a disease by its ease of recall rather than by its true prevalence. Human memory is particularly biased toward the recall of recent events, atypical presentations, and contradictory or shocking cases, leading to probability estimates that are far out of proportion to the actual prevalence of the disease.[2,39,42] For instance, a clinician who correctly diagnoses pheochromocytoma in one patient is likely to overestimate the probability of pheochromocytoma in the next hypertensive patient encountered, even though the overwhelming majority of such patients will have essential hypertension and the clinician is unlikely ever to see a case of pheochromocytoma again. Even the possibility of *becoming* a remarkable case (because of a dire outcome from a missed diagnosis) may lead the physician to substantially exaggerate the probability of rare but serious disorders.[48]

The *anchoring heuristic* leads clinicians to remain committed to their initial hypotheses even as contradictory evidence accumulates. A clinician who makes an initial diagnosis of nephrolithiasis (the anchor) has a tendency to adjust post-test probability inadequately (in comparison with Bayesian analysis) as new information (e.g., a negative urinalysis result) becomes available.[39,46]

Premature closure is a common mistake in which a physician settles upon a diagnosis without sufficient evidence or without seeking or carefully considering contradictory information.[49] For instance, a physician may be so certain that a patient with gastrointestinal symptoms has irritable bowel syndrome that further indicated evaluation (e.g., imaging studies or endoscopy) is not pursued. The application of a diagnostic label, however tentative, often curtails further evaluation and prematurely shifts the emphasis to treatment.

A related problem is *confirmation bias*, the tendency to look for evidence that supports an early working hypothesis, to ignore data that contradict it, and to misinterpret ambiguous evidence (by interpreting it to be in line with expectations).[2,3,41] This bias reflects the fact that physicians tend to struggle with discrepant information. It is particularly difficult late in the reasoning process to recognize the need to repeat early steps, such as the history and physical examination, and to invoke a new diagnosis. The result is a failure to fully consider and evaluate alternative diagnostic possibilities, thereby leading (as in premature closure) to an incorrect treatment course.

Since Bayes's theorem does not describe or reflect how learning occurs or how memory is formed, structured, or accessed in the human mind, there is little reason to suspect that it would accurately describe real-time clinical reasoning.[50] Rather, Bayesian analysis remains an accurate model of normative decision-making that complements the physician's diagnostic process as a decision-support tool. It provides instruction in how data *should* be integrated in the diagnostic process, and it is a particularly attractive alternative to human calculation when complex or abundant numerical data are available.[51]

METHODS TO IMPROVE DIAGNOSIS

Understanding both the cognitive processes and the cognitive errors of diagnosis is more than a theoretical pursuit. Armed with this insight, physicians have the opportunity to improve their own diagnostic abilities and their teaching of others.

Teaching students detailed and prototypical cases of common diseases — and requiring them to explicitly discriminate among such cases, as they will in practice — may enable them to form more accurate and rich illness scripts with which subsequent cases can be compared and contrasted. Since patients do not typically walk into the office reporting dysfunction in a particular organ system, trainees may benefit from being introduced to diseases in the context of presenting symptoms rather than in the context of a defined organ unit, lecture, or book chapter. As a result, their knowledge (illness scripts) may be formed in the same way that it is accessed — with an undiagnosed patient — facilitating problem representation and the formulation of hypotheses.[52]

An essential (but not sufficient) element of achieving diagnostic success is experience. Experience makes it possible for physicians to recognize cases as similar to previous ones and to more readily identify likely diagnoses and indicated diagnostic tests. Expertise, however, does not come about passively, simply as a result of taking care of patients[53,54]; rather, it requires ongoing attention to clinical decision-making, for example, by reflecting on previous decisions, seeking feedback and patient follow-up information from colleagues,[55] and taking the opportunity to learn from cases managed by other clinicians, as presented in rounds and clinical conferences and as described in the scientific literature.

Experience alone does not change a clinician's predilection to make cognitive errors.[49,56,57] However, knowledge about cognitive errors in diagnosis and the limitations of human judgment can help clinicians to be more thoughtful in making decisions.[39,58] Knowing the tendency to overestimate the probabilities of uncommon diseases may minimize the ordering of tests for which positive results are unlikely (and, when found, are likely to be false positives). Recognizing the predilection to cling to initial diagnoses and to favor confirmatory evidence may force clinicians to routinely ask, "What else could this be?" This type of mindful practice (metacognition, or thinking about thinking) may ultimately help to guard against diagnostic pitfalls.[58-60]

REFERENCES

1.
McCormick JS. Diagnosis: the need for demystification. Lancet 1986;2:1434-5.
2.
Leape LL. Error in medicine. JAMA 1994;272:1851-7.
3.
Bergus GR, Hamm RM. How physicians make medical decisions and why medical decision making can help. Prim Care 1995;22:167-80.
4.
Elstein AS, Schwarz A. Clinical problem solving and diagnostic decision making: selective review of the cognitive literature. BMJ 2002;324:729-32.
5.
Schmidt HG, Norman GR, Boshuizen HP. A cognitive perspective on medical expertise: theory and implication. Acad Med 1990;65:611-21. [Erratum, Acad Med 1992;67:287.]
6.
Regehr G, Cline J, Norman GR, Brooks L. Effect of processing strategy on diagnostic skill in dermatology. Acad Med 1994;69:Suppl:S34-S36.
7.
Elstein AS, Shulman LS, Sprafka SA. Medical problem solving: an analysis of clinical reasoning. Cambridge, Mass.: Harvard University Press, 1978.
8.
Kassirer JP, Kopelman RI. Cognitive errors in diagnosis: instantiation, classification, and consequences. Am J Med 1989;86:433-41.
9.
Kassirer JP, Gorry GA. Clinical problem solving: a behavioral analysis. Ann Intern Med 1978;89:245-55.
10.
Barrows HS, Bennett K. The diagnostic (problem solving) skill of the neurologist: experimental studies and their implications for neurological training. Arch Neurol 1972;26:273-7.
11.
Barrows HS, Norman GR, Neufeld VR, Feightner JW. The clinical reasoning of randomly selected physicians in general medical practice. Clin Invest Med 1982;5:49-55.
12.
Gruppen LD, Woolliscroft JO, Wolf FM. The contribution of different components of the clinical encounter in generating and eliminating diagnostic hypotheses. Proc Annu Conf Res Med Educ 1988;27:242-7.
13.
Miller GA. The magical number seven plus or minus two: some limits on our capacity for processing information. Psychol Rev 1956;63:81-97.
14.
Joseph GM, Patel VL. Domain knowledge and hypothesis generation in diagnostic reasoning. Med Decis Making 1990;10:31-46.
15.
Neufeld VR, Norman GR, Feightner JW, Barrows HS. Clinical problem-solving by medical students: a cross-sectional and longitudinal analysis. Med Educ 1981;15:315-22.
16.
Sisson JC, Donnelly MB, Hess GE, Woolliscroft JO. The characteristics of early diagnostic hypotheses generated by physicians (experts) and students (novices) at one medical school. Acad Med 1991;66:607-12.
17.
Kassirer J. Diagnostic reasoning. Ann Intern Med 1989;110:893-900.
18.
Price RB, Vlahcevic ZR. Logical principles in differential diagnosis. Ann Intern Med 1971;75:89-95.
19.
Coderre S, Mandin H, Harasym PH, Fick GH. Diagnostic reasoning strategies and diagnostic success. Med Educ 2003;37:695-703.
20.
Mandin H, Jones A, Woloschuk W, Harasym P. Helping students learn to think like experts when solving clinical problems. Acad Med 1997;72:173-9.
21.
Pauker SG, Kassirer JP. The threshold approach to clinical decision making. N Engl J Med 1980;302:1109-17.
22.
Idem. Therapeutic decision making: a cost-benefit analysis. N Engl J Med 1975;293:229-34.
23.
Gruppen LD, Woolliscroft JO, Kolars JC. Diagnostic accuracy and likelihood estimations of attending physicians and house officers. Acad Med 1996;71:Suppl:S4-S6.
24.
Joseph GM, Patel VL. Domain knowledge and hypothesis generation in diagnostic reasoning. Med Decis Making 1990;10:31-46.
25.
Patel VL, Groen CJ, Patel YC. Cognitive aspects of clinical performance during patient workup: the role of medical expertise. Adv Health Sci Educ Theory Pract 1997;2:95-114.
26.
Patel VL, Groen GJ, Frederiksen CH. Differences between medical students and doctors in memory for clinical cases. Med Educ 1986;20:3-9.
27.
Coughlin LD, Patel VL. Processing of critical information by physicians and medical students. J Med Educ 1987;62:818-28.
28.
Norman GR, Brooks LR, Allen SW. Recall by expert medical practitioners and novices as a record of processing attention. J Exp Psychol Learn Mem Cogn 1989;15:1166-74.
29.
Schmidt HG, Norman GR, Boshuizen HP. A cognitive perspective on medical expertise: theory and implication. Acad Med 1990;65:611-21.
30.
Bordage G, Zacks R. The structure of medical knowledge in the memories of medical students and general practitioners: categories and prototypes. Med Educ 1984;18:406-16.
31.
Custers EJ, Regehr G, Norman GR. Mental representations of medical diagnostic knowledge: a review. Acad Med 1996;71:Suppl:S55-S61.

32.
Custers EJ, Boshuizen HP, Schmidt HG. The influence of medical expertise, case typicality, and illness script component on case processing and disease probability estimates. Mem Cognit 1996;24:384-99.
33.
Larkin J, McDermott J, Simon DP, Simon HA. Expert and novice performance in solving physics problems. Science 1980;208:1335-42.
34.
Bordage G. Why did I miss the diagnosis? Some cognitive explanations and educational implications. Acad Med 1999;74:Suppl:S138-S143.
35.
Idem. Elaborated knowledge: a key to successful diagnostic thinking. Acad Med 1994;69:883-5.
36.
Bordage G, Lemieux M. Which medical textbook to read? Emphasizing semantic structures. Acad Med 1990;65:Suppl:S23-S24.
37.
Chang RW, Bordage G, Connell KJ. The importance of early problem representation during case presentations. Acad Med 1998;73: Suppl:S109-S111.
38.
Bordage G, Lemieux M. Some cognitive characteristics of medical students with and without diagnostic reasoning difficulties. Proc Annu Conf Res Med Educ 1986;25:185-90.
39.
Elstein AS. Heuristics and biases: selected errors in clinical reasoning. Acad Med 1999;74:791-4.
40.
Eddy DM, Clanton CH. The art of diagnosis: solving the clinicopathological exercise. N Engl J Med 1982;306: 1263-8.
41.
Hamm RM, Zubialde J. Physicians' expert cognition and the problem of cognitive biases. Prim Care 1995;22: 181-212.
42.
Richardson WS. Five uneasy pieces about pre-test probability. J Gen Intern Med 2002;17:881-2.
43.
Redelmeier DA, Tversky A. On the belief that arthritis pain is related to the weather. Proc Natl Acad Sci U S A 1996;93:2895-6.
44.
Patel VL, Kaufman DR, Arocha JF. Emerging paradigms of cognition in medical decision-making. J Biomed Inform 2002;35: 52-75.
45.
Tversky A, Kahneman D. Availability: a heuristic for judging frequency and probability. Cognit Psychol 1973;5:207-32.
46.
Idem. Judgment under uncertainty: heuristics and biases. Science 1974;185: 1124-31.
47.
Redelmeier DA, Ferris LE, Tu JV, Hux JE, Schull MJ. Problems for clinical judgement: introducing cognitive psychology as one more basic science. CMAJ 2001;164: 358-60.
48.
Thibault GE. The appropriate degree of diagnostic certainty. N Engl J Med 1994;331:1216-20.
49.
Voytovich AE, Rippey RM, Suffredini A. Premature conclusions in diagnostic reasoning. J Med Educ 1985;60:302-7.
50.
Norman GR. The epistemology of clinical reasoning: perspectives from philosophy, psychology, and neuroscience. Acad Med 2000;75: Suppl:S127-S135.
51.
Plante DA, Kassirer JP, Zarin DA, Pauker SG. Clinical decision consultation service. Am J Med 1986;80:1169-76.
52.
Eva KW. What every teacher needs to know about clinical reasoning. Med Educ 2005;39:98-106. [Erratum, Med Educ 2005;39:753.]
53.
Choudhry NK, Fletcher RH, Soumerai SB. Systematic review: the relationship between clinical experience and quality of health care. Ann Intern Med 2005;142: 260-73.
54.
Ericsson KA. Deliberate practice and the acquisition and maintenance of expert performance in medicine and related domains. Acad Med 2004;79:Suppl:S70-S81.
55.
Redelmeier DA. Improving patient care: the cognitive psychology of missed diagnoses. Ann Intern Med 2005;142:115-20.
56.
Friedman MH, Connell KJ, Olthoff AJ, Sinacore JM, Bordage G. Medical student errors in making a diagnosis. Acad Med 1998;73: Suppl:S19-S21.
57.
Chimowitz MI, Logigian EL, Caplan LR. The accuracy of bedside neurological diagnoses. Ann Neurol 1990;28: 78-85.
58.
Bradley CP. Can we avoid bias? BMJ 2005;330:784.
59.
Graber M, Gordon R, Franklin N. Reducing diagnostic errors in medicine: what's the goal? Acad Med 2002;77:981-92.
60.
Croskerry P. The importance of cognitive errors in diagnosis and strategies to minimize them. Acad Med 2003;78:775-80.

In each of the following *Clinical Problem-Solving*
exercises, information about a real patient
is presented in stages (boldface type)
to an expert clinician,
who responds to the information,
sharing his or her reasoning with the reader (regular type).
The authors' commentary follows.

High Time for Action

ASHA R. KALLIANPUR, M.D., KATHERINE A. POEHLING, M.D.,
AND ROBERT S. DITTUS, M.D., M.P.H.

A 58-year-old man receiving hemodialysis after failed renal transplantation was admitted with unstable angina. He had a history of hypertension, diabetes mellitus, ischemic heart disease, and transplant-related immunosuppression of several years' duration. Less than four weeks earlier, he had undergone repair of an intraabdominal aortic aneurysm and removal of the renal graft.

Cardiac catheterization was deferred because the prothrombin time and activated partial-thromboplastin time were prolonged, at 88.0 seconds (international normalized ratio [INR], 7.2) and 77 seconds (normal range, 28 to 40), respectively. He reported malaise, fevers, abdominal pain, nausea, and vomiting but no increase in bleeding since the surgery.

The abnormal results of the coagulation tests could be due to an inappropriate method of blood collection or to laboratory error. If the results are valid, the uneventful abdominal surgery indicates a recently acquired coagulopathy. Confirmation of normal preoperative coagulation tests is important. Prolongation of both the prothrombin time and the activated partial-thromboplastin time could be due to a deficiency of one or more factors in the pathway common to both tests (factor V, factor X, fibrinogen, and prothrombin), a circulating anticoagulant, or vitamin K deficiency. I would inquire about the patient's diet, the use of anticoagulants, and the recent use of antibiotics that might lead to low vitamin K levels.

The patient's wife reported that his oral intake had been "minimal" for the past month. His medications included isosorbide dinitrate, lovastatin, atenolol, prednisone given at a tapered dose since the removal of the graft (10 mg daily), aspirin (325 mg daily), insulin, lansoprazole, iron, and multivitamins. In response to a question, the patient stated that he had not taken oral anticoagulants or antibiotics. However, heparin was used regularly during dialysis.

On physical examination, the patient appeared to be chronically ill. His weight was 84 kg, which was 6 kg below his preoperative dry weight (the postdialysis weight). The

oral temperature was 37.7°C, respirations were 18, the pulse was 67 and regular, and the blood pressure was 172/78 mm Hg. Bleeding was absent. Heart sounds were normal. The surgical wound was well healed. Bowel sounds were decreased, and the right lower quadrant was tender. Distention, organomegaly, rebound, and guarding were absent, and there was no palpable mass. A stool guaiac test was negative for occult blood.

The abdominal pain, nausea, and fever are worrisome because they suggest the possibility of an abscess or bleeding in the region of the aortic graft or the renal-graft bed. Chronic disseminated intravascular coagulation complicating an aortic aneurysm or its repair has been well described.[1] A computed tomographic (CT) scan of the abdomen and pelvis would be helpful. Fever, chronic nausea, and abdominal pain also raise the possibility of adrenal insufficiency, pancreatitis, or a bowel infection. The aspirin treatment should be stopped pending evaluation of the coagulopathy. Oral iron treatment, which may contribute to nausea, should also be discontinued. Measurement of the prothrombin time and activated partial-thromboplastin time should be repeated.

The patient did not undergo dialysis the day the tests were performed, and the sample was obtained by peripheral venipuncture. The results of repeated coagulation tests were similarly abnormal. Levels of serum electrolytes, amylase, lipase, and liver enzymes were normal; the albumin level was 2.9 g per deciliter. The white-cell count was 5300 per cubic millimeter, with a normal differential count; the hematocrit was 33 percent; the platelet count was 172,000 per cubic millimeter. The chest film and electrocardiogram showed no acute abnormalities, and an abdominopelvic CT scan obtained after the oral administration of contrast material was unremarkable. The prothrombin time and activated partial-thromboplastin time had been tested four weeks earlier; the values at that time were 12.8 seconds (INR, 1.1) and 32 seconds, respectively.

The patient has an acquired coagulopathy. Vitamin K deficiency, exposure to warfarin or heparin, and liver disease are common causes of elevations in both the prothrombin time and the activated partial-thromboplastin time. In this case, however, the much greater increase in the prothrombin time than in the activated partial-thromboplastin time rules out heparin as the sole cause of the coagulopathy, and there is no evidence of intrinsic liver disease. A normal platelet count makes the diagnosis of disseminated intravascular coagulation unlikely, although the blood smear should be reviewed for the presence of schistocytes, and the levels of fibrinogen and of fibrin- and fibrinogen-degradation products should be measured. The patient did not report the use of warfarin, but a careful review of his medications is nonetheless important. His extended illness, hypoalbuminemia, and postoperative anorexia are consistent with a nutritional vitamin K deficiency. Vitamin K deficiency is an underrecognized complication of prolonged illness and malnutrition, especially in hospitalized patients who have undergone surgery.[2] There is no evidence of extrahepatic biliary obstruction or intestinal malabsorption, which are less common causes of vitamin K deficiency.

The blood smear showed no microangiopathic changes. The D-dimer level was more than 0.50 mg per deciliter (normal value, <0.25). The fibrinogen level was 654.4 mg per deciliter (normal range, 180 to 350). Inspection of the contents of available medication bottles and a review of the entire list of medications were unrevealing.

With bed rest, the patient had no further chest pain. However, he reported increased lower abdominal pain and diarrhea. His oral temperature remained in the range of 37.3 to 37.9°C. The results of an abdominal examination and an electrocardiogram were unchanged. Adrenal insufficiency was considered unlikely, since the patient reported that he had been taking three 2.5-mg tablets of prednisone daily before admission. Aspirin and iron were withdrawn.

An acquired inhibitor of coagulation should be ruled out by performing the prothrombin-time assay on a 1:1 incubation mixture of the patient's plasma and normal plasma. Measurement of the thrombin clotting time would be useful to determine whether heparin is contributing to the coagulopathy. Another possibility is the postoperative development of antibodies to topical bovine thrombin, a surgical hemostatic agent, or to the bovine factor V contained in the agent. These antibodies may cross-react with human factor V in the prothrombin-time assay and may react with thrombin in the thrombin-clotting-time assay. Reported in vitro elevations of the prothrombin time, activated partial-thromboplastin time, and thrombin clotting time due to such antibodies may not always be clinically significant.[3]

The patient had no abnormal bleeding. The thrombin clotting time was obtained after hemodialysis. The result of the prothrombin-time assay performed on a 1:1 dilution of the patient's plasma and control plasma was completely normal.

Rapid and complete correction of the prothrombin time in the 1:1 mixture makes an acquired inhibitor of coagulation unlikely. The thrombin clotting time is more sensitive for the detection of antithrombin antibodies. The administration of aqueous vitamin K

(5 to 10 mg daily) subcutaneously or by mouth is appropriate. Parenteral administration is possible but carries an increased risk of anaphylaxis. Fresh-frozen plasma, 2 to 4 units every 12 hours as needed, combined with ultrafiltration to prevent volume overload, should be administered to treat active bleeding. The use of heparin should be avoided.

Aqueous vitamin K (5 mg daily) was administered subcutaneously, and the dialysis unit was instructed to discontinue heparin treatment. The prothrombin time and activated partial-thromboplastin time returned to normal values within 48 hours after the first dose of vitamin K. The thrombin clotting time was normal. Stool samples were negative for white cells and *Clostridium difficile.*

On the eighth hospital day, the patient underwent coronary angioplasty and placement of a stent. A hematoma in the groin and hypotension complicated the procedure, despite correction of the coagulation times. At discharge, four days later, the patient was afebrile, with improved oral intake and a hematocrit that was stable at 30.6 percent. The medications were unchanged except for the addition of clopidogrel for stent protection; treatment with aspirin and iron was resumed. The patient was instructed to eat plenty of green, leafy vegetables. Close follow-up was scheduled.

Rapid correction of the prothrombin time with a low total dose of vitamin K (10 mg) is reassuring. Much larger doses are often needed to counteract warfarin toxicity. However, close follow-up to identify any further bleeding and thrombotic thrombocytopenic purpura, which is associated with the use of clopidogrel, is essential.[4]

Ten days later, the patient was readmitted with atypical chest pain, epistaxis, hemoptysis, recurrent fever, and nausea. The prothrombin time on admission was 83.0 seconds (INR, 8.6), and the activated partial-thromboplastin time was 109.3 seconds. The physical examination was unchanged except for an oral temperature of 37.9°C, blood in the nares, and a resolving hematoma in the groin. The platelet count was normal; the hematocrit was 27.7 percent.

The patient should be treated immediately with plasma and vitamin K. Platelet transfusions may be indicated because of the use of potent antiplatelet agents. The rapid recurrence of the coagulopathy strongly suggests an extrinsic cause of vitamin K antagonism. It is critically important to inspect all the pills that the patient is taking at home and to consider measuring blood levels of warfarin and brodifacoum (rat poison). The fever may be related to retroperitoneal bleeding or infection due to his immunocompromised state. In the absence of localizing signs of infection, relative adrenal insufficiency deserves reconsideration.

The patient's wife brought in all his medication bottles for review. Warfarin (2.5 mg) was found in a bottle labeled "prednisone, 2.5 mg." The prescription for prednisone had been written two months earlier in the dialysis unit, two days after a prescription for prednisone (10 mg daily) had been given at the clinic. As a cost-saving strategy, a three-month supply of 2.5-mg pills was dispensed, instead of the one-month supply prescribed. The patient had begun taking three of these tablets daily immediately after the repair of his aneurysm, and he had resumed taking the tablets after the recent hospital discharge. An investigation revealed that the prescription had been hand-filled by a pharmacy technician and that the error had not been detected, despite a review by a senior pharmacist. The close proximity of the warfarin and prednisone containers at the pharmacy technician's work station was thought to have contributed to this apparently isolated error.

The patient had a good response to treatment with fresh-frozen plasma and large doses of vitamin K. Treatment with prednisone was resumed at a dose of 10 mg daily, with resolution of his fever and gastrointestinal symptoms.

COMMENTARY

A recent report by the Institute of Medicine states that preventable medical errors (including medication errors) are far more common than previously thought, although the exact numbers continue to be debated.[5-7] Errors in the ordering and administration of medications for hospitalized patients have been studied more extensively than errors in the dispensing of outpatient prescriptions.[8,9]

The error in this case could have been detected during the patient's first hospitalization had his wife been asked to retrieve all medication bottles from their home, a three-hour drive from the hospital. However, the existence of a rational explanation for vitamin K deficiency and the easy correction of clotting times with treatment lowered the clinical suspicion of warfarin toxicity below a critical threshold. The rapid recurrence of the coagulopathy after the patient had been discharged prompted the consultants to reconsider this possibility.

With regard to results, dispensing errors mimic factitious drug ingestion or poisoning. They should be part of any differential diagnosis that includes noncompliance with medication or variations of Munchausen's syndrome.

Furthermore, dispensing errors may lead to reciprocal errors of equal or greater import. In this case, prednisone was inadvertently withheld from a patient with chronic suppression of the pituitary–adrenal axis when warfarin was substituted for it.

Pharmacy policies that alter the prescribing physician's instructions may have important ramifications for patient safety. Sending a patient a three-month supply of pills reduces the pharmacy's mailing costs but can worsen the effect of a dispensing error by delaying its detection. A patient who is instructed to complete a course of medication within a given period may assume that extra medication indicates a change in the prescribed dose. A nonselective policy of dispensing large quantities of prescription drugs that may soon be changed or discontinued increases the likelihood of medication-related errors.

In addition to increased attention to human factors, several system changes may reduce the frequency of dispensing errors. These include automated dispensing mechanisms, bar coding of drugs in the pharmacy, and computerized prescription entry.[9-11] Improved recording of medication changes and better communication between physicians and the pharmacy are needed. The challenge in the future will be to develop prescribing, dispensing, and information and tracking systems that make errors more visible and that minimize their effect. The recognition of errors only after the onset of clinical and laboratory abnormalities (the elevated prothrombin time and activated partial-thromboplastin time in this case) constitutes a system failure.[12]

Physicians usually check medications by reviewing a list or the container labels, not by examining the actual contents of the containers. In this case, "Coumadin" was inscribed on the tablets, which were green, and the physicians caring for the patient knew that prednisone tablets are not green. However, it would be impossible for most physicians to recognize the myriad pills patients take by appearance alone. Many pills look similar, and some do not have identifiable markings. Patients, on the other hand, frequently know their medications solely by their appearance, and they should be encouraged to ask the provider or pharmacist to check any discrepancies that might reflect dispensing errors.[13] Patients and caregivers might also be empowered to detect dispensing errors themselves.

The technology is available to scan a digital color photograph of each pill, with a complete description of its appearance, into every pharmacy's computer. The scanned image and description of the pill (linked to the bar code) can then be printed automatically on the container label. Contracts between pharmacies and drug manufacturers may ultimately require that, for all oral medications, such information be placed in a central computerized database to which health care professionals and patients have access. This strategy could potentially be cost-effective, given the cost of hospitalizations and acute care visits estimated to result from medication errors.[14,15]

Although system changes can and should result from the identification of avoidable medical errors, caregivers must also bear in mind that these errors may occur.[16,17] When the clinical presentation can be explained by an unintended drug effect, it is time to look at the patient's pills.

Supported in part by an unrestricted gift from the Pfizer Foundation.

The views expressed in this article do not necessarily represent the views of the Department of Veterans Affairs or of the U.S. government.

This article first appeared in the January 4, 2001, issue of the New England Journal of Medicine.

REFERENCES

1.
Aboulafia DM, Aboulafia ED. Aortic aneurysm-induced disseminated intravascular coagulation. Ann Vasc Surg 1996;10:396-405.

2.
Ansell JE, Kumar R, Deykin D. The spectrum of vitamin K deficiency. JAMA 1977;238:40-2.

3.
Ortel TL, Charles LA, Keller FG, et al. Topical thrombin and acquired coagulation factor inhibitors: clinical spectrum and laboratory diagnosis. Am J Hematol 1994;45:128-35.

4.
Bennett CL, Connors JM, Carwile JM, et al. Thrombotic thrombocytopenic purpura associated with clopidogrel. N Engl J Med 2000;342:1773-7.

5.
Kohn LT, Corrigan JM, Donaldson MS, eds. To err is human: building a safer health system. Washington, D.C.: National Academy Press, 2000.

6.
McDonald CJ, Weiner M, Hui SL. Deaths due to medical errors are exaggerated in Institute of Medicine report. JAMA 2000;284:93-5.

7.
Leape LL. Institute of Medicine medical error figures are not exaggerated. JAMA 2000;284:95-7.

8.
Brennan TA, Leape LL, Laird NM, et al. Incidence of adverse events and negligence in hospitalized patients: results of the Harvard Medical Practice Study I. N Engl J Med 1991;324:370-6.

9.
Allan EL, Barker KN, Malloy MJ, Heller WM. Dispensing errors and counseling in community practice. Am Pharm 1995;35(12):25-33.

10.
Allnutt MF. Human factors in accidents. Br J Anaesth 1987;59:856-64.

11.
Davis NM, Cohen MR. Slips and mistakes in dispensing. Am Pharm 1994;34(4):18.

12.
Leape LL. Error in medicine. JAMA 1994;272:1851-7.

13.
Davis NM, Cohen MR. Ten steps for ensuring dispensing accuracy. Am Pharm 1994;34(7):22-3.

14.
Johnson JA, Bootman JL. Drug-related morbidity and mortality: a cost-of-illness model. Arch Intern Med 1995;155:1949-56.

15.
Einarson TR. Drug-related hospital admissions. Ann Pharmacother 1993;27:832-40.

16.
Leape LL, Bates DW, Cullen DJ, et al. Systems analysis of adverse drug events. JAMA 1995;274:35-43.

17.
Langley GJ, Nolan KM, Nolan TW, Provost LP, Norman CL. The improvement guide: a practical approach to enhancing organizational performance. San Francisco: Jossey-Bass, 1996.

Of Nicks and Time

BRAHMAJEE K. NALLAMOTHU, M.D., M.P.H.,
SANJAY SAINT, M.D., M.P.H., THEODORE J. KOLIAS, M.D.,
AND KIM A. EAGLE, M.D.

A 32-year-old man with a history of asthma and "crack" cocaine use presented to the emergency department after an episode of syncope. Earlier that evening, he had smoked crack cocaine several times. Shortly after his last use, he began to have sharp chest pain, which radiated to his shoulders and was associated with dizziness and diaphoresis, followed by a sudden loss of consciousness. His wife, who witnessed the event, described him as "foaming at the mouth" and having involuntary trembling of his arms and legs. He was brought immediately to the emergency department.

The patient reported no shortness of breath, nausea, or vomiting. He had no history of intravenous drug use, coronary artery disease, hypertension, diabetes mellitus, or hypercholesterolemia and no family history of sudden death or cardiac disease. He took no medications. He smoked cigarettes and marijuana regularly but stated that he had used crack cocaine only once before.

The differential diagnosis includes acute coronary insufficiency leading to a tachyarrhythmia or bradyarrhythmia, low cardiac output as a result of profound myocardial ischemia, or an acute tachyarrhythmia caused by the effects of cocaine. Additional possibilities include a seizure, which might occur with a cocaine-induced hypertensive crisis, vasodepressor syncope or bradyarrhythmia, and acute dissection of the ascending aorta. It would be useful to know whether the onset of chest pain was sudden. In cocaine-related acute coronary insufficiency, symptoms generally evolve over a period of minutes. In the case of an arrhythmia or aortic dissection, in contrast, the onset is typically more sudden.

In the emergency department, the patient was alert but in mild distress from chest discomfort. He was afebrile, with a blood pressure of 116/77 mm Hg, a pulse of 112 beats per minute, and a respiratory rate of 16 per minute. Examination of the head and neck revealed no signs of trauma. There was no jugular venous distention or carotid bruits. An examination of the lungs revealed scattered wheezes. Heart sounds were normal, and there were no murmurs, rubs, or gallops. There was no cyanosis, clubbing, or edema of the arms or

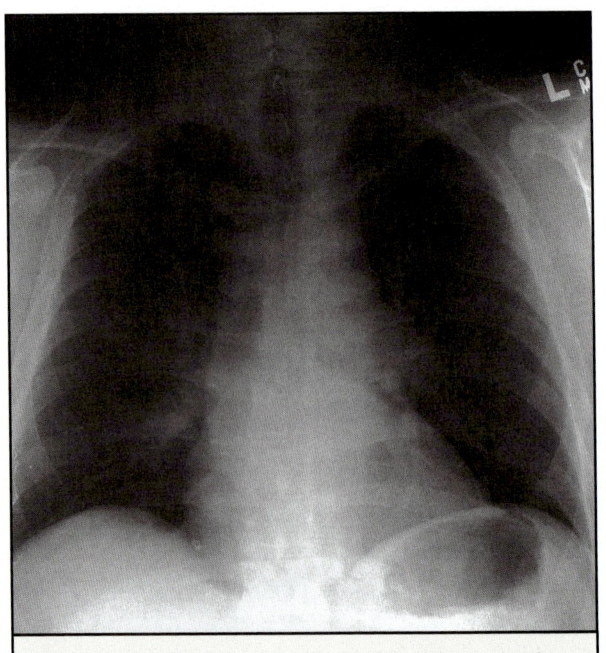

Figure 1. Chest Film Showing Fullness of the Pulmonary Hilar Vessels and Prominence of the Ascending Aorta.

legs. The results of the neurologic examination were normal. Initial laboratory studies showed a leukocyte count of 18,200 per cubic millimeter. The hematocrit and levels of serum electrolytes, serum creatinine, blood urea nitrogen, and cardiac enzymes were normal. Urinary drug screening was positive for cannabinoids and cocaine. Electrocardiography showed sinus tachycardia with a short PR interval, a vertical axis, mild respiratory variation in the QRS complex, and subtle elevation of the ST-segment leads in V2, III, and aVF. Chest radiography was performed (Figure 1). A computed tomographic (CT) examination of the head, obtained without the administration of contrast medium, showed no abnormalities.

It would be useful to know whether all the arterial pulses were carefully examined and whether the blood pressure was measured in each arm. The increased white-cell count is consistent with the occurrence of a myocardial infarction or aortic dissection. The chest film shows fullness of the pulmonary hilar vessels, and the ascending aorta appears somewhat prominent.

Acute coronary insufficiency and myocardial infarction are by far the most common cardiac diagnoses in someone presenting with chest discomfort after cocaine use. However, the subtle abnormalities on the electrocardiogram and chest film raise the possibility of aortic dissection with pericardial bleeding.

The proper approach in this case is challenging. If acute coronary insufficiency is present, antiplatelet and anticoagulant therapies are indicated. However, the use of anticoagulants is contraindicated in patients with aortic dissection. A beta-blocker is the preferred approach to the treatment of elevated blood pressure in patients with aortic dissection, whereas in patients with acute coronary insufficiency as a result of cocaine use, there is concern that isolated beta-blocker therapy may increase coronary vasoconstriction in response to unopposed α-adrenergic stimulation. Additional information is needed to clarify the diagnosis. A spiral CT scan of the chest, a transesophageal echocardiogram, or both should be obtained immediately to rule out aortic dissection. A transesophageal echocardiogram might also be useful in the diagnosis of acute coronary insufficiency if it showed abnormalities in regional wall motion.

The patient was given aspirin, ketorolac, intravenous fluids, and nebulized albuterol and ipratropium. His chest discomfort decreased substantially. He was admitted for overnight observation with telemetric monitoring. Approximately six hours after admission, he again reported mild discomfort in his chest and upper back. His blood pressure was 98/67 mm Hg, his pulse was 120 beats per minute, and his respiratory rate was 22 per minute. He was given a sublingual nitroglycerin tablet and subsequently became dizzy and briefly lost consciousness. No seizure activity was noted. After he recovered consciousness, his blood pressure was unmeasurable with a noninvasive blood-pressure cuff, his pulse was 140 beats per minute and regular, and his respiratory rate was 28 per minute.

The patient was immediately transferred to the coronary care unit, where treatment with intravenous fluids and dopamine hydrochloride was begun. Systolic blood pressure, measured with use of a radial arterial catheter, was 70 mm Hg; an electrocardiogram showed sinus tachycardia with no acute changes suggestive of ischemia. On examination, the patient was somnolent and reported occasional sharp pains in his chest, upper shoulders, and back. While sitting upright, he had marked jugular venous distention. The heart sounds were rapid and faint, with no murmurs, rubs, or gallops. The lungs were clear. The patient's hands and feet were cool and clammy, with faint peripheral pulses. The results of the neurologic examination remained normal.

There has been a serious deterioration in the patient's condition. If coronary ischemia was the cause of this syndrome, marked electrocardiographic changes and pulmonary congestion would be expected. The presence of clear lung fields argues against left ventricular failure as the primary cause of his worsening status. The low-output state and elevated jugular venous pressure suggest that right ventricular function is poor. At this point, the differential diagnosis includes an acute right ventricular infarction or subacute cardiac rupture as a result of myocardial infarction with pericardial tamponade. Another possibility is pulmonary embolism; however, there is no clear predisposing condition. Aortic dissection of the ascending aorta with cardiac tamponade would explain all of the clinical findings. Although aortic dissection occurs much less often than coronary insufficiency in patients with cocaine-related chest pain, the electrocardiographic findings in this case are not suggestive of an acute myocardial infarction of the inferior wall, a right ventricular myocardial infarction, or an extensive ventricular injury.

Emergency transthoracic echocardiography revealed a moderate-sized pericardial effusion with evidence of right atrial and right ventricular diastolic collapse, dramatic respiratory changes in mitral inflow velocity, a dilated aortic root (54 mm), and minimal aortic insufficiency. Hyperechoic areas suggestive of thrombus were noted in the pericardial space. Pulmonary-artery catheterization revealed a right atrial pressure of 20 mm Hg, a pulmonary-artery pressure of 30/22 mm Hg, and a pulmonary-capillary wedge pressure of 22 mm Hg.

The presence of presumed thrombus in the pericardial space and equalization of the diastolic pressures in the right atrium, pulmonary artery, and pulmonary-capillary wedge confirm the diagnosis of acute hemopericardium. The most likely cause is cardiac rupture or acute dissection of the ascending aorta. Given the continued hypotension, the patient is at high risk for death in the next few minutes or hours. The patient must go to the operating room immediately. Delaying surgery for the sake of further diagnostic testing would be a mistake.

The patient was taken to the operating room, where an urgent median sternotomy was performed. A tense pericardium was noted. After the patient was placed on cardiopulmonary bypass, the pericardium was opened, revealing a substantial amount of organized thrombus and blood. Further examination revealed a short, circumferential dissection of the proximal ascending aorta (Figure 2). The aortic root and valve were replaced with a stentless bioprosthetic composite graft. The patient recovered without complications and was discharged in good condition nine days after admission. He declined any formal substance-abuse counseling. Four months after hospitalization, he remained well and denied any further use of cocaine.

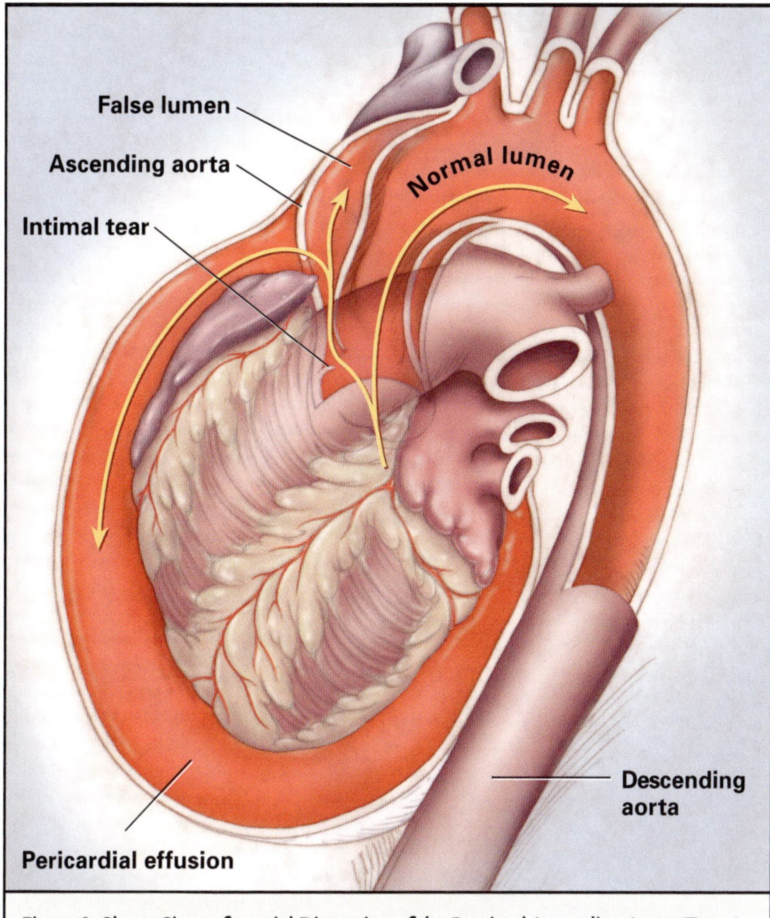

Figure 2. Short, Circumferential Dissection of the Proximal Ascending Aorta (Type A Dissection), with Organized Thrombus and Blood in the Pericardium.

Presumably, a rapid elevation in blood pressure induced by cocaine use precipitated the destabilization of medial disease present throughout the aorta. It is important to realize that the patient's aortic problem has not been cured. There is a likelihood of 25 to 35 percent that he will subsequently require reoperation for aortic aneurysm, dissection, or rupture. Follow-up CT scanning may be useful. Transthoracic echocardiography should be performed in follow-up to assess the function of the bioprosthetic valve. His outcome may be improved by careful control of his blood pressure, with aggressive beta-blockade to maintain a low blood pressure and pulse rate. He is also at increased risk for infective endocarditis and will require antibiotic prophylaxis. Perhaps most important, he must avoid cocaine use.

COMMENTARY

This patient presented to the emergency department with sharp chest pain and syncope after the use of crack cocaine. Initially, he was treated as a low-risk patient with cocaine-associated chest pain and admitted for overnight observation to rule out myocardial infarction. Although subtle, several symptoms and signs present on his initial evaluation suggested the existence of a more dangerous pathophysiologic process, but these were either minimized or missed in the emergency department. They included unexplained syncope, sinus tachycardia, and minor electrocardiographic and radiographic abnormalities. Although none of these point specifically to an acute aortic dissection, they do imply that a more dangerous clinical situation exists and, as the discussant states, warrant urgent additional testing. Early diagnosis is essential in this situation, since the treatment of aortic dissection, which includes urgent surgical evaluation, possible beta-blocker therapy, and avoidance of anticoagulants, differs dramatically from the treatment of acute coronary syndromes after cocaine use, the conditions with which aortic dissection is most often confused.[1,2]

Twenty-five million Americans have used cocaine at least once, and 1.5 million are current users.[3] It is estimated that chest pain, a common symptom related to cocaine use,[4] results in more than 64,000 evaluations in the emergency department per year at a cost of $83 million.[5] The diagnostic and therapeutic approach to a patient with cocaine-associated chest pain is difficult, given the wide spectrum of diseases associated with the recreational use of this drug.[6] Although life-threatening conditions such as acute coronary insufficiency, acute myocarditis, ventricular arrhythmia, and aortic dissection have all been reported in association with cocaine use,[2,3] most patients who present to the emergency department with chest pain after cocaine use do well, with a reported one-year survival rate of 98 percent.[7]

The initial evaluation of a patient with cocaine-related chest pain is usually focused — as it was in this case — on ruling out myocardial infarction, since this is the most common cardiovascular complication associated with the use of cocaine.[5] Like myocardial infarction, aortic dissection after cocaine use is thought to be due to a rapid increase in blood pressure and heart rate as a result of sympathetic stimulation caused by inhibited reuptake of epinephrine and norepinephrine at neuronal synapses.[2] These sudden changes increase shear stress in the thoracic aorta, resulting in small "nicks," or tears, of the intima, which can then propagate in both an antegrade fashion along the aorta and a retrograde fashion into the coronary vessels and pericardium. In addition to sudden changes in shear stress, an inherent structural weakness of the arterial wall, such as that resulting from Marfan's syndrome or mild connective-tissue abnormalities, is also thought to be necessary for the initiation of dissection.[8,9] Aortic dissections are classified according to their location; the commonly used Stanford classification labels those involving the ascending aorta as type A and those involving the descending aorta (i.e., distal to the left subclavian artery) as type B.

The clinical presentation of aortic dissection is highly variable, depending on its location, extent, and the presence or absence of end-organ complications; severe, sharp pain in the chest and upper back is the most common presenting symptom.[10] Syncope is also frequent and is present in about 9 percent of patients.[10] Reliance on classic findings on physical examination and chest radiography is of limited value in aortic dissection, since pulse deficits, regurgitation murmurs, and a widened mediastinum or abnormal aortic contour are often absent or are not recognized. Although the findings on electrocardiography are nonspecific for dissection, electrocardiography should be performed to rule out myocardial ischemia.

Once aortic dissection is suspected, time is critical. Rapid diagnosis and an awareness of its complications are essential, and appropriate treatment including surgical repair must be instituted immediately. In-hospital mortality is approximately 27 percent, with most deaths occurring soon after the onset of symptoms.[10] Transthoracic echocardiography appears to be helpful as an initial screening test, particularly in patients with type A dissections, for which its sensitivity ranges from 78 to 100 percent.[11] In addition, the test can uncover important complications such as valvular regurgitation and pericardial effusions. Although typical echocardiographic criteria for aortic dissection — an undulating intimal flap or central displacement of intimal calcification — were absent in the patient under discussion, a hemopericardium with tamponade and a dilated aortic root were present and suggested dissection.

Percutaneous drainage of pericardial fluid, a common treatment for hemodynamically unstable tamponade, was not performed, since drainage could have led to a rapid restoration of blood pressure as well as extension of the dissection and pericardial bleeding.[12] Instead, urgent surgical exploration, pericardiotomy, and repair of the ascending aortic valve and root were performed.

In this patient, the strict avoidance of further cocaine use is just as important as careful medical care and follow-up. However, cocaine users frequently have serious psychological and cognitive issues that require highly specialized therapy programs.[13] Treatment is further complicated in this group of patients by the high frequency of abuse of other types of substances, especially alcohol.[3] There are high rates of recidivism even with the optimal use of pharmacotherapy, psychotherapy, and behavioral therapy.[13] This patient's long-term prognosis will ultimately depend in large part on whether he continues to use cocaine or other drugs.

We are indebted to Camilla Payne, R.N., and Padma Nallamothu, M.D., for their careful review of the manuscript and helpful suggestions.

This article first appeared in the August 2, 2001, issue of the New England Journal of Medicine.

REFERENCES

1.
Isner JM, Estes NAM III, Thompson PD, et al. Acute cardiac events temporally related to cocaine abuse. N Engl J Med 1986;315: 1438-43.

2.
Kloner RA, Hale S, Alker K, Rezkalla S. The effects of acute and chronic cocaine use on the heart. Circulation 1992;85:407-19.

3.
Lange RA, Hillis LD. Cardiovascular complications of cocaine use. N Engl J Med 2001;345:351-8.

4.
Rich JA, Singer DE. Cocaine-related symptoms in patients presenting to an urban emergency department. Ann Emerg Med 1991;20:616-21.

5.
Hollander JE. The management of cocaine-associated myocardial ischemia. N Engl J Med 1995;333:1267-72.

6.
Cregler LL, Mark H. Medical complications of cocaine abuse. N Engl J Med 1986;315:1495-500.

7.
Hollander JE, Hoffman RS, Gennis P, et al. Cocaine-associated chest pain: one-year follow-up. Acad Emerg Med 1995;2:179-84.

8.
Pretre R, Von Segesser LK. Aortic dissection. Lancet 1997;349:1461-4.

9.
Eagle KA, DeSanctis RW. Aortic dissection. Curr Probl Cardiol 1989;14:225-78.

10.
Hagan PG, Nienaber CA, Isselbacher EM, et al. The International Registry of Acute Aortic Dissection (IRAD): new insights into an old disease. JAMA 2000;283:897-903.

11.
Cigarroa JE, Isselbacher EM, DeSanctis RW, Eagle KA. Diagnostic imaging in the evaluation of suspected aortic dissection: old standards and new directions. N Engl J Med 1993;328: 35-43.

12.
Isselbacher EM, Cigarroa JE, Eagle KA. Cardiac tamponade complicating proximal aortic dissection: is pericardiocentesis harmful? Circulation 1994;90:2375-8.

13.
Mendelson JH, Mello NK. Management of cocaine abuse and dependence. N Engl J Med 1996;334: 965-72.

More Than Your Average Wheeze

CAREY CONLEY THOMSON, M.D., ANDREW M. TAGER, M.D.,
AND PETER F. WELLER, M.D.

A 59-year-old man presented to a pulmonary clinic with a two-month history of rapidly progressive shortness of breath. At the onset of his dyspnea, prednisone (60 mg per day) relieved his symptoms, but dyspnea recurred when the dose was tapered after three weeks. He had had postnasal drip and a nonproductive cough for four years. Asthma had been diagnosed three years earlier, because of occasional wheezing, and inhaled albuterol and fluticasone and oral theophylline were prescribed. He had also been treated for sinusitis with antibiotics and a nasal septotomy and had received omeprazole for esophageal reflux, but he continued to wheeze. The only treatment that relieved his symptoms was multiple short courses of prednisone. His history was notable only for adult-onset diabetes and hyperlipidemia. He had no history of other lung diseases, fever, allergies, tobacco use, recent travel, a change in his job or home environment, or a new pet in his home.

If the patient does have asthma, the presence of dyspnea suggests that it is not well controlled. Potential reasons for lack of control include poor adherence to therapy, improper use of inhalers, or the presence of exacerbating factors. Potential exacerbating factors, including sinusitis and esophageal reflux, had been treated, but this failed to improve his symptoms. Still, the possibility of these or other asthma triggers should be reconsidered. I would obtain a chest radiograph to rule out infiltrates and perform pulmonary-function tests to evaluate the type and severity of impairment.

One month earlier, he had gone to the emergency department because of chest tightness, shortness of breath, and asymmetric edema of the legs. The oxygen saturation was 92 percent while he was breathing room air. A chest radiograph revealed atelectasis of the right lower lobe, and an elevated right hemidiaphragm.

He was hospitalized, and a myocardial infarction was ruled out. He was treated with aspirin and furosemide, with no improvement in symptoms. Cardiac catheterization was negative for coronary artery disease. A ventilation–perfusion scan found "no evidence of pulmonary embolism."

It is important to consider diagnoses other than asthma. Ischemic heart disease has been ruled out. Noninvasive studies of the legs would have been reasonable given the presence of asymmetric edema, but the results of ventilation–perfusion scanning make pulmonary embolism unlikely. The findings on radiography of the chest do not suggest heart failure as the cause of dyspnea, and the patient's symptoms did not respond to furosemide.

The dyspnea progressed, and the patient went to the pulmonary clinic for evaluation. His medications included salmeterol, fluticasone, theophylline, fexofenadine, furosemide, omeprazole, glyburide, rosiglitazone, atenolol, and gemfibrozil. On examination, he was in mild respiratory distress. The respiratory rate was 16 per minute, the blood pressure was 150/85 mm Hg, and the pulse was 80 beats per minute and regular. Examination of the sinuses and oral cavity was normal, as were cardiac and abdominal examinations. Examination of the lungs revealed diffuse wheezing with diminished breath sounds bilaterally. There were several small, papular lesions on the medial aspects of the legs and bilateral edema of the legs, which was worse on the right leg.

A radiograph of the chest revealed an elevated right hemidiaphragm and atelectasis of the right lower lobe. The oxygen saturation was 93 percent while the patient was breathing room air and 89 percent after two minutes of exertion; in an arterial-blood sample the partial pressure of oxygen was 62 mm Hg, the pH was 7.4, and the partial pressure of carbon dioxide was 39 mm Hg. The results of pulmonary-function tests were consistent with the presence of severe, partially reversible airflow obstruction (Table 1). The patient had a good response to a bronchodilator, as assessed by comparing the results of spirometry obtained before and five minutes after the administration of two puffs of albuterol.

His symptoms and the findings on examination of the lungs and pulmonary-function testing are consistent with the presence of asthma. However, the atelectasis and elevated hemidiaphragm evident on radiography of the chest are not expected with this condition.

The patient was questioned about his use of bronchodilators and admitted that he rarely used them because they "never helped." He was unable to demonstrate the proper use of an inhaler. The use of an inhaler with a spacer was reviewed, and he was instructed to begin using inhalers daily.

A vital step in the management of asthma is to teach patients the importance of the use of inhalers in controlling the disease, as well as how to use these devices effectively. The

Table 1. Results of Pulmonary-Function Tests.

Variable	Value
Forced expiratory volume in one second	
Liters	1.50
% of predicted value	38
Forced vital capacity	
Liters	2.63
% of predicted value	52
Forced expiratory volume in one second:forced vital capacity	0.57
Peak expiratory flow	
Liters/sec	4.64
% of predicted value	51
Response to bronchodilator (% increase over baseline value)	16
Total lung capacity	
Liters	6.61
% of predicted value	93
Residual volume	
Liters	3.98
% of predicted value	160
Residual volume:total lung capacity	
Value	0.6
% of predicted value	172
Carbon monoxide diffusing capacity	
ml/min/mm Hg	29.4
% of predicted value	111

condition of patients may improve dramatically once they learn how to use inhalers correctly and consistently.

Because severe symptoms developed in late adulthood in this patient, diagnoses other than or in addition to asthma remain a possibility. I would check the results of routine laboratory tests for evidence of inflammation. In addition, computed tomography (CT) of the chest would be important to determine whether infiltrates or bronchiectasis is present. Such findings would be associated with disorders distinct from asthma.

The white-cell count was 15,500 per cubic millimeter, with 44 percent eosinophils; the hematocrit was 35.7 percent; and the platelet count was 188,000 per cubic millimeter. The erythrocyte sedimentation rate was 70 mm per hour. Noninvasive studies of the legs were negative for deep venous thromboses. Spiral CT of the chest with contrast medium revealed minimal atelectasis in the right lower lobe, several small mediastinal lymph nodes, and a moderate pericardial effusion; there were no infiltrates and no evidence of pulmonary embolism.

Although eosinophilia may accompany asthma, the levels rarely exceed 800 per cubic millimeter even in severe cases. In addition, the patient's erythrocyte sedimentation rate is markedly elevated, a finding not seen in asthma. I am concerned about the possibility of systemic eosinophilic syndromes associated with asthma.

The patient was hospitalized. The eosinophil count and erythrocyte sedimentation rate remained markedly elevated. The level of IgE was 3130 IU per milliliter (normal range, 0 to 100), the IgG level was 2620 mg per deciliter (normal range, 614 to 1295), and the IgA level was 397 mg per deciliter (normal range, 69 to 309). The urinalysis was negative for blood. An echocardiogram revealed a small pericardial effusion with no evidence of tamponade, a dilated and hypertrophied left ventricle, and no wall-motion abnormalities or intraventricular thrombi. Tests for antineutrophil cytoplasmic antibodies (ANCA) and antinuclear antibody were negative. CT of the sinus revealed long-term changes in the right ethmoidal sinuses and minimal, new-onset changes in the maxillary sinuses. The patient was treated empirically with amoxicillin–clavulanate for sinusitis, without improvement in his symptoms. Gemfibrozil, furosemide, and atenolol were discontinued, but the eosinophil count remained elevated.

The triad of asthma, sinus disease, and marked eosinophilia is very suggestive of the Churg–Strauss syndrome. The test for ANCA is positive in 50 to 70 percent of cases, and a negative test thus does not rule out the diagnosis. The elevated erythrocyte sedimentation rate would also be compatible with the presence of this syndrome. Other possible diagnoses include allergic bronchopulmonary aspergillosis, eosinophilic pneumonia, hypersensitivity pneumonitis, cancer, and helminthic infection. However, the chest CT did not show central bronchiectasis (as is often seen in patients with allergic bronchopulmonary aspergillosis), infiltrates, or interstitial changes. I would ask the patient about his travel history to assess the risk of infections and inflammatory lung diseases associated with nonnative pathogens.

The patient reported no history of sputum plugs. He noted that he had lived in Asia for six years in the 1960s. Skin tests revealed minimal reactions to typical allergens, and a serologic test for aspergillus-specific antibodies was negative. Stool specimens were negative for ova and parasites, as was a serologic test for antibodies against strongyloides. The findings on endoscopy, sigmoidoscopy, and CT of the abdomen were unremarkable.

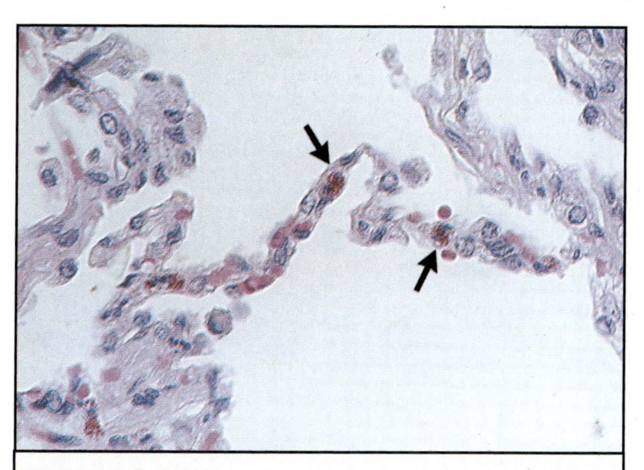

Figure 1. Transbronchial-Biopsy Specimen Showing an Alveolus Infiltrated by Eosinophils (Arrows) (Hematoxylin and Eosin, ×1000).

The evaluation was negative for allergic bronchopulmonary aspergillosis. The patient's travel history raises the possibility of strongyloides, which can remain dormant for decades and subsequently lead to eosinophilia, eosinophilic infiltrates, and asthma. Treatment with corticosteroids can unmask a parasitic infection and lead to enterocolitis and gram-negative sepsis. The fact that the patient received several cycles of treatment with prednisone without progression makes strongyloides an unlikely diagnosis, and tests for this parasite were negative.

A review of outpatient records revealed that the proportion of eosinophils on a complete blood count had been 7 percent eight years earlier and 33 percent on a more recent count. The patient recalled that he had had similar skin lesions on his legs two years earlier, but they had resolved when he was treated with prednisone.

Bronchoscopy was performed and revealed clear airways without mucosal obstruction. The bronchoalveolar-lavage fluid contained 70 percent eosinophils. Transbronchial biopsy revealed diffuse eosinophilic infiltrates (Figure 1). Staining, cultures, and cytologic examinations of the lavage fluid and biopsy specimens for microorganisms were negative. A biopsy of a skin lesion from the leg revealed eosinophilic infiltration but not vasculitis.

The results of bronchoscopy show eosinophilic infiltration of the lungs, which arouses concern about the possibility of infiltration of other organs. The documented history of eosinophilia indicates a chronic disorder.

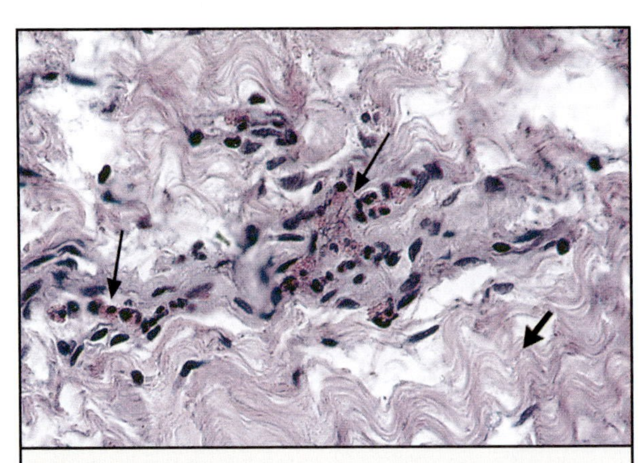

Figure 2. Pericardial-Biopsy Specimen Showing Eosinophilic Infiltration (Thin Arrows) and Fibrosis (Thick Arrow) (Hematoxylin and Eosin, ×400).

The patient's symptoms improved during treatment with bronchodilators and inhaled corticosteroids, and he was discharged. Two days later, follow-up pulmonary-function tests demonstrated decreased airflow obstruction, with a forced expiratory volume in one second of 3.09 liters (78 percent of the predicted value). The eosinophil count, erythrocyte sedimentation rate, and immunoglobulin levels remained elevated.

Although the patient's symptoms and the results of pulmonary-function tests improved during treatment with inhaled corticosteroids and bronchodilators, the elevated levels of inflammatory markers and eosinophil count indicate continued disease activity.

Because the diagnosis remained uncertain, a pericardial biopsy and open-lung biopsy were performed. The pericardial-biopsy specimen showed eosinophilic infiltration (Figure 2). Inflammation and fibrosis were seen on both biopsy specimens, but there was no evidence of cancer, infection, or vasculitis.

Treatment with 60 mg of prednisone per day was begun, and the dose was tapered over a period of several months to 5 mg per day. The patient's cough, shortness of breath, wheeze, and sinus congestion resolved completely. He was able to return to work and exercise within two weeks, and he has remained free of symptoms with normal or nearly normal laboratory values and pulmonary-function tests.

COMMENTARY

The patient's presentation, which ultimately proved consistent with the presence of the Churg–Strauss syndrome, illustrates some of the difficulties in recognizing this condition. When the patient was first seen, his dyspnea appeared to be due to adult-onset asthma; this impression was supported by the documentation of partially reversible airflow obstruction on pulmonary-function testing. He had sinusitis, which can accompany asthma as well as the Churg–Strauss syndrome. In retrospect, clues to his evolving Churg–Strauss syndrome included the increasing level of eosinophilia and episodes of pruritic skin lesions that were responsive to corticosteroid therapy. In combination with his increasing dyspnea, the findings of profound eosinophilia[1] and a markedly elevated erythrocyte sedimentation rate[2] distinguished his illness from usual asthma. The prominent eosinophilic infiltrates of the skin, lung, and pericardium confirmed the presence of a systemic eosinophilic syndrome.

The Churg–Strauss syndrome is a rare disease, occurring in an estimated two to four patients per million patient-years.[2,3] Since most affected patients have asthma, patients who present with asthma and marked eosinophilia may have underlying Churg–Strauss syndrome and the syndrome may be unmasked when the dose of prednisone used for asthma is reduced. This may be why the Churg–Strauss syndrome is diagnosed in some patients who are receiving inhaled corticosteroids or leukotriene antagonists.[2] Whether leukotriene inhibitors cause the syndrome remains uncertain.[2]

Though its presentation can be quite variable, the Churg–Strauss syndrome is often a triphasic illness.[1] The phases consist of allergic rhinitis and asthma of variable severity (often developing in adulthood); eosinophilia and infiltration of tissue by eosinophils; and potentially life-threatening vasculitis that may involve multiple organs but often includes the skin, lungs, heart, gastrointestinal tract, and nervous system.

The Churg–Strauss syndrome remains primarily a clinical rather than a pathological diagnosis. Six features[4] — asthma, more than 10 percent eosinophils in blood, mononeuropathy or polyneuropathy, nonfixed pulmonary infiltrates, abnormalities of the paranasal sinuses, and extravascular eosinophils — are commonly present.[1] However, the diagnostic usefulness of these features has been validated only in patients with documented vasculitis; hence, they should be considered as guides for clinicians rather than rigid criteria.

Of the diseases that are characterized by eosinophilia, the hypereosinophilic syndrome is also consistent with some aspects of this patient's presentation. The hypereosinophilic syndrome is uncommon and is not a single disorder, but rather includes many distinct, as yet largely idiopathic, clinical entities associated with eosinophilia. Consequently, the

Table 2. Clinical Characteristics of the Churg–Strauss Syndrome and the Hypereosinophilic Syndrome.*

Characteristic	Churg–Strauss Syndrome	Hypereosinophilic Syndrome
Cardiac findings	Microvascular vasculitis; pericardial involvement; myocardial thickening	Endocardial fibrosis; mural thrombus; restrictive cardiomyopathy; mitral and tricuspid regurgitation
Lung involvement	Asthma almost always present; infiltrates common	Asthma rare; infiltrates rare; pulmonary edema rare
Sinus involvement	Common	Rare
Neurologic abnormalities	Mononeuropathy or polyneuropathy common	Mononeuropathy or polyneuropathy possible
Skin lesions	Palpable purpura; macular or papular rashes; hemorrhagic lesions; nodules	Varied rashes
Eosinophilia	Present	Present
Erythrocyte sedimentation rate	Commonly elevated	May be elevated
IgE levels	Commonly elevated	May be elevated
Antineutrophil cytoplasmic antibodies	Commonly present	Rare
Vasculitis	Present in late phase	Absent

*Data are from Allen and Davis[6] and Weller and Bubley.[7]

syndrome is heterogeneous in presentation and widely variable in outcome. The original defining criteria were the presence of more than 1500 eosinophils per cubic millimeter for longer than six months; the absence of parasites, allergies, or other causes; and the presence of signs and symptoms of organ involvement.[5]

The hypereosinophilic syndrome and the Churg–Strauss syndrome have many overlapping features (Table 2).[6-9] However, several features that are common in the Churg–Strauss syndrome are rare in the hypereosinophilic syndrome,[7] including asthma and elevated IgE levels, making the latter disorder less likely in the patient described.

In most patients with the Churg–Strauss syndrome, the eosinophilia and symptoms respond quickly to corticosteroid therapy, and some may benefit from interferon alfa.[10] Because a delay in the diagnosis and treatment of the syndrome increases the risk of death from vasculitic complications involving the heart, gastrointestinal tract, or other organs,[11] physicians should consider this diagnosis when a patient's symptoms and signs are atypical of asthma alone.

This article first appeared in the February 7, 2002, issue of the New England Journal of Medicine.

REFERENCES

1. Lanham JG, Elkon KB, Pusey CD, Hughes GR. Systemic vasculitis with asthma and eosinophilia: a clinical approach to the Churg-Strauss syndrome. Medicine (Baltimore) 1984;63:65-81.
2. Weller PF, Plaut M, Taggart V, Trontell A. The relationship of asthma therapy and Churg Strauss syndrome: NIH workshop summary report. J Allergy Clin Immunol 2001;108: 175-83.
3. Watts RA, Lane SE, Bentham G, Scott DG. Epidemiology of systemic vasculitis: a ten-year study in the United Kingdom. Arthritis Rheum 2000;43: 414-9.
4. Masi AT, Hunder GG, Lie JT, et al. The American College of Rheumatology 1990 criteria for the classification of Churg-Strauss syndrome (allergic granulomatosis and angiitis). Arthritis Rheum 1990;33:1094-100.
5. Chusid MJ, Dale DC, West BC, Wolff SM. The hypereosinophilic syndrome: analysis of fourteen cases with review of the literature. Medicine (Baltimore) 1975;54:1-27.
6. Allen JN, Davis WB. Eosinophilic lung diseases. Am J Respir Crit Care Med 1994;150:1423-38.
7. Weller PF, Bubley GJ. The idiopathic hypereosinophilic syndrome. Blood 1994;83:2759-79.
8. Schwartz RA, Churg J. Churg-Strauss syndrome. Br J Dermatol 1992;127: 199-204.
9. Churg J, Strauss L. Allergic granulomatosis, allergic angiitis, and periarteritis nodosa. Am J Pathol 1951;27:277-301.
10. Tatsis E, Schnabel A, Gross WL. Interferon-alpha treatment of four patients with Churg-Strauss syndrome. Ann Intern Med 1998;129:370-4.
11. Chen KR, Ohata Y, Sakurai M, Nakayama H. Churg-Strauss syndrome: report of a case without preexisting asthma. J Dermatol 1992;19:40-7.

Where Are You From?

KEVIN C. KATZ, M.D., SHARON L. WALMSLEY, M.D.,
ANNE G. McLEOD, M.D., JAY S. KEYSTONE, M.D.,
AND ALLAN S. DETSKY, M.D., PH.D.

A 54-year-old man of Guyanese origin with human immunodeficiency virus (HIV) infection was hospitalized in Toronto with a one-week history of low-grade fever (temperature, <38°C). He had had a temperature of 38.5°C on each of the two days preceding hospitalization, in association with rigors.

The combination of fever, HIV infection, and the patient's country of origin evokes a broad range of differential diagnoses. I would be most concerned about conditions related to his HIV infection. Opportunistic infections obviously come to mind, but non-Hodgkin's lymphoma or a drug reaction (such as sulfonamide hypersensitivity) may also cause fever. The patient's history of emigration from Guyana suggests the possibility of tuberculosis, malaria, and other tropical diseases.

At this point I would want to know whether he has any localizing symptoms. It would also be important to know the CD4 cell count, the HIV viral load, and whether he is taking antiretroviral medications and other agents for prophylaxis against opportunistic infections. I wonder when he was last in Guyana.

The patient's only localizing symptom was a two-month history of loose bowel movements (two to three per day) with no blood or mucus. There was no history of weight loss, night sweats, rash, headache, shortness of breath, cough, neck stiffness, or joint pain. He had not had abdominal pain, nausea, or vomiting.

The HIV infection was diagnosed in 1995 and was most likely acquired through unprotected anal intercourse. The CD4 cell count was 80 per cubic millimeter three months before presentation, and the viral load was undetectable. The patient had been receiving highly active antiretroviral therapy since 1996.

His history of two to three loose bowel movements per day may indicate the presence of infectious diarrhea. Infection with giardia and *Entamoeba histolytica* can occur at any stage of HIV infection. With a CD4 cell count of less than 100 per cubic millimeter, he is at risk for water- or food-borne infections with agents such as cryptosporidia, cyclospora, *Isos-*

pora belli, and microsporidia. Disseminated mycobacterial infection and cytomegalovirus infection are less likely, since they tend to occur when the CD4 cell count is less than 50 per cubic millimeter. His diarrhea might alternatively be related to medications or other noninfectious causes. In many patients with advanced HIV disease and diarrhea, the cause of diarrhea is never determined.

The low CD4 cell count also arouses concern that *Pneumocystis carinii* infection is the cause of fever, but the absence of respiratory symptoms makes this possibility less likely. Toxoplasmosis and cryptococcosis are also unlikely, since the patient has no headache or other neurologic symptoms.

The patient had no history of opportunistic infections or cancer. He did, however, have chronic anemia, which required intermittent transfusions, and a history of thrombocytopenia dating back at least five years that was associated with frequent nosebleeds. He had received prednisone for the thrombocytopenia but had not taken this medication for the past six months.

Chronic anemia and thrombocytopenia are common in patients with HIV disease. The medications that the patient is taking for HIV might contribute to these conditions, but his thrombocytopenia, at least, appears to have begun before these medications were started. Opportunistic infections, especially those due to histoplasma, *Mycobacterium avium* complex, and leishmania, can also suppress bone marrow function.

The patient had moved from Guyana to Canada 15 years earlier but had visited Guyana in 1995. He had no known exposure to tuberculosis or hepatitis and no history of recent travel.

Given the long interval since he was last in Guyana, any infection acquired there would need to have a long latency period. Tuberculosis is the first disease that comes to mind, given its frequency and the high risk of reactivation in a patient with HIV infection. In people who have been repeatedly infected, falciparum malaria can present up to three years after the acquisition of the infection. *Plasmodium vivax*, *P. ovale*, and *P. malariae* often have a longer period of latency and cause an illness that is less severe. Leishmaniasis usually has an incubation period of three to eight months but, in some cases, may remain dormant for years. Melioidosis, caused by infection with *Burkholderia pseudomallei*, has been described in Guyana. It has been termed the "Vietnamese time bomb" because it has occurred in war veterans more than two decades after their return from Vietnam. Other diseases that occur in Guyana and have long latency periods are schistosomiasis, trichinosis, and bancroftian filariasis. Chronic schistosomiasis can first be manifested by anemia and thrombocytopenia relating to hypersplenism and portal hypertension. Trichinosis frequently produces subclinical infections, but late presentations often include muscle aches, cardiac symptoms, and eye disturbances that are absent in this patient. Although filariasis is frequent in Guyana, fever without lymphangitis would be a very unusual presentation of this infection.

At this point, I would perform a physical examination to look for findings suggestive of the presence of one of these infections or other diseases.

The patient had a blood pressure of 150/90 mm Hg, a pulse of 90, a respiratory rate of 24 breaths per minute, and a temperature of 38.7°C. His conjunctivae were pale but anicteric. His neck was supple, and there was no evidence of lymphadenopathy. Jugular venous pressure was elevated, at 7 cm of water above the sternal angle, and S_1 and S_2 were normal. Lung examination revealed bibasilar crackles. There was no clubbing. The liver span was 14 cm, and the spleen was palpable below the umbilicus. Digital rectal examination was negative for blood.

The presence of massive splenomegaly focuses the diagnostic possibilities. Hepatosplenomegaly has multiple causes, but splenomegaly that extends below the umbilicus is uncommon and greatly reduces the possibilities. Possible neoplastic causes, unrelated to HIV infection, include chronic myelogenous leukemia, myelofibrosis, and lymphoproliferative disorders, especially hairy-cell leukemia. Gaucher's disease might present this late in life in the form of massive splenomegaly, although this condition is less likely given the patient's other clinical features. I would focus on infectious causes. Tuberculosis, malaria, and schistosomiasis can cause splenomegaly. Visceral leishmaniasis, or kala-azar, and infection with *M. avium* complex are other possibilities that cause particular concern, given this patient's immunocompromised state. I would obtain a complete blood count, routine chemical analyses, and three blood films to look for parasites. An abdominal imaging study should also be performed.

The patient's white-cell count was 2200 per cubic millimeter (1500 neutrophils and 400 lymphocytes per cubic millimeter), the hemoglobin level was 80 g per liter, and the platelet count was 32,000 per cubic millimeter. The reticulocyte count was 1 percent. The serum creatinine level was 1.2 mg per deciliter (104 μmol per liter), and the blood urea nitrogen level was 21 mg per deciliter (7.6 mmol per liter). The results of liver-function tests were normal. A chest x-ray film showed cardiomegaly and mild interstitial edema. Tests for hepatitis B and C viruses were negative.

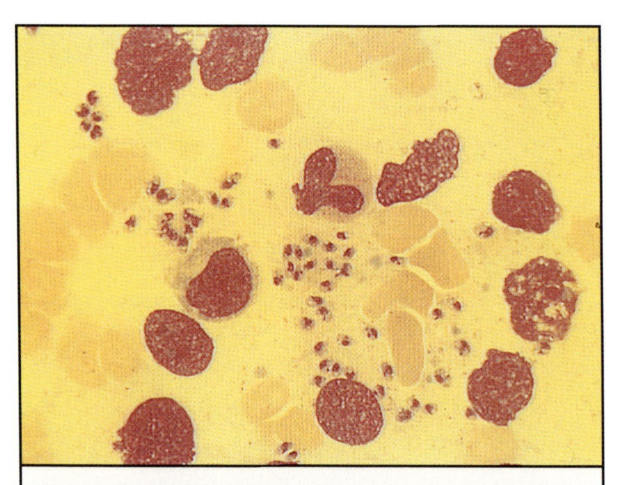

Figure 1. Amastigotes Released from Macrophages in Bone Marrow (Giemsa Stain, ×1000).

Cultures of blood, urine, stool, and sputum were negative for bacteria. Blood cultures were also negative for *M. avium* complex. Monospot and cytomegalovirus antigen tests were negative. The blood film did not reveal either intracellular parasites (such as malaria or leishmania) or extracellular parasites. A lumbar puncture was deferred owing to the thrombocytopenia. Abdominal ultrasonography confirmed that the liver (18.1 cm) and spleen (18.5 cm) were enlarged.

Given the presence of massive splenomegaly and chronic anemia, a bone marrow biopsy and aspiration, including cultures, would be the next step.

Bone marrow biopsy revealed macrophages filled with organisms whose appearance was consistent with that of leishmania (Figure 1). Within 10 days, a culture of the bone marrow confirmed the presence of leishmaniasis. The patient was treated with a lipid formulation of amphotericin B. His clinical condition improved, and the size of his spleen decreased.

COMMENTARY

Visceral leishmaniasis is caused by an infection of the reticuloendothelial system with leishmania species, usually *Leishmania donovani*. The clinical presentation of infection with leishmania can range from no symptoms to the syndrome of kala-azar, which includes

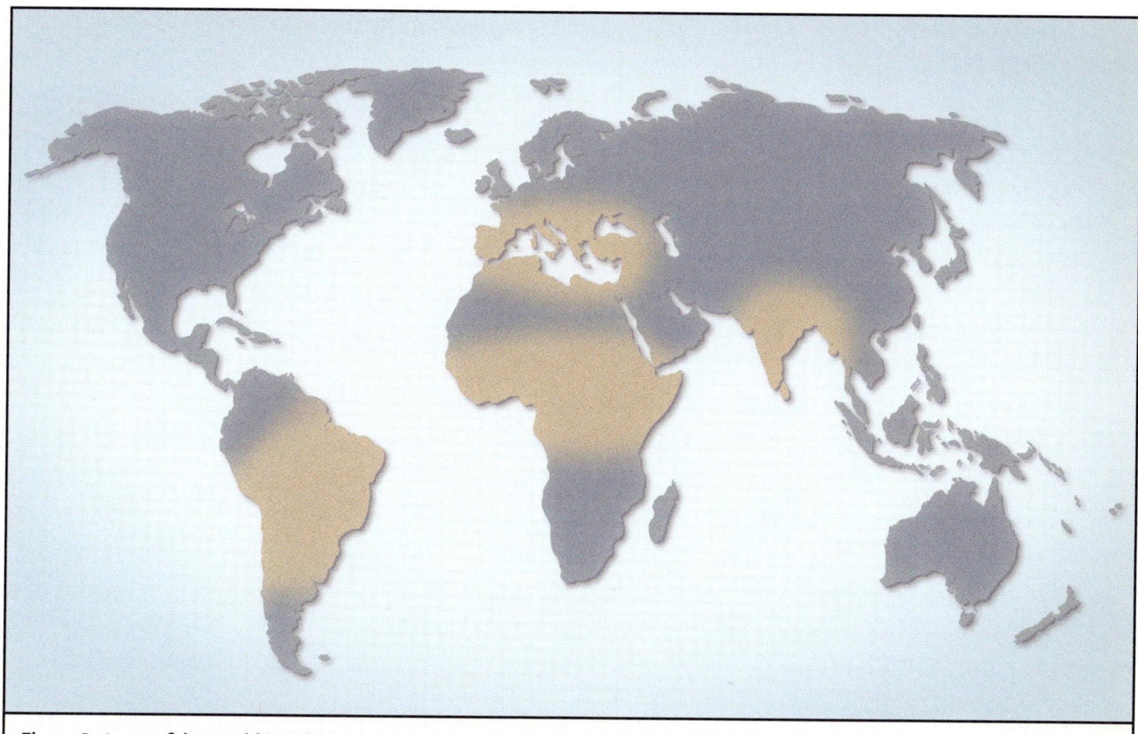

Figure 2. Areas of the World in Which Visceral Leishmaniasis Occurs.

fever, weight loss, hepatosplenomegaly, anemia, and leukopenia. Visceral leishmaniasis occurs in South America, the area surrounding the Mediterranean Sea, and parts of Asia (Figure 2).

Visceral leishmaniasis may be the presenting opportunistic infection in HIV-infected patients but more frequently complicates advanced HIV disease. Case series of HIV-infected patients with leishmaniasis indicate that 75 percent present with fever, hepatomegaly, splenomegaly, and pancytopenia.[1] The digestive and respiratory tracts can also be affected. However, some HIV-infected patients have no symptoms or organomegaly and have negative serologic tests for leishmania. Leishmaniasis may remain latent for years and then first become apparent when the patient becomes immunocompromised.

Although the differential diagnosis of fever in patients with HIV infection is extremely broad,[2] in this case, the correct diagnosis was reached by focusing on the finding with the narrowest differential diagnosis — that is, massive splenomegaly. Although leishmaniasis is an unlikely cause of splenomegaly among patients presenting for care in the United States or Canada, the intersection of the conditions that cause splenomegaly and the other findings (in particular chronic HIV infection and a remote history of travel to Guyana) led the consultant to consider this possibility early, averting many unnecessary tests.

This case emphasizes that unexplained symptoms or signs in patients who have emigrated from or traveled to a developing country may be related to an infectious agent acquired there many years earlier. This possibility is a particular concern in immunocompromised patients.

Presented as part of the Summer Case Series at Mount Sinai Hospital, Toronto.

We are indebted to Dr. Andrew Morris, the patient's attending physician, for bringing this case report to our attention.

This article first appeared in the March 7, 2002, issue of the New England Journal of Medicine.

REFERENCES

1.
Alvar J, Canavate C, Gutierrez-Solar B, et al. Leishmania and human immunodeficiency virus coinfection: the first 10 years. Clin Microbiol Rev 1997;10:298-319.

2.
Barat LM, Gunn JE, Steger KA, Perkins CJ, Craven DE. Causes of fever in patients infected with human immunodeficiency virus who were admitted to Boston City Hospital. Clin Infect Dis 1996;23:320-8.

Diagnosis Still in Question

ASHISH K. JHA, M.D., HAROLD R. COLLARD, M.D.,
AND LAWRENCE M. TIERNEY, M.D.

A 59-year-old banker was referred for the evaluation of fevers that had started three weeks earlier, shortly after his arrival in western Texas on business. The fevers were associated with dyspnea on exertion. A physician prescribed an inhaled beta-agonist and clarithromycin, which had no effect. The patient's fevers worsened, as did the dyspnea on exertion. A nonproductive cough, a sore throat, a nonpruritic erythematous rash over his trunk, and right-sided pleurisy developed. Another physician prescribed levofloxacin.

Many diagnoses might explain these symptoms. Coccidioidomycosis is endemic in some parts of far western Texas. Exertional dyspnea can occur with this disorder and would not respond to the treatment administered. The subsequent events are less in keeping with this disease, and other causes of pleuritic chest pain should be considered, as well as conditions causing fever and rash. Toxicogenic strains of streptococcus, staphylococcus, and in rare cases, pneumococcus are all possible causes. I would determine whether the patient had risk factors for pulmonary emboli and whether he had had chills or associated joint symptoms. More information is needed.

The patient was admitted for the evaluation of fever of unknown origin in association with night sweats, rigors, and myalgias. His chest pain and cough had resolved, and the dyspnea was decreased. The patient lived on a ranch in the San Joaquin Valley in California. He enjoyed pitching hay and cleaning his barn, which housed cows, pigs, and horses, and also had mice. He had recently visited Idaho on a fishing trip. He had borderline hypertension, took no regular medications, and had no drug allergies. He occasionally drank alcohol but did not smoke cigarettes or use illicit drugs.

Night sweats and rigors are the physiological adaptations to rapidly changing body temperatures. The patient's dyspnea had resolved, so a community-acquired pneumonia could have been responsible. His unusual history, including the site of his home, exposure to animals, and history of travel suggest other possibilities. Living in the San Joaquin Valley, he would have been exposed to coccidioidomycosis. Pitching hay suggests the possibility of hypersensitivity pneumonitis due to thermophilic actinomycetes. The mouse-infested barn could harbor many pathogens, including leptospira, which is ordinarily transmitted by contact with rat urine. Though these possibilities should be included in the broad differential diagnosis, I would proceed in a different direction and evaluate the high, spiking fever. The disappearance of pleurisy may indicate that a pleural effusion has developed. I would think broadly about the likelihood of cancer, autoimmune disease, and infection in particular. The findings on the physical examination should be helpful.

The temperature was 39.2°C, the blood pressure was 135/99 mm Hg, the heart rate was 98 beats per minute, the respiratory rate was 16, and the oxygen saturation was 97 percent while the patient was breathing room air. His neck was supple, his conjunctivae and fundi were normal, his oropharynx was erythematous without an exudate, and his teeth were in good condition. Bilateral, small, rubbery inguinal lymph nodes were palpable. The chest, cardiovascular, abdominal, and genitourinary examinations revealed no abnormalities. A stool specimen was negative for blood. The patient had an erythematous maculopapular eruption on his trunk, which was more pronounced with fever spikes. He also had an erythematous, nontender nodule measuring 5 by 5 mm on the palmar aspect of the distal phalanx of the second digit of his left hand. The results of the neurologic examination were normal.

The electrocardiogram and chest x-ray film were unremarkable. The white-cell count was 31,500 per cubic millimeter, with 29,200 neutrophils per cubic millimeter; the hematocrit was 37 percent; and the platelet count was 265,000 per cubic millimeter. The electrolyte levels were normal. The following laboratory values were obtained: aspartate aminotransferase, 96 U per liter; alanine aminotransferase, 64 U per liter; alkaline phosphatase, 154 U per liter; total bilirubin, 0.8 mg per deciliter (14 μmol per liter); lactate dehydrogenase, 314 U per liter; creatine kinase, 28 U per liter; and erythrocyte sedimentation rate, 125 mm per hour. The results of urinalysis were normal.

There is no mention of systemic toxicity. Plague occurs in western Texas, and affected persons appear severely ill. The phalangeal nodule might be the site of inoculation, but there is no evidence of lymphadenopathy, as would be expected with plague. A herpetic whitlow may have a similar appearance, and patients with primary herpes simplex infection typically appear ill, but marked leukocytosis is unusual. A truncal rash in a patient with a hectic fever (i.e., characterized by a daily spike in the temperature) suggests the possibility of adult Still's disease, but this is a diagnosis of exclusion. Given the patient's history of living on a ranch, *Nocardia brasiliensis* infection should be considered. This infection causes an ascending lymphangitis proximal to the point of inoculation but does not cause systemic symptoms such as those of this patient. I would consider a systemic condition to be a more likely cause. The initial studies should include blood cultures, a biopsy of the digital lesion, and perhaps serologic tests for hepatitis, although only infection with hepatitis A virus causes such striking fever. Tests for human immunodeficiency virus type 1 (HIV-1) and infectious mononucleosis are reasonable. Radiographic studies such as computed tomography (CT) are unlikely to be helpful.

The levofloxacin was discontinued, and multiple blood cultures were obtained. The cultures remained sterile at seven days. Tests were negative for antibody against HIV-1; heterophil antibodies; hepatitis A, B, and C viruses; cold agglutinins; IgG antibodies against coccidioides; IgM and IgG antibodies against *Coxiella burnetii* and *Borrelia burgdorferi*; antinuclear antibodies; and rheumatoid factor. A Venereal Disease Research Laboratory test was nonreactive. Serum and urine protein electrophoreses did not reveal monoclonal gammopathy. Histoplasma antigen was undetectable in urine. A biopsy of the skin lesion disclosed granuloma annulare, and cultures of the lesion remained negative. An abdominal CT scan showed thickening of the ascending colon but no other abnormalities. Colonoscopy was performed, and random biopsy specimens were obtained.

I am not sure that all these studies were needed, but it was prudent to obtain blood cultures after discontinuing antibiotics. The absence of growth after seven days of culture does not exclude an indolent case of endocarditis. Infections with HIV-1, cytomegalovirus, and Epstein–Barr virus seem unlikely. The absence of IgG antibodies against coccidioides indicates a lack of immunity, making coccidioidomycosis a distinct possibility. Q fever is possible given the patient's exposure to animals, but he would need to have had direct contact with sheep to make this illness a serious consideration. Moreover, in this disorder, rash does not usually occur in conjunction with fever. An autoimmune disorder other than adult Still's disease remains possible. Though systemic lupus erythematosus can cause fevers, the absence of other features of lupus, such as antinuclear antibodies, makes this condition unlikely. The finding of granuloma annulare on biopsy is interesting because the histologic appearance of this lesion is similar to that of vasculitis and the lesion can appear to be identical to a rheumatoid nodule. However, this benign, self-limited dermatosis is often found in patients with diabetes mellitus and would not account for the systemic symptoms. If the thickening of the ascending colon on the CT scan is a legitimate finding, other conditions should also be considered. Typhoid fever usually causes leukopenia, not leukocytosis, unless there is perforation. Ameboma of the cecum is found sporadically throughout the United States, but it is more likely to form a mass than an area of thickening. *Mycobacterium tuberculosis* infection is possible. Inflammatory bowel disease, especially Crohn's disease, can cause fevers. Cancer, chronic infection, and autoimmune disease still remain in the picture. I would next look for IgM antibodies against coccidioides.

The patient had daily, nocturnal temperature elevations up to 40.3°C but was otherwise afebrile. The rash persisted but did not spread. The results of colonic biopsy were negative. On the fourth day of hospitalization, the patient reported right-knee pain. On examination, the knee was warm and erythematous and had a normal range of motion. Joint aspiration yielded 30 ml of straw-colored fluid, with a white-cell count of 30,450 per cubic millimeter (87 percent neutrophils). The results of Gram's staining and polarizing microscopy were normal. Fluid was sent for bacterial, fungal, and mycobacterial cultures.

Sequential observation of a patient often narrows the differential diagnosis. The development of arthritis of the knee, in addition to the fever and rash, suggests various possibilities. In rare cases, gout causes high fever, but fever is present at the onset of illness. Adult Still's disease remains a strong possibility, but again, this diagnosis is one of exclusion; the development of arthritis well into the course of the illness is characteristic, although the patient's age of 59 years is rather advanced for this disorder. Tuberculosis remains a concern. The third most common site of tuberculous infection is skeletal, and the knee is typically involved. Pulmonary disease is encountered in half of such cases. Tuberculous arthritis has an indolent course, however, and the onset of arthritis in this patient was relatively soon in the course of his disease. I would consider performing both a synovial biopsy to look for granuloma and a skin test with purified protein derivative; this test is generally positive in patients with tuberculous arthritis. I doubt that septic arthritis is the cause, because the synovial-fluid white-cell count is typically higher than 30,000 per cubic millimeter in affected patients, and it should not appear five days after hospitalization, unless bacteremia was caused by a diagnostic procedure.

The knee pain improved within 48 hours. Bacterial and fungal cultures of synovial fluid were negative. The serum ferritin level was 23,200 ng per milliliter on the fifth day of hospitalization. Indomethacin therapy was initiated, and the fevers decreased (maximal temperature, 38°C), the white-cell count fell to 12,000 per cubic millimeter, and the patient felt better. He was discharged with a presumptive diagnosis of Still's disease.

The improvement without antituberculosis therapy and in response to indomethacin is surely in keeping with a diagnosis of adult Still's disease. Much has been made of the dramatic elevation of serum ferritin levels in this disorder, but this abnormality may be present in many chronic inflammatory illnesses. I would still be concerned about the possibility of tuberculosis or even coccidioidomycosis, but at this point I would pursue these further only if the test for IgM antibodies against coccidioides was positive or if fever recurred.

The patient returned for a follow-up visit four weeks after discharge. Cultures of synovial fluid were negative for mycobacteria, and the dose of indomethacin was decreased. His fevers had ceased, other symptoms had abated, and his condition was markedly improved. He returned to his primary physician for ongoing care.

COMMENTARY

The lack of a specific diagnostic test for and specific features of Still's disease, as well as its relative infrequency, makes this diagnosis challenging. The classic triad of Still's disease is fever, oligoarticular arthritis, and an evanescent salmon-colored rash (which typically appears with the fever spikes),[1,2] although the rash is persistent in up to one third of patients.[3] A sore throat is characteristic, and elevated ferritin levels, leukocyte counts, liver-enzyme levels, and erythrocyte sedimentation rates are common. Still's disease typically occurs in patients younger than 35 years of age, but it has been described in older adults. Men and women are affected in equal proportions. Treatment consists of nonsteroidal antiinflammatory drugs, though corticosteroids are also effective.[4] The condition of many patients improves spontaneously, but long-term symptoms, especially articular symptoms, are not uncommon.[5]

When a diagnosis is not readily apparent, a surfeit of symptoms can become distracting. The discussant considered some unusual conditions on the basis of the patient's potential exposure to certain agents. However, he focused on the common causes of the main finding — fever of unknown origin.

When can a patient be classified as having fever of unknown origin? In 1961, Petersdorf and Beeson[6] defined fever of unknown origin as the finding of a body temperature of more than 38.3°C on several occasions over a period of more than three weeks, whose cause remains uncertain after one week of in-hospital investigation. Today, the requirement for hospitalization has been replaced by the completion of an aggressive evaluation.[7]

Fever of unknown origin is due to infection in 30 to 50 percent of cases, to cancer in 25 to 30 percent, and to autoimmune disease in 15 to 25 percent.[8-12] Drug fever remains an important, underrecognized cause.[10] The incidence of cancer as a cause has declined in recent years, probably as a result of improved methods of detection.[11] Although many physicians reflexively order multiple tests when they are dealing with a patient with a fever of unknown origin, a delay in diagnosis rarely jeopardizes the patient's condition, and a more measured approach is justified except in suspected cases of intraabdominal abscess, miliary tuberculosis, disseminated fungal infections, or recurrent pulmonary emboli, all of which can be rapidly fatal if left undiagnosed.[10]

The approach to the patient with a fever of unknown origin should be individualized. After the history-taking and physical examination, simple laboratory studies, chest radiography, and blood cultures are warranted. When the fever is hectic, active tuberculosis or other systemic inflammatory conditions should be considered. Ordering multiple additional diagnostic tests and abdominal CT scans in patients at low risk for the conditions these studies evaluate increases the chance of false positive results. In this case, the abdominal CT scan revealed a thickened ascending colon, which turned out to be a red herring.

When life-threatening conditions are deemed unlikely, a sensible approach to diagnosis is to permit the disease to reveal itself. The appearance of monoarticular arthritis led to the more serious consideration of Still's disease and tuberculosis. The extreme elevation in serum ferritin levels — although nonspecific — further suggested the diagnosis of Still's disease.[13] Because the diagnosis of Still's disease is one of exclusion, careful follow-up is indicated to confirm the clinical impression and the response to therapy.

Clinicians organize information into recognizable patterns and then find a diagnosis that can explain these patterns. By keeping the differential diagnosis broad and by following the patient's clinical trail, the discussant was able to arrive at the most likely diagnosis.

We are indebted to Dr. Tom Baudendistel for assistance with data collection.

This article first appeared in the June 6, 2002, issue of the New England Journal of Medicine.

REFERENCES

1.
Ohta A, Yamaguchi M, Kaneoka H, Nagayoshi T, Hiida M. Adult Still's disease: review of 228 cases from the literature. J Rheumatol 1987;14: 1139-46.

2.
Yamaguchi M, Ohta A, Tsunematsu T, et al. Preliminary criteria for classification of adult Still's disease. J Rheumatol 1992;19: 424-30.

3.
Kaur S, Bambery P, Dhar S. Persistent dermal plague lesions in adult onset Still's disease. Dermatology 1994;188:241-2.

4.
Larson EB. Adult Still's disease: evolution of a clinical syndrome and diagnosis, treatment, and follow-up of 17 patients. Medicine (Baltimore) 1984;63:82-91.

5.
Sampalis JS, Esdaile JM, Medsger TA Jr, et al. A controlled study of the long-term prognosis of adult Still's disease. Am J Med 1995;98:384-8.

6.
Petersdorf RG, Beeson PB. Fever of unexplained origin: report on 100 cases. Medicine (Baltimore) 1961;40:1-30.

7.
Petersdorf RG. Fever of unknown origin: an old friend revisited. Arch Intern Med 1992;152:21-2.

8.
de Kleijn EM, van der Meer JW. Fever of unknown origin (FUO): report on 53 patients in a Dutch university hospital. Neth J Med 1995;47:54-60.

9.
Iikuni Y, Okada J, Kondo H, Kashiwazaki S. Current fever of unknown origin 1982-1992. Intern Med 1994;33: 67-73.

10.
Arnow PM, Flaherty JP. Fever of unknown origin. Lancet 1997;350:575-80.

11.
Knockaert DC, Vanneste LJ, Vanneste SB, Bobbaers HJ. Fevers of unknown origin in the 1980s: an update of the diagnostic spectrum. Arch Intern Med 1992;152:51-5.

12.
Larson EB, Featherstone HJ, Petersdorf RG. Fever of undetermined origin: diagnosis and follow-up of 105 cases, 1970-1980. Medicine (Baltimore) 1982;61:269-92.

13.
Lee MH, Means RT Jr. Extremely elevated serum ferritin levels in a university hospital: associated diseases and clinical significance. Am J Med 1995;98:566-71.

The Unusual Suspect

SANDRA BLISS, M.D., STEVEN WEINBERGER, M.D., MARK MEIER, M.D., AND SANJAY SAINT, M.D., M.P.H.

A previously healthy 17-year-old boy awoke with left-sided pleuritic chest pain. He also noticed mild dyspnea on exertion during track-and-field practice but reported no sputum production, fever, chills, or recent trauma.

Pleuritic chest pain reflects inflammation, irritation, or stretching of sensory-nerve fibers in the parietal pleura. Often, the process primarily involves the pleura, as in the case of pneumothorax, a pleural inflammatory or infectious process, or a tumor with pleural involvement. Alternatively, pleuritic pain can result from a pulmonary parenchymal process that extends to the visceral pleural surface and secondarily involves the parietal pleura, especially in the case of pneumonia or pulmonary embolus. The acute onset of pleuritic chest pain in an otherwise healthy teenager suggests spontaneous pneumothorax or the relatively acute onset of pneumonia, although the absence of fever, chills, or sputum production makes the latter diagnosis less likely.

The patient was evaluated by his primary care provider and told that chest radiography revealed a dislocated rib but was otherwise normal. Over the course of the next four months, progressive exertional dyspnea developed; dyspnea then occurred when the patient was at rest and was accompanied by three-pillow orthopnea.

I am uncertain what is meant by a "dislocated rib" and would explore the rib finding to confirm whether an abnormality is really present. Progressive dyspnea has become the predominant symptom, and its severity and progression are quite striking. Pulmonary disorders that might progress at this rate include pulmonary parenchymal disease (a broad spectrum, ranging from disseminated tumor to pulmonary alveolar proteinosis and Goodpasture's syndrome), airway disease (e.g., asthma or obliterative bronchiolitis), or pulmonary vascular disease (e.g., primary pulmonary hypertension or occult thromboembolic disease). The presence of orthopnea raises the possibility of underlying cardiac disease associated with high left atrial pressure, as might be seen with mitral-valve disease or a cardiomyopathy.

On the day of admission to his local hospital, the patient had lightheadedness on standing that was followed by an episode of syncope when he was leaving the bathroom. At the time of hospital admission, he also reported having had an intermittent dry cough for two years with occasional hemoptysis and was noted to have lost 9 kg (20 lb) over a period of several months.

Lightheadedness and syncope are not typical symptoms of either pulmonary parenchymal disease or airway disease. Rather, I would lean toward either pulmonary vascular or cardiac disease, leading to obstruction of forward flow, diminished cardiac output, and impaired systemic perfusion. The intermittent dry cough and hemoptysis are more suggestive of pulmonary vascular than cardiac pathology, with the possible exceptions of mitral stenosis or a disorder mimicking mitral stenosis (such as cor triatriatum or left atrial myxoma). Although it is uncommon, any primary pulmonary vascular disorder associated with pulmonary hypertension could produce this constellation of symptoms, including chronic (or recurrent) pulmonary thromboembolism, tumor embolism, primary pulmonary hypertension, pulmonary venoocclusive disease, or mediastinal fibrosis producing pulmonary venous obstruction, pulmonary arterial obstruction, or both. The coexistence of orthopnea with the other symptoms suggests a postcapillary rather than precapillary origin of pulmonary hypertension and might therefore favor a diagnosis of pulmonary venoocclusive disease or mediastinal fibrosis with pulmonary venous obstruction.

The patient was not receiving any medications and indicated that he did not use tobacco or recreational drugs. He reported occasional alcohol use. He had not received a blood transfusion and said he had not engaged in sexual activity. He lived on a farm in Michigan with his mother and brother. He was a junior in high school, played football, and competed in the discus throw for the track-and-field team. His great-aunt had had a pulmonary embolism at 40 years of age.

The patient's temperature was 36.7°C, his heart rate was 110 beats per minute, his respiratory rate was 24 per minute, his blood pressure was 101/67 mm Hg, and his oxygen saturation was 88 percent while he was breathing room air. He had an athletic build and appeared to be in no acute distress. On cardiovascular examination, he was noted to have tachycardia, with a prominent S_2. He had no murmurs and no jugular venous distention. His lungs were clear bilaterally, and he had no clubbing. The remainder of the physical examination was normal.

The physical examination is helpful, with major findings being abnormal vital signs accompanied by a prominent S_2. This pattern of findings is consistent with pulmonary hypertension, although there are no other findings on examination to suggest a specific cause. However, additional historical information provides some tantalizing clues. Causes related to drugs or the human immunodeficiency virus seem unlikely. Residence on a farm in the Midwest raises the specter of either chronic hypersensitivity pneumonitis or histoplasmosis (a potential cause of fibrosing mediastinitis). Although a great-aunt is a rather distant relative, the possibility of one of the inherited thrombophilias should also be considered.

In addition to basic laboratory tests, I would initially order chest radiography, pulmonary-function tests, electrocardiography, and echocardiography. He will also need computed tomography (CT) of the chest — preferably CT angiography that would allow us not only to view his pulmonary parenchyma, but also to assess his pulmonary vessels and the possibility of subclinical, recurrent thromboembolism.

The white-cell count was 8100 per cubic millimeter, the hematocrit 47 percent, the platelet count 288,000 per cubic millimeter, the partial-thromboplastin time 39 seconds (normal range, 19 to 30), and the international normalized ratio for the prothrombin time 1.6. The serum aspartate aminotransferase level was 35 U per liter, the serum alanine aminotransferase level 81 U per liter, and the serum albumin level 3.3 g per deciliter. Electrocardiography revealed a pattern of right ventricular strain, and chest radiography demonstrated mild cardiomegaly and clear lung fields. Surface echocardiography suggested pulmonary hypertension, with an estimated right ventricular systolic pressure of 76 mm Hg, right ventricular enlargement, diminished right ventricular function, and slightly diminished left ventricular function.

The echocardiogram confirms the presence of pulmonary hypertension. The demonstration of clear lung fields on chest radiography and the absence of substantial cardiac pathology suggest that we should focus on primary pulmonary vascular disease. The differential diagnosis now revolves around precapillary and postcapillary forms of pulmonary hypertension. The presence of orthopnea is suggestive of a postcapillary form of pulmonary hypertension (such as pulmonary venoocclusive disease), whereas the finding of clear lung fields on chest radiography is suggestive of a precapillary origin (such as primary pulmonary hypertension or recurrent thromboembolic disease). The patient also has mildly abnormal results on coagulation studies that are currently unexplained and that warrant further characterization.

A spiral CT scan of the chest demonstrated multiple acute pulmonary emboli in the posterobasilar and anterior segments of the right lower lobe and left upper lobe, a nonocclusive thrombus in the left upper lobe, and prominent pulmonary arteries.

The spiral CT scan confirms the presence of thromboembolic disease as the cause of pulmonary hypertension. In the absence of any underlying reason for thrombosis in the arms or abdomen, large veins of the legs are the likely source of thromboemboli. Pulmonary emboli are quite unusual in adolescents and, in the absence of trauma or pregnancy, suggest an underlying thrombophilic state. Apart from antiphospholipid antibodies (of the lupus-anticoagulant type), inherited or acquired thrombophilic states generally are not associated with prolongation of either the prothrombin time or the partial-thromboplastin time. Because both are slightly prolonged, I would consider the possibility that a lupus anticoagulant is present. Although the lupus-anticoagulant phenomenon traditionally causes prolongation only of the partial-thromboplastin time, the prothrombin time may also be affected in some cases.

CT scans of the head, abdomen, and pelvis did not reveal evidence of cancer. Doppler ultrasonography of the veins in the arms and legs did not reveal thrombus. An evaluation for hypercoagulability (including measurement of the level or activity of protein C, protein S, antithrombin III, plasminogen, fibrinogen, heparin cofactor II, and homocysteine), gene analysis for factor V Leiden, prothrombin gene 20210, and methylenetetrahydrofolate reductase mutations, and immunologic analysis for antinuclear antibodies, anticardiolipin antibodies, and lupus anticoagulant were negative.

Heparin therapy was initiated, and the patient also received thrombolytic therapy with reteplase. He was transferred to the pediatric intensive care unit at a tertiary care hospital for further evaluation of the cause of pulmonary emboli.

When dealing with an unusual case of pulmonary embolic disease, the clinician is faced with two issues: where are the clots coming from, and is there any predisposition to clot formation? In this case, the usual suspects have been rounded up, but none of them has yet been proved guilty. Even though the ultrasonographic examination of the arms and legs was negative, it is still possible that the arms or, more likely, the legs were the source of the emboli but that all identifiable clots had already embolized. Alternatively, ultrasonography could have missed a clot that was either too proximal or too distal to be detected, or a clot could still be originating from an intraabdominal source or from the right atrium or

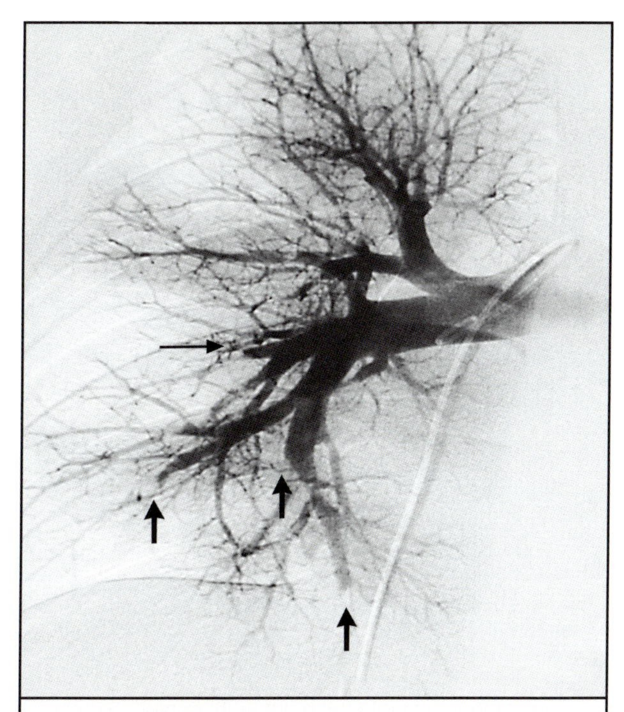

Figure 1. Initial Pulmonary Angiogram Demonstrating Occlusions in the Right Middle Lobe (Thin Arrow) and the Right Lower Lobe (Thick Arrows).

ventricle. Finally, we may be dealing with another type of embolic disease — specifically, tumor emboli.

A pulmonary angiogram was obtained that demonstrated elevated pulmonary arterial pressures (67/33 mm Hg). Multiple bilateral diffuse segmental and subsegmental filling defects consistent with the presence of acute and subacute pulmonary emboli were found (Figure 1). The inferior vena cava was patent, with normal anatomy. Evaluation of the right subclavian vein demonstrated wall irregularities and a nonocclusive thrombus underlying the clavicle and first rib, without collateral flow (Figure 2). The patient's dyspnea and oxygenation improved over the next several days, and he was weaned to room air. He continued to receive heparin while warfarin therapy was initiated, and he was discharged from the hospital with a therapeutic prothrombin time; he was given oxygen for home use during activity, and a plan was made for him to return in three months for surgical decompression of the thoracic outlet.

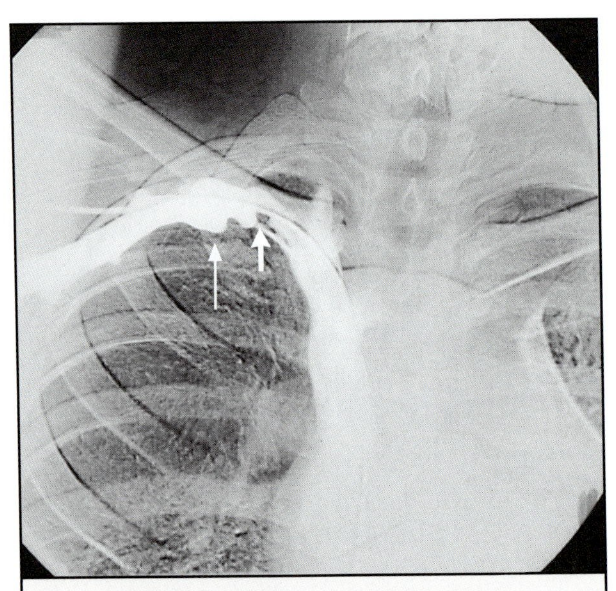

Figure 2. Right Subclavian Angiogram Revealing Chronic Nonocclusive Thrombus (Thick Arrow) and Irregularities and Aneurysmal Dilatation (Thin Arrow) in the Subclavian Vein.

Imaging studies confirm the presence of "spontaneous" thrombosis of the axillary subclavian veins, also called the Paget–Schroetter syndrome. This syndrome has been associated with exertion of the arms, and hence the term "effort thrombosis" has also been used. The patient's track-and-field activities could certainly have contributed to the thrombosis in his arms. However, the additional feature often present is extrinsic venous compression by the first rib or by a cervical rib. In retrospect, the "dislocated rib" seen on initial chest radiograph might have provided a clue if the anomaly was in the region of the thoracic outlet. Surgical decompression, typically including resection of the first rib, is an important component of treatment when venous compression is present.

One week after the patient was discharged from the hospital, vomiting and abdominal pain developed, and readmission was required. He had an oxygen saturation of 95 percent when breathing 5 liters of supplemental oxygen and appeared to be moderately ill. Echocardiography revealed a right ventricular systolic pressure of 100 mm Hg. Pulmonary angiography revealed a marked increase in filling defects in both pulmonary arteries as compared with the previous study (Figure 3). Mechanical thrombectomy was performed and intraarterial reteplase administered without improvement in pulmonary-artery flow. After the procedure was terminated because of hypotension and increasing hypoxemia, cardiac arrest

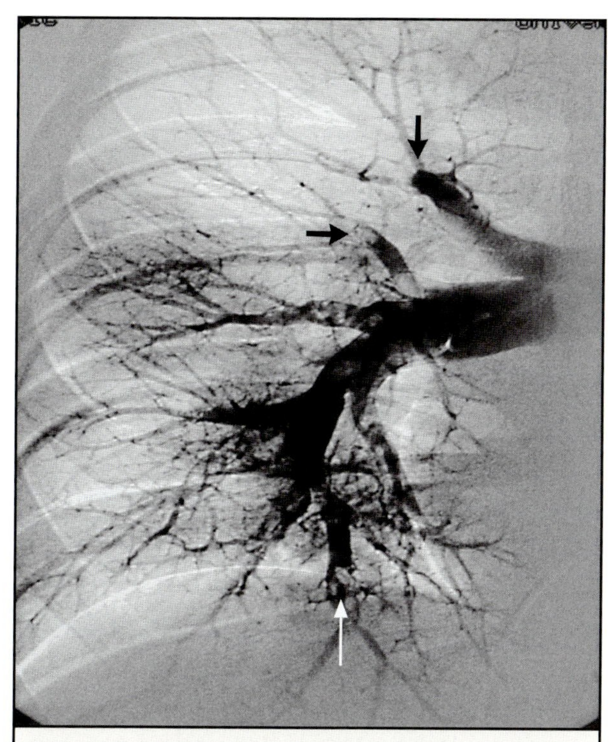

Figure 3. Repeated Pulmonary Angiogram Revealing New Filling Defects in the Right Upper Lobe (Black Arrows) and Right Lower Lobe (White Arrow).

This angiogram was obtained just before the patient's death.

occurred. The patient was resuscitated, and a circuit for extracorporeal membrane oxygenation was established. However, the patient had inadequate tissue perfusion, and when extracorporeal membrane oxygenation was discontinued, he died. Autopsy revealed numerous recent and organizing pulmonary emboli bilaterally, hypertensive changes in the pulmonary arteries, a large organizing infarct in the right lower lobe, and right ventricular hypertrophy and dilatation without mural thrombi or evidence of endocarditis. The inferior vena cava and superior vena cava were patent and without thrombi.

COMMENTARY

When a patient unexpectedly dies of a catastrophic illness, it is natural to review the clinical decisions that were made in order to verify that they were sound. Retrospectively, the physician tries to reaffirm that he or she made no errors in judgment that might have contributed to the death. This inspection is conducted with even greater scrutiny when the death was, at least in theory, preventable.

A possible misstep in this case was the delay in suspecting and confirming the diagnosis of pulmonary thromboembolic disease. Four months elapsed from the time the patient first sought medical attention for pleuritic chest pain to the hospital admission leading to appropriate studies and interventions. Many adolescents, especially boys, are reluctant to seek medical attention; often, our only interactions with members of this population come when physical examinations are required for participation in sports or school enrollment. Male adolescents may be more stoic than other patients and less likely to report symptoms; in addition, they may have an inflated sense of their own invincibility. This patient, however, sought medical attention early in the course of his illness, and therefore the delay in diagnosis cannot be attributed to procrastination in seeking care.

The physical examination may have been misleading. The patient was noted to have no jugular venous distention even at a time when his right ventricular and pulmonary arterial pressures were markedly elevated. Clinical assessment of jugular venous pressure is notoriously poor. In three studies comparing the prediction by physicians of central venous pressure with simultaneous pressure measurements obtained with an indwelling central venous catheter, the overall accuracy was only 56 percent.[1] Connors and colleagues reported a sensitivity of 49 percent for the detection of elevated central venous pressure.[2] When the clinical assessment is inaccurate, central venous pressure is more frequently underestimated than overestimated.[3]

The physician may harbor a presumption that adolescent athletes are healthy. Although athletic activity may exacerbate or unmask serious conditions such as hypertrophic cardiomyopathy or asthma, athletic participation is not usually harmful in a healthy teenager. The notion that athletic participation may cause catastrophic illness is foreign to most of us.

The diagnosis was most likely delayed because a physically robust patient presented in an atypical fashion with an uncommon disease. Although the incidence of pulmonary embolism among adults is estimated at 1 in 1000 per year,[4] it is rare among children and adolescents. Bernstein and colleagues have estimated that 7.8 per 10,000 hospital admissions of adolescents or young adults are the result of pulmonary embolism — an incidence much lower than that among older adults.[5] The incidence does appear to be higher among adolescents than among younger children.[6] In addition, although the signs and symptoms of pulmonary embolism are similar in children and adults, adolescents may present with less dyspnea and tachypnea than adults,[7] possibly reflecting better physiological tolerance.

Primary thrombosis of the axillary subclavian vein was described in 1875 by Sir James Paget and in 1884 by Leopold von Schroetter.[8] The term "effort thrombosis" was later coined to acknowledge the role of unusual exertion of the arms. Paget–Schroetter syndrome usually develops in young, healthy persons with a history of repetitive motion of the arms. Spontaneous thromboses in the arms have been reported in athletes such as golfers, football players, weight lifters, baseball players, wrestlers, tennis players, and cheerleaders, as well as in painters and beauticians.[8,9] The majority of patients are affected in the dominant arm. Unlike this athlete, most patients present with symptoms of venous obstruction such as pain, swelling, bluish discoloration, and venous collaterals.[10] Nonocclusive thromboses, as seen in this patient, may not present with local symptoms, instead becoming symptomatic only after embolization.[9]

Repetitive shoulder–arm motion, extrinsic compression of the subclavian vein, and in some patients, a hypercoagulable state may contribute to the development of primary thrombosis of the subclavian vein. Repetitive motion of the shoulder and arm predisposes persons to thrombosis by a number of mechanisms. Lateral abduction of the arm leads to compression of the subclavian vein, causing turbulence or obstruction of flow.[9,11] In addition, microscopic intimal damage may occur, stimulating the coagulation cascade. Repetitive motion may also contribute to anatomical stricture of the thoracic outlet through hypertrophy of the tendon of the subclavian muscle, the anterior scalene muscles, or both. Other possible sites of external compression include the first rib, complete or incomplete cervical ribs, fibromuscular bands, and callus from old clavicular fracture (Figure 4).[12] Lifting of heavy objects may lead to depression of the shoulder, which further narrows the costoclavicular space.[11] Although most patients with Paget–Schroetter syndrome have isolated vascular compression, some also have classic symptoms of thoracic outlet syndrome, including paresthesias, numbness, and muscle weakness. Factors associated with hypercoagulability appear to increase risk; for example, it is hypothesized that exposure to exogenous estrogen in female athletes predisposes them to this syndrome.[11] Furthermore, patients with an underlying hypercoagulable state may have more refractory thrombosis.[13] In this patient, the abnormal coagulation results on presentation, the family history, and the progression of thromboemboli despite adequate anticoagulation all suggest a superimposed, yet unidentified, thrombophilia.

Historically, treatment of this syndrome consisted of elevation and anticoagulation, but long-term complications were common. More recently, catheter-directed thrombolytic therapy followed by decompression of the thoracic outlet has become the standard of care.[14] The rates of vessel patency and of symptom-free survival approach 100 percent,

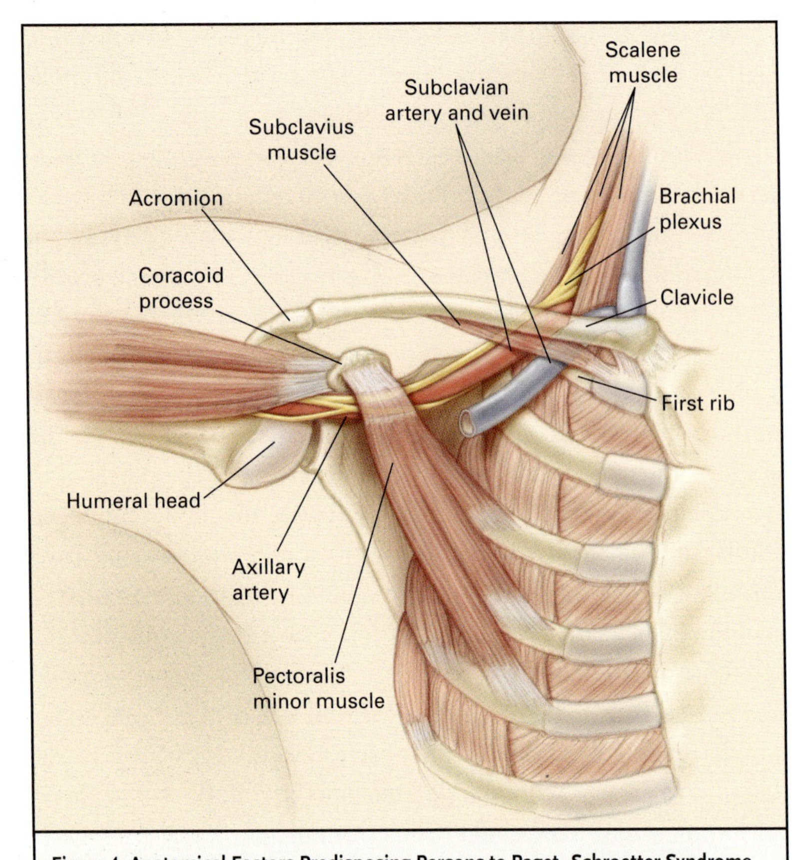

Figure 4. Anatomical Factors Predisposing Persons to Paget–Schroetter Syndrome.

Venous compression may occur as a result of abnormality or hypertrophy of the anterior scalene or subclavian muscles, complete or incomplete cervical ribs, fibromuscular bands, and callus from old clavicular fractures.

although patients who do not undergo thrombolysis early have worse outcomes.[8,11] The incidence of pulmonary embolism in patients with Paget–Schroetter syndrome varies from 10 to 30 percent, depending on how the diagnosis is made[11]; most emboli are probably clinically silent.

Once this patient presented with pulmonary hypertension and syncope, the diagnosis of pulmonary thromboembolic disease secondary to Paget–Schroetter syndrome was made expeditiously. Despite thrombolysis and anticoagulation, new thromboemboli, progressive pulmonary hypertension, and right heart failure developed. Although management was consistent with the known standards of care, the outcome was disastrous. Although rare, the unusual suspect known as Paget–Schroetter syndrome should be considered whenever a person with repetitive arm motion presents with pulmonary hypertension or thromboembolic disease.

Dr. Saint is supported by a Career Development Award from the Health Services Research and Development Program of the Department of Veterans Affairs and a Patient Safety Development Center Grant (P20-HS11540) from the Agency for Healthcare Research and Quality.

We are indebted to Camilla Payne, R.N., for assistance in the preparation of the manuscript.

This article first appeared in the December 5, 2002, issue of the New England Journal of Medicine.

REFERENCES

1.
Cook DJ, Simel DL. Does this patient have abnormal central venous pressure? JAMA 1996;275:630-4.

2.
Connors AF Jr, McCaffree DR, Gray BA. Evaluation of right-heart catheterization in the critically ill patient without acute myocardial infarction. N Engl J Med 1983;308:263-7.

3.
Eisenberg PR, Jaffe AS, Schuster DP. Clinical evaluation compared to pulmonary artery catheterization in the hemodynamic assessment of critically ill patients. Crit Care Med 1984;12:549-53.

4.
Goldhaber SZ. Pulmonary embolism. N Engl J Med 1998;339:93-104.

5.
Bernstein D, Coupey S, Schonberg SK. Pulmonary embolism in adolescents. Am J Dis Child 1986;140:667-71.

6.
David M, Andrew M. Venous thromboembolic complications in children. J Pediatr 1993;123:337-46.

7.
Green RM, Meyer TJ, Dunn M, Glassroth J. Pulmonary embolism in younger adults. Chest 1992;101:1507-11.

8.
Urschel HC Jr, Razzuk MA. Paget-Schroetter syndrome: what is the best management? Ann Thorac Surg 2000;69:1663-9.

9.
Kommareddy A, Zaroukian MH, Hassouna HI. Upper extremity deep venous thrombosis. Semin Thromb Hemost 2002;28:89-99.

10.
Nichols AW. The thoracic outlet syndrome in athletes. J Am Board Fam Pract 1996;9:346-55.

11.
Adelman MA, Stone DH, Riles TS, Lamparello PJ, Giangola G, Rosen RJ. A multidisciplinary approach to the treatment of Paget-Schroetter syndrome. Ann Vasc Surg 1997;11:149-54.

12.
Makhoul RG, Machleder HI. Developmental anomalies at the thoracic outlet: an analysis of 200 consecutive cases. J Vasc Surg 1992;16:534-45.

13.
Kreienberg PB, Chang BB, Darling RC III, et al. Long-term results in patients treated with thrombolysis, thoracic inlet decompression, and subclavian vein stenting for Paget-Schroetter syndrome. J Vasc Surg 2001;33:Suppl:S100-S105.

14.
Machleder HI. Evaluation of a new treatment strategy for Paget-Schroetter syndrome: spontaneous thrombosis of the axillary-subclavian vein. J Vasc Surg 1993;17:305-17.

Easy to See but Hard to Find

BRENDAN M. REILLY, M.D., PETER CLARKE, M.D.,
AND PETROS NIKOLINAKOS, M.D.

A 46-year-old woman from the Philippines with no history of serious medical conditions was hospitalized with fatigue, body aches, and a weight loss of 4.5 kg (10 lb) over the previous three months. She did not have fever, sweats, or a cough and had not recently traveled outside Chicago. She did not smoke cigarettes or use any drugs. Her family history was unremarkable.

Physical examination showed no abnormalities except for pallor, orthostatic hypotension, and moderate tenderness on palpation of the patient's upper arms, anterior thorax, and lower spine. The results of laboratory studies were as follows: hemoglobin, 8.0 g per deciliter; white-cell count, 8500 per cubic millimeter, with a normal differential count; platelet count, 177,000 per cubic millimeter; mean corpuscular volume, 89 μm^3; reticulocyte count, 5.6 percent; blood urea nitrogen, 59 mg per deciliter (21.1 mmol per liter); creatinine, 2.8 mg per deciliter (247.5 μmol per liter); calcium, 13.2 mg per deciliter (3.3 mmol per liter); phosphate, 3.8 mg per deciliter (1.2 mmol per liter); total protein, 7.5 g per deciliter; and albumin, 4.6 g per deciliter. Liver-function tests, urinalysis, and a chest radiograph showed no abnormalities.

This patient has several problems, all apparently new: hypercalcemia, anemia, renal failure, and orthostatic hypotension. There is most likely a single unifying diagnosis to explain all the findings. Multiple myeloma comes to mind first, despite her age.

Most patients presenting with serum calcium levels of 13 mg per deciliter (3.2 mmol per liter) or higher have a malignant condition. The anemia and elevated reticulocyte count might at first glance suggest hemolysis or blood loss, but the reticulocyte-production index (calculated by dividing the patient's hemoglobin value by the normal value, multiplying the result by the reticulocyte count, and then dividing by 2) is only 1.9, indicating underproduction by the bone marrow. The elevated ratio of blood urea nitrogen to creatinine and the orthostatic hypotension suggest prerenal azotemia, perhaps as a result of hypercalcemic diuresis. Obstructive uropathy due to bilateral calculous disease and myeloma kidney are less likely possibilities.

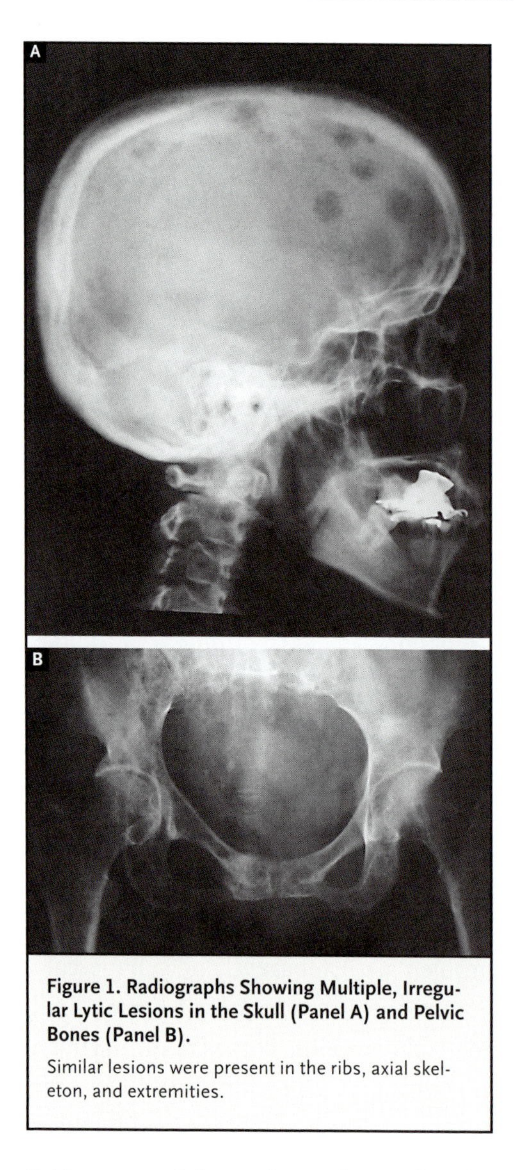

Figure 1. Radiographs Showing Multiple, Irregular Lytic Lesions in the Skull (Panel A) and Pelvic Bones (Panel B).

Similar lesions were present in the ribs, axial skeleton, and extremities.

I would perform careful breast, pelvic, and rectal examinations; review the peripheral blood smear; and order a serum parathyroid hormone assay. I would then observe the patient's clinical response to intravenous rehydration.

Pelvic and breast examination showed no abnormalities. A stool specimen was negative for occult blood. The blood smear was unremarkable except for normocytic anemia. After rehydration with saline, the patient's orthostatic hypotension resolved and her serum creatinine level fell to 1.2 mg per deciliter (106.1 μmol per liter). However, her serum

calcium level remained high (12.3 mg per deciliter [3.1 mmol per liter]), with an intact serum parathyroid hormone level of 3.5 pg per milliliter (normal range, 10 to 55).

A skeletal bone survey revealed multiple lytic bone lesions in the axial skeleton, skull, bilateral ribs, pelvis, both femurs, and both humeri (Figure 1). Compression fractures were noted in the T12, L2, and L4 vertebral bodies. The patient was given intravenous pamidronate, and her serum calcium level returned to normal.

The low parathyroid hormone level and the radiographic findings strongly suggest cancer. Such extensive bone lesions would be most unusual in a patient with hypercalcemia due to a nonmalignant condition that was unassociated with parathyroid hormone production, such as sarcoidosis, hyperthyroidism, or the milk-alkali syndrome. The patient's neurologic status deserves careful attention in view of the spinal lesions. The possibility of pathologic fractures in her arms and legs should also be considered.

A targeted evaluation for myeloma and metastatic carcinomas commonly associated with lytic bone metastases (tumors in the breast, lung, and kidney) is warranted now. An elevated parathyroid hormone–related protein level might argue against myeloma, but this finding is not entirely specific. A high 1,25-dihydroxyvitamin D level would suggest lymphoma or granulomatous disease, but these diagnoses seem unlikely.

The findings on bilateral mammography were normal. Computed tomographic (CT) studies of the neck, thorax, abdomen, and pelvis showed no abnormalities except for the previously described bone lesions. The results of serum and urinary protein electrophoresis and the serum 1,25-dihydroxyvitamin D level were also normal.

Serum was obtained for quantitative immunoglobulin assays, and bone marrow aspiration and biopsy were performed. Pending the results, the patient was discharged from the hospital while taking oral opiates for pain control, and arrangements were made for her to be seen in the oncology clinic the following week.

The bone marrow aspirate and biopsy specimen were normal (<3 percent plasma cells). The IgG level was 822 mg per deciliter (normal range, 694 to 1618), the IgA level was 100 mg per deciliter (normal range, 68 to 378), and the IgM level was 29 mg per deciliter (normal range, 77 to 220). At the clinic visit the week after her discharge, the patient reported that her pain was adequately controlled. Examination revealed mild, diffuse weakness but no focal neurologic deficit. The serum calcium level was 10.2 mg per deciliter (2.6 mmol per liter).

The normal bone marrow findings and normal results of protein electrophoresis make the diagnosis of myeloma much less likely. Isolated suppression of the IgM level raises the question of nonsecretory myeloma, but this disorder is very uncommon, and it is characterized by plasmacytosis in the bone marrow.

The common cancers that cause diffuse lytic bone lesions also seem highly unlikely in this case. In this regard, thyroid carcinoma also should be considered. Was the thyroid gland examined carefully? At this point, one could repeat the bone marrow aspiration and biopsy in search of myeloma, but it seems more prudent to perform a biopsy of an accessible bone lesion.

The results of repeated serum and urinary protein electrophoresis were normal. Repeated bone marrow aspiration and biopsy revealed no abnormal cells, infiltrates, or fibrosis. Breast and thyroid examinations by a surgical consultant showed no abnormalities. A bone scan revealed increased uptake in multiple ribs, the thoracic and lumbar spine, the sternum, and both scapulae.

At this point, a bone biopsy is mandatory. Myeloma or metastatic cancer from an unknown primary site is the most likely diagnosis, because nonmalignant disorders that cause widespread bone lesions in adults — granulomatous diseases, mastocytosis, Gaucher's disease, and histiocytosis disorders — all seem very unlikely.

The patient was readmitted to the hospital with worsening pain, generalized weakness, and new dyspnea. Examination revealed a temperature of 40°C; crackles in the lower lung fields bilaterally; diffuse skeletal tenderness, which was greatest in the right iliac fossa; and bilateral proximal leg weakness.

The white-cell count was 4700 per cubic millimeter, the hemoglobin level was 6.2 g per deciliter, the calcium level was 16.3 mg per deciliter (4.1 mmol per liter), the blood urea nitrogen level was 58 mg per deciliter (20.7 mmol per liter), and the creatinine level was 4.1 mg per deciliter (362.4 μmol per liter). A chest radiograph revealed patchy infiltrates in both lower lung fields. Cultures, a tuberculin skin test, and a repeated serum parathyroid hormone test were performed.

The patient was treated with intravenous saline, ceftriaxone and erythromycin, morphine, packed red cells, and pamidronate.

Mycobacterial, fungal, and chronic salmonella infections can cause lytic bone lesions with lung involvement. However, the extensive nature of the bone lesions, the absence of prior fever, and the temporal course of the illness make these highly unlikely explanations for the patient's entire illness. Cancer, now complicated by pneumonia, remains most likely.

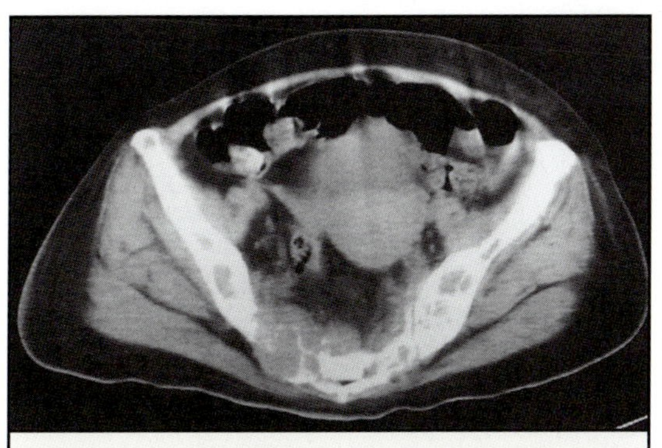

Figure 2. Large Destructive Lesion in the Right Iliac Bone, the Site of Two CT-Guided Bone Biopsies.

The leg weakness is alarming. Given the known spinal involvement, magnetic resonance imaging (MRI) should be performed to rule out epidural compression by a tumor or, less likely, infection.

In any event, we need a tissue diagnosis. If a bony lesion in the pelvis is the most symptomatic area and is accessible to CT-guided biopsy, I would obtain tissue from that site after the patient's condition has been stabilized.

The patient's fever and dyspnea improved rapidly with antibiotic therapy. All cultures and a tuberculin skin test were negative. The serum parathyroid hormone level again was low. After rehydration, the serum creatinine level fell to 2.2 mg per deciliter (194.5 μmol per liter), and the serum calcium level fell to 10.7 mg per deciliter (2.7 mmol per liter).

MRI of the spine showed compression deformities in multiple thoracic and lumbar vertebral bodies. There was a slight deformity of the ventral aspect of the thecal sac at L4, but there was no epidural compression or evidence of disk-space infection. A bone marrow biopsy again showed no abnormalities; stains for acid-fast bacilli and fungi were negative.

CT-guided biopsy of a large lytic lesion in the right iliac bone (Figure 2) was performed, during which the patient had severe pain in her right upper arm. Radiographs revealed a pathologic nondisplaced fracture of the humerus (Figure 3). Pending the results of the bone biopsy, an orthopedic consultant recommended nonoperative treatment of the fracture. Cytologic analysis of the specimen from the iliac-bone biopsy was nondiagnostic, and there was insufficient tissue for a definitive histopathological evaluation.

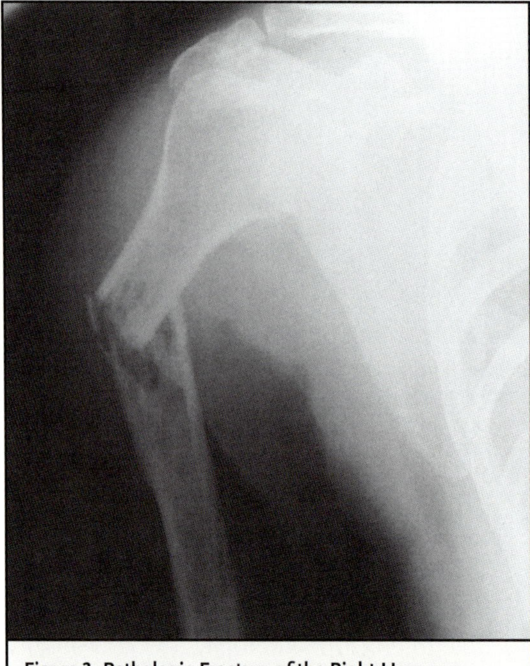

Figure 3. Pathologic Fracture of the Right Humerus, Sustained during the First Bone Biopsy.

Again, we need a tissue diagnosis. Another bone biopsy should be performed. Options include a repeated CT-guided biopsy of the lesion in the pelvic area or of a symptomatic, accessible lesion at another site; surgical biopsy of the humerus by the orthopedist; or surgical biopsy of the lower lumbar spine (with definitive exclusion of the possibility of epidural disease).

A second CT-guided biopsy of the bone lesion in the pelvis was performed, complicated by sustained local bleeding and pain. An oncologist recommended that treatment for myeloma be initiated if this second biopsy was also inconclusive, because "the patient's condition is deteriorating, and myeloma is almost certainly the diagnosis." The bone biopsy revealed nonspecific inflammatory cells and small areas of fibrosis.

At this point, we must weigh the risks of delayed treatment and morbidity from further diagnostic testing against the risks of treatment under conditions of slight uncertainty. I would continue to pursue a tissue diagnosis. Establishing a diagnosis of an atypical presentation of myeloma by the process of elimination makes me uncomfortable. It would be a serious error to give the patient toxic therapy for myeloma if that diagnosis turned out to be wrong, and I would not underestimate the suffering the patient might experience by receiving only presumptive confirmation of such a grave diagnosis.

I would favor an open biopsy after discussing the options with the patient. There is no shortage of lesions available in this case, and the risks of a minimally invasive procedure seem acceptable.

The patient reported increasing weakness in both legs. Neurologic examination revealed decreased strength diffusely in the legs, with normal deep-tendon reflexes and no sensory deficit or sphincter dysfunction.

Neither the neurologic findings nor the previous MRI studies suggest compression of the epidural cord or cauda equina. Nevertheless, given the need for a tissue diagnosis, surgical exploration and biopsy of the lesions in the lumbosacral spine seem to be the best option at this point.

Surgical laminectomy, foraminectomy, and biopsy of the L4 vertebral body were performed. Histopathological examination of the biopsy specimen revealed diffuse plasma-cell infiltration (Figure 4). Immunocytochemical staining showed extensive cytoplasmic staining for kappa immunoglobulin light chains, with no staining for lambda light chains.

The patient was treated with intravenous dexamethasone and four cycles of vincristine and doxorubicin. Her pain gradually subsided, and her neurologic function returned to normal. The pathologic fracture of the humerus healed, and the other bone lesions gradually improved. The patient is currently awaiting bone marrow transplantation.

COMMENTARY

Patients with nonsecretory myeloma, a rare disease, have undetectable monoclonal immunoglobulins in serum and urine, but the clinical findings are otherwise typical of myeloma, including bone marrow plasmacytosis.[1] This case is very unusual — an uncommon presentation of a rare disease. Why, then, did our discussant pursue this particular diagnosis so doggedly? And why, before the diagnosis was confirmed, did the oncology consultant recommend (potentially toxic) chemotherapy for myeloma?

In an adult with widespread lytic bone lesions and hypercalcemia that is not mediated by parathyroid hormone, diagnostic testing for myeloma and metastatic cancer is the

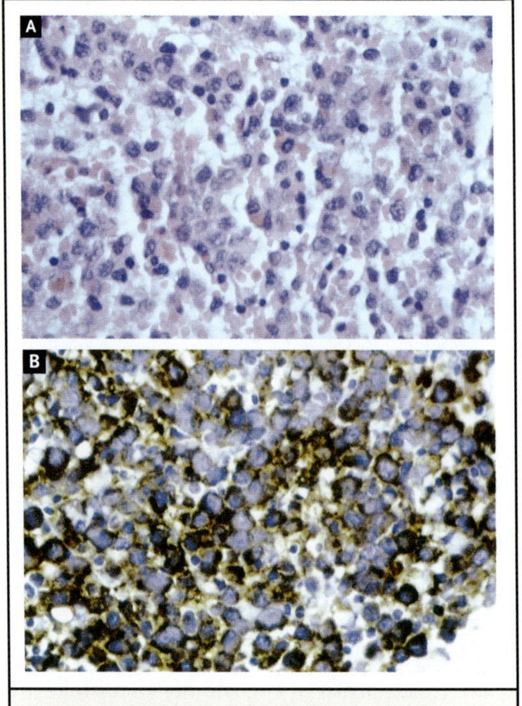

Figure 4. Surgical Biopsy Specimen from the L4 Vertebral Body.

Panel A shows a diffuse plasma-cell infiltrate (hematoxylin and eosin, ×100). Panel B shows immunocytochemical staining for kappa light chains (×100).

obvious strategy. But in our patient, this strategy seemed to fail, since all the tests were unrevealing. If the pretest probability of myeloma is 90 percent, negative results of immunoglobulin and bone marrow studies together reduce this probability to less than 5 percent. If the pretest probability of metastatic cancer is 10 percent, normal imaging studies (mammography and extensive CT scanning) reduce this probability to less than 1 percent.[2] The combined post-test probability of myeloma or metastatic cancer is only about 5 percent, suggesting that some other diagnosis is highly likely. But what other diagnosis? No other possibilities make clinical sense.

Paradoxically, therein lies the solution to the problem. If the only reasonable diagnostic possibilities are myeloma and metastatic cancer, then the sum of their probabilities must equal 1. Under these conditions, tests targeted at one diagnosis, when negative, reciprocally act as "positive" tests for the alternative diagnosis (Table 1). The absence of monoclonal immunoglobulins decreases the odds of myeloma by a factor of approximately 20 (a

Table 1. Diagnostic Probabilities and Odds of Myeloma during the Testing Sequence.*

Test†	Result	Probability of Myeloma	Probability of Nonmyeloma Cancer	Odds of Myeloma
Pretest		0.90	0.10	9:1
Post-test 1: measurement of immunoglobulins	Negative‡	0.31	0.69	5:11
Post-test 2: imaging studies	Negative§	0.90	0.10	9:1
Post-test 3: bone marrow biopsy	Negative¶	0.64	0.36	9:5

* The odds is the probability divided by 1 minus the probability. It is assumed that disorders other than myeloma and nonmyeloma cancer have been excluded from diagnostic consideration.

† Tests are considered in sequence, with the post-test probability after each test serving as the pretest probability for the next test.

‡ The negative likelihood ratio — calculated as 1 minus the sensitivity, divided by the specificity — is 0.05 for myeloma, assuming that the sensitivity of immunoglobulin studies is 0.95 for myeloma and that the specificity is 0.99 for nonmyeloma cancer.

§ The negative likelihood ratio is 0.05 for nonmyeloma cancer, assuming that the sensitivity of mammography plus computed tomography (of the neck, chest, abdomen, and pelvis) is 0.95 for nonmyeloma cancer and that the specificity is 0.99 for myeloma.

¶ The negative likelihood ratio is 0.20 for myeloma, assuming that the sensitivity of bone marrow aspiration and biopsy is 0.90 for myeloma and that the specificity is 0.50 for nonmyeloma cancer.

negative likelihood ratio — calculated as 1 minus the sensitivity, divided by the specificity — of 0.05)[3] but also increases the odds of metastatic cancer by the same amount. Normal imaging studies have the opposite effect. As a result, if immunoglobulin and imaging studies are negative, the post-test odds of myeloma remain the same as the pretest odds (9:1). Normal findings on bone marrow examination change these odds (to 9:5) by decreasing the probability of myeloma relative to metastatic cancer. But nonsecretory myeloma remains the most likely diagnosis, despite its rarity.

However, does this justify the oncologist's recommendation to initiate treatment for myeloma before the diagnosis was confirmed? Even if the pretest probability of myeloma exceeded 90 percent (or the low IgM level was considered a positive test for myeloma), conventional wisdom holds that treatment of cancer requires definitive proof of the diagnosis. The answer depends on the "test–treatment threshold," the probability of myeloma above which treatment without further testing is the optimal course of action.[4] When deciding whether to initiate treatment or delay it until further studies have been performed, few clinicians quantify the threshold probability, but most consider its determinants: the risks and accuracy of further testing, the likely benefit of treatment if the diagnosis is correct, and the potential harm of treatment if the diagnosis is incorrect.

There are two principal reasons why, as a rule, the test–treatment threshold in patients with suspected cancer is 1.0 (in other words, testing is preferable to treatment until the diagnosis is 100 percent certain). First, tests to diagnose cancer (tissue biopsies) usually have low risk and high accuracy. Second, the potential harm of cancer treatment given to a patient without cancer is usually considered so unacceptable that it seems greatly to outweigh the likely benefit of that treatment given to a patient with cancer.

But this patient's case is an exception to the rule on both counts. The diagnostic accuracy of bone biopsy has not been well studied, but its sensitivity is certainly less than perfect,[2] and its risk cannot be discounted in a patient who has had serious complications from previous biopsies. In addition, the likely benefit of treatment for myeloma if our patient has myeloma[5] outweighs its potential harm if she does not have myeloma. Why? Because the only other reasonable diagnosis is widely metastatic cancer, in which case the patient's life expectancy is likely to be short no matter how she is treated.[2,6]

For these reasons, the test–treatment threshold for this patient was less than 1.0, at least in terms of life expectancy. From that perspective, the oncologist's unorthodox recommendation to initiate treatment for myeloma before there was definitive proof of the diagnosis may make good sense. But, as the discussant noted, it is essential to work with the patient in arriving at a final decision. Even when communication between the patient and the physician is optimal, some patients will favor unconventional options,[7] just as physicians sometimes do.

We are indebted to Arthur Evans, M.D., M.P.H., for his insightful comments about this case.

This article first appeared in the January 2, 2003, issue of the New England Journal of Medicine.

REFERENCES

1.
Blade J, Kyle RA. Nonsecretory myeloma, immunoglobulin D myeloma, and plasma cell leukemia. Hematol Oncol Clin North Am 1999;13:1259-72.

2.
Katagiri H, Takahashi M, Inagaki J, Sugiura H, Ito S, Iwata H. Determining the site of primary cancer in patients with skeletal metastasis of unknown origin: a retrospective study. Cancer 1999;86:533-7.

3.
Sackett DL, Richardson WS, Rosenberg W, Haynes RB. Evidence-based medicine: how to practice and teach EBM. New York: Churchill Livingstone, 1997.

4.
Sox HC, Blatt MA, Higgins MC, Marton KI. Medical decision making. Boston: Butterworths, 1988.

5.
Munshi NC, Tricot G, Barlogie B. Plasma cell neoplasms. In: DeVita VT Jr, Hellman S, Rosenberg SA, eds. Cancer: principles & practice of oncology. 6th ed. Philadelphia: Lippincott Williams & Wilkins, 2001:2465-99.

6.
Greco FA, Hainsworth JD. Cancer of unknown primary site. In: DeVita VT Jr, Hellman S, Rosenberg SA, eds. Cancer: principles & practice of oncology. 6th ed. Philadelphia: Lippincott Williams & Wilkins, 2001: 2537-60.

7.
Gearin-Tosh M. Living proof: a medical mutiny. New York: Scribner, 2002.

A Gut Feeling

JESSICA HABERER, M.D., NEIL N. TRIVEDI, M.D.,
JEFFREY KOHLWES, M.D., M.P.H., AND LAWRENCE TIERNEY, JR., M.D.

A 79-year-old man was referred to our hospital because of an 18-kg weight loss over the previous six months. Seven months before admission, his house burned down, and insomnia, anorexia, and anhedonia developed. One month before admission, he began having diffuse, episodic, dull abdominal pain without radiation, relation to food or position, or improvement with the use of a proton-pump inhibitor. The patient had several yellow, watery stools per day. He said he did not have melena, fever, chills, night sweats, or dysphagia.

The main issue is involuntary weight loss, and the amount should be verified. Depression is understandable after a fire and is an often-overlooked cause of weight loss. The presence of abdominal pain leads to additional considerations, particularly when the pain is associated with abnormal bowel habits. Has the patient been using alcohol, which may cause recurrent pancreatitis and associated malabsorption? The abdominal pain should also trigger consideration of an intraabdominal neoplasm, particularly of the pancreas and colon. My line of inquiry would focus on features of depression or additional gastrointestinal symptoms suggestive of these diagnoses.

The patient repeatedly denied being depressed and expressed a desire to resume his usual routine. He reported having a good appetite but could not maintain his usual weight of 64 kg. Initial investigation elsewhere had revealed leukocytosis (white-cell count, 31,000 per cubic millimeter) and a urinary tract infection that was treated with levofloxacin. Esophagogastroduodenoscopy revealed multiple gastric ulcerations, a hiatal hernia, and esophagitis. No cancer was detected on biopsy. A colonoscopic examination performed with suboptimal preparation showed left-sided diverticula. The patient was subsequently transferred to our hospital for further evaluation.

The patient has the unusual combination of marked leukocytosis and gastric ulcers. Gastric ulcers, whether benign or malignant, are typically associated with weight loss. Duodenal ulcers classically result in weight gain, because most such ulcers hypersecrete acid and produce pain, which is relieved by the buffering effect of food. The negative biopsy results do not rule out cancer and should be reviewed. The leukocytosis is striking in a patient with a urinary tract infection, unless the infection is associated with sepsis or a perinephric abscess. Abdominal pain caused by pyelonephritis has resulted in more than one visit to the operating room. A rare condition, phlegmonous gastritis, is a type of gastric cellulitis with interruption of the gastric mucosa that occurs in poorly nourished patients. Oral flora enters the gastric media, resulting in a thick, nondistensible stomach with severe clinical illness. Depression itself may have caused anorexia, stress-related ulcers, and subsequent bacterial gastritis, but this is extremely unlikely.

The patient had a history of chronic obstructive pulmonary disease, peptic ulcer disease, mycosis fungoides, and peripheral vascular disease. He said he had not had any previous episodes of pancreatitis. He underwent an aortofemoral bypass and left carotid endarterectomy in the 1990s. He is a former leather worker without known exposure to toxic solvents. He had a history of 50 pack-years of smoking and did not consume alcohol. His medications included lansoprazole, dietary supplements, and levofloxacin.

The history adds complexity to the case. The hypoxemia that results from chronic obstructive pulmonary disease is associated with a higher incidence of peptic ulcer disease. Testing for *Helicobacter pylori* should be performed, and the patient should be asked about the use of over-the-counter nonsteroidal antiinflammatory drugs, since many patients take such drugs without their physician's knowledge. Mycosis fungoides is a T-cell lymphoma, and its stage should be established before the clinician speculates about visceral involvement. A most promising clue to the diagnosis is the peripheral vascular disease. The patient is a smoker and clearly has aortic atherosclerosis, suggesting another often-overlooked cause of weight loss — chronic mesenteric ischemia. The absence of the typical postprandial discomfort is not unusual. Patients learn to avoid food because it produces pain and become unaware of their anorexia. A calorie count provides a simple test of this hypothesis. Calorie counts are underused in the care of inpatients, despite the accuracy provided by hospital dietitians. The extent of the patient's vascular disease on examination will be important.

Next, I would look for cancer. With this degree and rapidity of weight loss, the cause is usually obvious at first evaluation. Other common causes of profound weight loss, such as hyperthyroidism, should also be quite apparent.

The patient was markedly cachectic. His temperature was 36°C (97°F), the blood pressure was 116/68 mm Hg, the heart rate was 81 beats per minute, the respiratory rate was 16 breaths per minute, and the oxygen saturation was 96 percent while he was breathing ambient air. His weight was 46 kg, and his height was 1.67 m. No icterus was present; the oropharynx was clear. The patient's neck was supple without bruits or lymphadenopathy and had a well-healed surgical scar. The cardiopulmonary examination was normal. The abdomen was scaphoid with normal bowel sounds but no organomegaly or tenderness. The patient had guaiac-positive stool and an enlarged, smooth prostate. He had no peripheral edema, distal pulses were faintly present bilaterally, and a well-healed scar was present in the right groin. The neurologic examination was normal. Laboratory studies revealed a white-cell count of 31,000 per cubic millimeter with 87 percent neutrophils, a platelet count of 647,000 per cubic millimeter, and a hematocrit of 42 percent. Electrolytes, liver-function tests, and amylase and coagulation studies were normal, except for a serum albumin concentration of 3.4 g per deciliter. Urinalysis showed 25 to 50 white cells per high-power field and bacteria. A chest radiograph revealed hyperinflated lungs with a new 1-cm nodule in the left lower lobe.

This patient has lost an extraordinary 30 percent of his body weight. It is unusual for such a patient to have cancer without focal findings on physical examination. A major exception, however, is pancreatic carcinoma. The thrombocytosis is interesting; a review of unselected cases suggests that visceral cancer is the most common cause. Chronic infection, rheumatoid arthritis, and iron deficiency should also be considered. The marked leukocytosis without fever or the appearance of infection continues to puzzle me. Chronic intestinal ischemia becomes more likely as we garner further information. In addition, patients with severe chronic obstructive pulmonary disease or end-stage congestive heart failure may have cachexia, although in such cases, the weight loss generally occurs over a period of years rather than months.

What to do next? Imaging of the abdomen, which might expose hidden causes of weight loss, is appropriate. A periappendiceal or peridiverticular abscess could account for the hematologic abnormalities and the weight loss. I would consider repeating upper and lower endoscopy to search for cancer, particularly in the stomach, where previous investigation resulted in nonspecific findings.

The patient was treated with levofloxacin for presumed prostatitis, and additional laboratory tests were performed on serum. These tests revealed a lactate dehydrogenase concentration of 157 U per liter, a thyrotropin concentration of 0.57 μU per milliliter, an erythro-

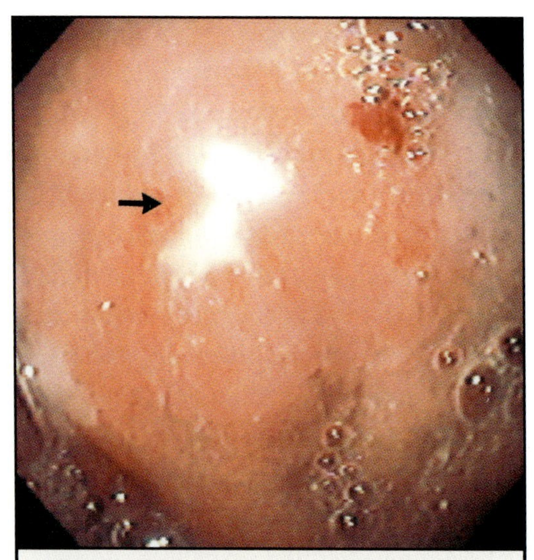

Figure 1. Endoscopic Image Showing Markedly Abnormal Gastric Mucosa with Multiple Malignant-Appearing Ulcerations (Arrow).

cyte sedimentation rate of 15 mm per hour, a prostate-specific antigen concentration of 2.4 ng per milliliter, and a gastrin concentration of 172 pg per milliliter (normal range, 95 to 140). Stool studies were negative for bacteria, ova, parasites, and fat. Tests for antigliadin and endomysial antibodies and human immunodeficiency virus (HIV); serum and urine protein electrophoresis; and a skin test with purified protein derivative were negative. A review of the gastric-biopsy report revealed no evidence of *Helicobacter pylori.* A three-day calorie count revealed a total intake of 1000 kcal. Review of the peripheral-blood smear indicated the presence of a reactive process. Computed tomography (CT) of the lungs showed severe diffuse emphysema and multiple scattered nodules, the largest of which was located in the left lower lung and measured 1.8 by 1.5 cm. Abdominal CT demonstrated a possible obstruction of the gastric outlet, mildly dilated small-bowel loops, and a distended bladder.

Although the pulmonary nodules cannot be overlooked, I do not believe that they could account for this much weight loss. The gastrin level is not as high as would be expected with a gastrin-producing neoplasm and probably reflects the use of a proton-pump inhibitor. Furthermore, the level of acid production is typically normal or decreased in patients who have a benign gastric ulcer, which is not the case in patients with a duodenal ulcer. Given a possible obstruction of the gastric outlet, repeated upper endoscopy is certainly

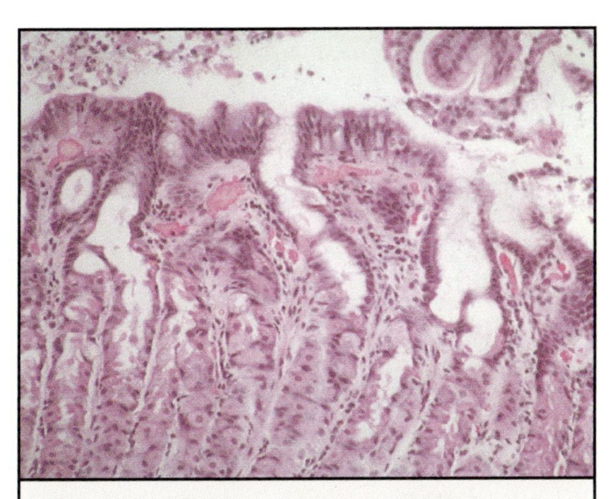

Figure 2. Gastric-Biopsy Specimen (Periodic Acid–Schiff with Diastase, ×400) Revealing Erosions with Focal Acute Inflammation and Reactive Changes but No Malignant Cells.

warranted. Reassessment of the CT scan may reveal calcification of the visceral arteries, suggesting the presence of intestinal ischemia.

The medical team believed that the pulmonary nodules were consistent with a previous inflammatory process and did not appear to be malignant. At this point, they were most concerned about a gastric neoplasm. Repeated endoscopy showed markedly abnormal gastric mucosa with multiple malignant-appearing ulcerations (Figure 1). Pathological analysis revealed erosions with focal acute inflammation and reactive changes but no malignant cells (Figure 2). Esophagogastroduodenoscopy was repeated with ultrasonography to assess the patient more definitively for any neoplasm, and a normal stomach-wall thickness was noted.

The absence of thickening of the gastric wall and the repeatedly negative biopsies rule out phlegmonous gastritis and the linitis plastica variant of gastric adenocarcinoma. Again, I would review the imaging studies to look for calcific lesions in the abdominal circulation. I would also review the histology with a pathologist in order to evaluate for gastric lymphoma, although this condition is usually associated with a thickening of the stomach wall. Unless the patient's lung disease is severe, we have ruled out the common causes of marked weight loss. I continue to be concerned about ischemia, even though gastric ischemia is extremely rare, given the rich arterial supply to the stomach. The weight loss might well be attributable to impaired blood flow in the superior-mesenteric-artery system. Food ingestion should be observed directly to see whether it causes pain.

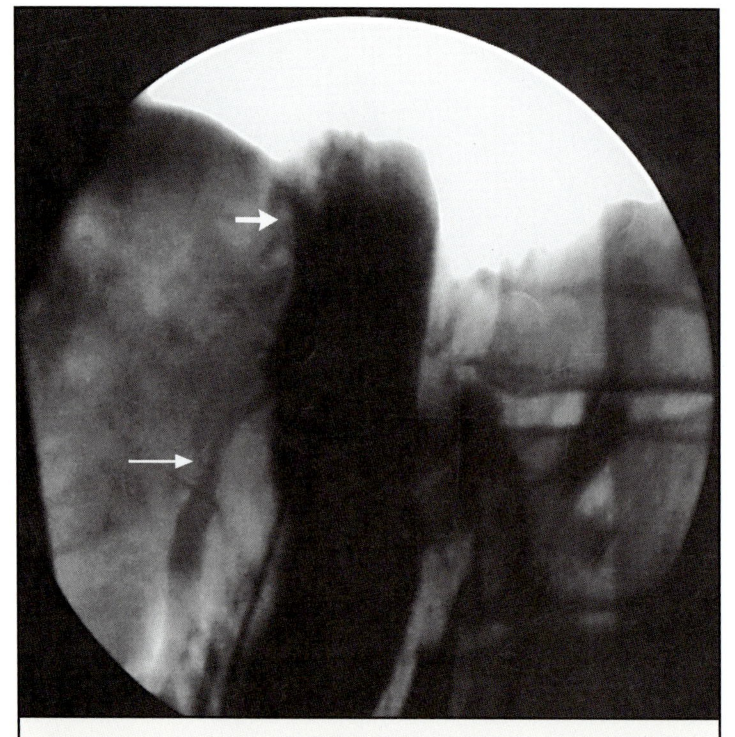

Figure 3. Intestinal Angiographic Image Demonstrating a Lack of Blood Flow through the Celiac Axis (Thick Arrow) and Tight Stenosis in the Superior Mesenteric Artery (Thin Arrow).

Later images (not shown) revealed a small inferior-mesenteric-artery filling through collaterals.

On review of the biopsy specimens, a few areas of erosion and atrophy in the lamina propria were seen, accompanied by regenerative epithelial changes. These subtle findings suggested a focal contact-type gastritis or possibly small-vessel disease, and it was recommended that a clinical correlation be sought. A more directed history was obtained from the patient, who then reported postprandial pain and indicated the location of the pain by clenching his fist over the epigastrium (an abdominal equivalent of the Levine sign). Because the initial colonoscopy was suboptimal, the medical team requested a repeated colonoscopy with adequate preparation to assess for focal signs of ischemic colitis or fibrosis. The gastroenterology consultants, however, thought that intestinal ischemia was too unlikely to warrant repeated colonoscopy. Vascular surgeons were consulted and also did not believe that further evaluation was warranted. Because the patient's extensive vascular calcification limited the interpretability of CT or magnetic resonance imaging, traditional intestinal angiography was performed. This study demonstrated an absence of blood flow

through the celiac axis, tight stenosis in the superior mesenteric artery, and flow through the inferior mesenteric artery only through collaterals (Figure 3).

These findings are exceptional. We must seriously consider an ischemic cause for the entire picture, particularly in view of the arteriographic findings. The patient is surviving on a minuscule portion of normal intestinal circulation, and any condition producing volume depletion could be devastating. He is at great risk for infarction in the distribution of the superior mesenteric artery because of the lack of patent collateral circulation. Consideration should be given to reconstruction of the superior mesenteric artery, which has met with some success in patients of this kind.

After evaluating the angiographic findings, the vascular surgeons thought that gastric ischemia was the likely cause of the patient's condition. The risks and benefits of revascularization were discussed extensively among the clinicians and with the patient, who elected to undergo repair of his celiac and superior mesenteric axis by anterograde bypass. He tolerated the surgery well and was discharged to his home. Six months later, he reported that his weight had returned to its base-line level, he could eat a normal diet, and he had resumed his hobby of fly-fishing.

This case is an excellent example of a rare manifestation of an extremely common disorder — atherosclerotic vascular disease. Ischemic gastritis is seldom diagnosed, but I believe there is no other explanation. Certainly, the reconstitution of the patient's weight and well-being after revascularization suggest that this very unusual combination was responsible for his clinical picture and the endoscopic findings.

COMMENTARY

Physicians should have no difficulty in diagnosing common illnesses. In the case of profound, unintentional weight loss, several conditions must always be considered: cancer, malabsorptive disorders, psychiatric illness, diabetes, hyperthyroidism, tuberculosis, and HIV disease.[1] Early in the evaluation of this patient, the clinicians appropriately ruled out these conditions with methodical history taking, physical examination, and laboratory tests.

Uncommon illnesses require a much higher index of suspicion, especially when the diagnosis is difficult to establish. Although encountered infrequently, chronic intestinal ischemia usually presents with postprandial abdominal pain and weight loss. Atherosclerosis of the celiac, superior mesenteric, and inferior mesenteric arteries accounts for the majority of cases, although other conditions, including vasculitis, fibromuscular dysplasia, radiation injury, and vascular malformations, have been implicated.[2] Even if chronic mesenteric ischemia is suspected, the symptoms associated with this condition may be attributed to other disorders, such as cancer and chronic pancreatitis.

CT and magnetic resonance angiography can identify atherosclerotic changes and collateral vessels, which suggest the presence of chronic ischemia, and these imaging techniques are associated with fewer complications than traditional angiography. With standard CT angiography, sensitivity for ischemia ranges from 64 percent to 82 percent; however, newer multidetector CT techniques may increase the sensitivity considerably.[3-6] The sensitivity and specificity of magnetic resonance angiography are estimated to be 100 percent and 95 percent, respectively.[7] Artifacts from extensive calcification, however, can limit the usefulness of these studies, as they did in this case. Other noninvasive techniques, such as duplex scanning and tonometry, may also aid in making the diagnosis.[2,8] Radiographic findings alone, however, do not establish the diagnosis of ischemia. Autopsy and angiographic studies have revealed the presence of severe three-vessel disease in asymptomatic persons.[2] For a secure diagnosis, a clinical response to revascularization is required.[9]

Although this patient had symptoms of chronic intestinal ischemia, the presence of gastric lesions deflected the clinicians from consideration of this possibility. The stomach has a more abundant vascular supply than the intestines, receiving blood primarily through the celiac axis and an extensive network of collateral vessels.[2] Gastric ischemia is therefore much less likely than intestinal ischemia and is rarely suspected. This case and others in the literature suggest that it may be more common than is typically believed.[10-13]

The differential diagnosis for multiple gastric lesions is short and includes lymphoma, the Zollinger–Ellison syndrome, contact-type gastritis, and linitis plastica, as well as ischemia. The fact that this list of conditions is so limited suggests that ischemia should have been considered earlier. Given the patient's cachexia and leukocytosis, however, the clinicians first focused on the possibility of a neoplasm. Furthermore, the other diagnoses were not suggested by the initial biopsy reports. Only when the clinicians personally reviewed the slides with the pathologist did she mention that the findings were suggestive of ischemia. She had not raised the possibility of gastric ischemia in her report because it is a rare condition. A review of primary information can prove vital in determining a difficult diagnosis.

Moreover, revisiting the patient's history and physical examination can clarify an uncertain clinical picture. Although the patient initially denied any relation between the pain and food, he ultimately reported postprandial discomfort when questioned more thoroughly. As suggested by the discussant, he may have had anorexia for so long that he had forgotten the initial cause. Furthermore, the probability of gastrointestinal ischemia was supported by his age, his history of vascular disease, and the abdominal Levine sign found on examination.

Because gastric ischemia is so uncommon, many of the consultants were initially dubious and did not believe that additional tests were warranted, given their attendant risks. Although the operative risk was high,[14] on balance, the attending vascular surgeon believed that the likelihood of the diagnosis and the benefits of intervention outweighed the risk associated with revascularization. Without such intervention, it seemed likely that the patient would die from malnutrition or intestinal infarction in the near term. Fortunately for this patient, this gut feeling was correct and led to a gratifying outcome.

This article first appeared in the July 3, 2003, issue of the New England Journal of Medicine.

REFERENCES

1. Bouras EP, Lange SM, Scolapio JS. Rational approach to patients with unintentional weight loss. Mayo Clin Proc 2001;76:923-9.

2. Brandt LJ, Boley SJ. Intestinal ischemia. In: Feldman M, Friedman LS, Sleisenger MH, eds. Sleisenger & Fordtran's gastrointestinal and liver disease. 7th ed. Vol. 2. Philadelphia: W.B. Saunders, 2002:2321-40.

3. Horton KM, Fishman EK. Multi-detector CT of mesenteric ischemia: can it be done? Radiographics 2001;21:1463-73.

4. Horton KM, Fishman EK. CT angiography of the GI tract. Gastrointest Endosc 2002;55:Suppl:S37-S41.

5. Kim TS, Chung JW, Park JH, Kim SH, Yeon KM, Han MC. Renal artery evaluation: comparison of spiral CT angiography to intra-arterial DSA. J Vasc Interv Radiol 1998;9:553-9.

6. Taourel PG, Deneuville M, Pradel JA, Regent D, Bruel JM. Acute mesenteric ischemia: diagnosis with contrast-enhanced CT. Radiology 1996;199:632-6.

7. Meaney JF, Prince MR, Nostrant TT, Stanley JC. Gadolinium-enhanced MR angiography of visceral arteries in patients with suspected chronic mesenteric ischemia. J Magn Reson Imaging 1997;7:171-6.

8. Moawad J, Gewertz BL. Chronic mesenteric ischemia: clinical presentation and diagnosis. Surg Clin North Am 1997;77:357-69.

9. Hojgaard L, Krag E. Chronic ischemic gastritis reversed after revascularization operation. Gastroenterology 1987;92:226-8.

10. Babu SC, Shah PM. Celiac territory ischemic syndrome in visceral artery occlusion. Am J Surg 1993;166:227-30.

11. Bakker RC, Brandjes DP, Snel P, Lawson JA, Lindeman J, Batchelor D. Malabsorption syndrome associated with ulceration of the stomach and small bowel caused by chronic intestinal ischemia in a patient with hyperhomocysteinemia. Mayo Clin Proc 1997;72:546-50.

12. Dunphy JE. Abdominal pain of vascular origin. Am J Med Sci 1936;192:109-13.

13. Van Damme H, Jacquet N, Belaiche J, Creemers E, Limet R. Chronic ischaemic gastritis: an unusual form of splanchnic vascular insufficiency. J Cardiovasc Surg (Torino) 1992;33:451-3.

14. McAfee MK, Cherry KJ Jr, Naessens JM, et al. Influence of complete revascularization on chronic mesenteric ischemia. Am J Surg 1992;164:220-4.

Anatomy of a Diagnosis

HAROLD R. COLLARD, M.D., MICHAEL P. GRUBER, M.D.,
STEVEN E. WEINBERGER, M.D., AND SANJAY SAINT, M.D., M.P.H.

A 33-year-old man presented for evaluation of hemoptysis. He had been in his usual state of health until the day of presentation, when he had a transient cough productive of one tablespoon (approximately 15 ml) of bright red blood. He did not have associated chest pain or dyspnea. He reported that he had not had recent weight loss, fever, illness, or trauma and that he did not have a history of bleeding.

The differential diagnosis of hemoptysis is effectively addressed from an anatomical point of view. True hemoptysis can originate from a process that primarily affects the airways, the pulmonary parenchyma, or the pulmonary vasculature, but blood coming from the upper airway or the upper gastrointestinal tract can also masquerade as blood coming from the lungs. I will assume for now that in this case the blood is originating from the lower respiratory tract. Many of the more common causes of hemoptysis may be suggested by historical clues to the diagnosis — for example, bronchitis or pneumonia may be suggested by cough, sputum production, and fever; lung cancer by cough, weight loss, and a history of smoking; and heart failure by dyspnea and orthopnea. The absence of additional symptoms in this case leads me to consider processes that can otherwise be clinically silent.

In a young adult, important considerations with regard to blood from an airway source include a carcinoid tumor or bronchiectasis; from a parenchymal source, an inflammatory or immune disorder (e.g., Goodpasture's syndrome or Wegener's granulomatosis) or a subclinical infection (e.g., tuberculosis); and from a pulmonary vascular source, an arteriovenous malformation. I would start the evaluation with chest radiography, knowing that I would probably then proceed to computed tomographic (CT) scanning of the chest. Although bronchoscopy may help localize a site of bleeding, I would perform the imaging studies first, since information obtained from a CT scan may preclude the need for bronchoscopy or may guide the bronchoscopist and improve the yield from the procedure.

The findings on physical examination and the complete blood count were normal. Chest radiography revealed scattered alveolar infiltrates. Empirical treatment with oral antibiotics for community-acquired pneumonia was prescribed. The patient felt well until five

weeks later, when he had a second episode of hemoptysis, described as "a full cup" (approximately 250 ml) of blood. This episode was preceded by acute shortness of breath and a sensation of "flooding" in the upper chest. The patient was admitted to the hospital.

The presence of scattered alveolar infiltrates on the initial chest radiograph suggests either that the blood is arising from a diffuse parenchymal process or that blood originating from another source is being distributed throughout the pulmonary parenchyma. In the absence of coexisting fever, leukocytosis, or the production of purulent sputum, the combination of hemoptysis and patchy alveolar infiltrates probably does not indicate the presence of community-acquired pneumonia. I would not have discharged the patient with a prescription for empirical antibiotics without a more definitive diagnosis.

At the time of the second episode of hemoptysis, the associated symptom of dyspnea is cause for concern because it may indicate the presence of significant bleeding, as is also suggested by the volume of coughed blood. Although there are no firm guidelines for admitting a patient with hemoptysis to the hospital, the presence of coexisting dyspnea, significant gas-exchange abnormalities, or a substantial increase in the volume of coughed blood all probably warrant hospitalization. The history since the first examination does not limit the earlier differential diagnosis, but I would focus on an episodic parenchymal source of hemorrhage and would expand the list of possibilities to include idiopathic pulmonary hemosiderosis and systemic lupus erythematosus.

The patient's medical history was notable for hypertension, gastroesophageal reflux disease, occasional cocaine use, heavy alcohol use, repair of an aortic coarctation in childhood, and tobacco use. His medications included verapamil and bupropion for smoking cessation. He was married and worked in sales. He said that he had not had any occupational exposures but that he had used rat poison (d-Con) on one occasion before his first episode of hemoptysis. He also said that he did not have risk factors for human immunodeficiency virus or tuberculosis infection. There was no family history of hemoptysis or bleeding disorders.

It would be important to know whether the patient had used cocaine before either of the episodes of hemoptysis, since inhalation of "crack" cocaine may lead to alveolar hemorrhage. Although the history of smoking raises the possibility of bronchogenic carcinoma, the patient's age argues against that diagnosis. Smoking is also known to increase the risk of alveolar hemorrhage in patients with anti–glomerular basement membrane antibodies, the underlying problem in Goodpasture's syndrome. A particularly intriguing (though probably coincidental) fact is that the patient was exposed to rat poison before his first episode of hemoptysis, since brodifacoum (an anticoagulant similar to warfarin) is the primary ingredient in this pesticide. A history of heavy alcohol use does not relate directly to hemoptysis, but it does raise the possibility of upper gastrointestinal bleeding that is mimicking hemoptysis or of a coagulation disorder related to underlying alcohol-induced liver disease.

The patient stated that he had not used cocaine recently. On physical examination, his temperature was 37.3°C, his blood pressure 167/86 mm Hg, his heart rate 109 beats per minute, his respiratory rate 18 breaths per minute, and his oxygen saturation 85 percent while he was breathing room air. Examination of his head and neck revealed no abnormalities. On examination of the chest, there was no dullness to percussion, and there were no adventitial sounds. Examination of the heart revealed tachycardia and normal heart sounds without murmurs. Abdominal, neurologic, and musculoskeletal examinations revealed no abnormalities. The white-cell count was 11,600 per cubic millimeter, the hematocrit 29 percent, the platelet count 373,000 per cubic millimeter, the prothrombin time 13.1 seconds (international normalized ratio, 1.1), and the partial-thromboplastin time 22.7 seconds. The serum levels of electrolytes, creatinine, aminotransferases, and total bilirubin were normal. Toxicologic screening of the urine on admission was negative for cocaine and other substances of abuse.

The absence of a recent history of cocaine use, along with the negative results on toxicologic screening of the urine, shifts the differential diagnosis away from cocaine-induced pulmonary hemorrhage. Additional useful information is provided by the patient's low hematocrit, which suggests either additional subclinical episodes of bleeding or an underlying process associated with anemia of chronic disease. The low oxygen saturation suggests a significant amount of intraparenchymal bleeding or, alternatively, substantial bleeding within the airways, resulting in a ventilation–perfusion mismatch. At this point, I am thinking mostly about disorders associated with diffuse parenchymal hemorrhage, such as Goodpasture's syndrome, idiopathic pulmonary hemosiderosis, and the less likely possibilities of systemic lupus erythematosus and Wegener's granulomatosis. Nevertheless, it still has not been confirmed that the bleeding does not have its origin in an airway and that it does not have a pulmonary vascular origin. Additional studies that would be useful at this point include a urinalysis, with examination for red cells or red-cell casts, and repeated chest radiography.

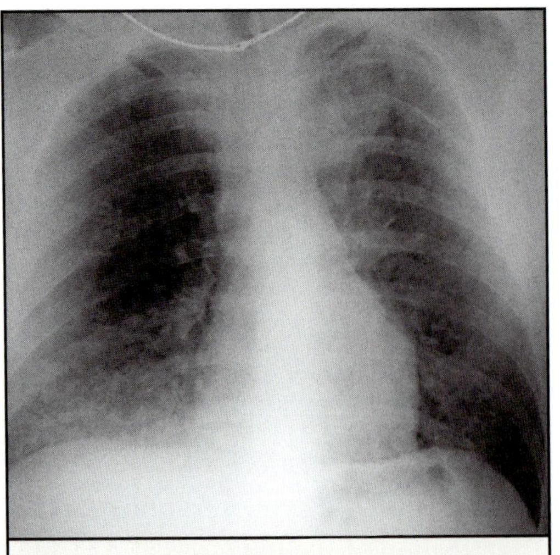

Figure 1. Radiograph of the Chest, Showing Bilateral Alveolar Opacities.

Repeated chest radiography revealed bilateral alveolar opacities (Figure 1). CT scanning of the chest revealed normal intraluminal filling of the pulmonary arteries and consolidation, predominantly in the left upper lobe. The results of urinalysis, the erythrocyte sedimentation rate, and the level of C-reactive protein were normal.

The chest radiograph shows patchy alveolar densities, presumably reflecting the presence of blood in the alveolar spaces. It is interesting that adventitial sounds were absent on examination of the chest, despite the prominent radiographic abnormality. This seeming incongruence is observed in many patients with diffuse lung disease and illustrates the poor sensitivity of physical examination in these patients. In this case, there is also an area of focal opacification in the left upper lobe; the opacification is unexplained but is confirmed by the CT scan. It could represent the source or primary site of the bleeding.

Given the location of the abnormality, which appears to be adjacent to the aorta, one important possibility would be a late complication of the repair of an aortic coarctation in childhood — namely, an aortopulmonary or aortobronchial fistula originating at the repair site, perhaps with pseudoaneurysm formation. In retrospect, the patient's sensation of "flooding" in the upper chest could have been a clue to bleeding in this region. An alternative, though less likely and less immediately life-threatening, possibility is that the patient has a bronchial carcinoid tumor, leading to recurrent bleeding and obstruction of the involved airway, with postobstructive infection or volume loss resulting in the appearance of consolidation in the lung. Diffuse pulmonary hemorrhage due to the conditions I mentioned earlier also remains a possibility.

Bronchoscopy revealed that the airways were normal, and culture of a bronchoalveolar-lavage specimen for bacteria and fungus was negative. Antinuclear antibodies, antineutrophil cytoplasmic antibodies, and anti–glomerular basement membrane antibodies were not present. Thoracoscopic biopsy of the left upper lobe revealed alveolar hemorrhage with abundant hemosiderin-laden macrophages but only minimal interstitial inflammation and fibrosis.

The absence of antineutrophil cytoplasmic antibodies argues against a diagnosis of Wegener's granulomatosis, and the absence of anti–glomerular basement membrane antibodies argues against a diagnosis of Goodpasture's syndrome. Given that bronchoscopy revealed no abnormalities, a bronchial carcinoid tumor becomes unlikely as an explanation for the hemoptysis and the left-upper-lobe abnormality. Even though bronchoscopy is a reasonable procedure in many if not most cases of unexplained hemoptysis — and it did provide some useful information here — I would probably have focused more on evaluation of the site of the previous aortic surgery and its relation to the abnormality in the left upper lobe. Careful review of the CT scan might suggest the presence of a fistula, a pseudoaneurysm, or both, although a fistula might be difficult to identify.

I do not think that thoracoscopic lung biopsy was indicated here, nor do I think it is a primary diagnostic procedure in most patients with hemoptysis. Even when blood is identified within the parenchyma, examination of the biopsy specimen does not necessarily confirm that the blood originated at the alveolar level, and it is not likely to identify the underlying cause of bleeding that is alveolar. The cause of parenchymal bleeding is more likely to be identified on the basis of the clinical history and the presence or absence of underlying diseases, associated abnormalities in renal function or the urinary sediment, and anti–glomerular basement membrane antibodies or antineutrophil cytoplasmic antibodies.

Administration of high-dose corticosteroids was started. The patient's condition improved, and he was discharged home while taking prednisone. Two weeks later, he was readmitted to the hospital after a third episode of hemoptysis, which he described as the production of "two large cups" (approximately 500 ml) of bright red blood.

The crescendo pattern of this illness, with increasingly short intervals between episodes of hemoptysis and increasing amounts of coughed blood, suggests that we are sitting on a

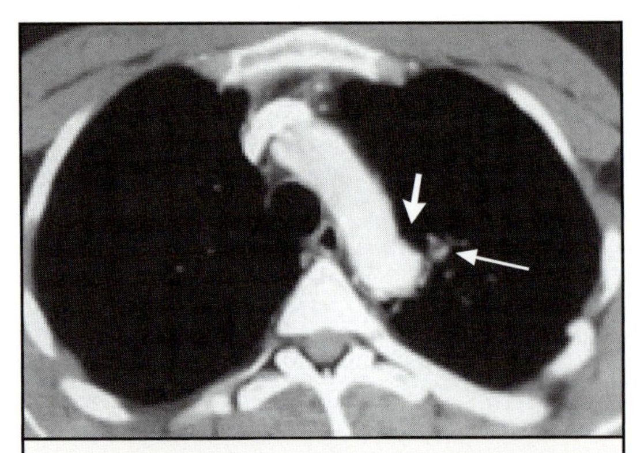

Figure 2. CT Scan of the Chest.
The scan reveals a focal irregularity in the posterolateral aortic arch (thick arrow) and a small area of consolidation in the adjacent left upper lobe, with an area of central contrast enhancement (thin arrow).

time bomb and that a definite diagnosis needs to be established quickly. Bronchoscopy did not reveal a primary source in an airway, and lung biopsy and serologic studies did not point to a disorder associated with diffuse alveolar (pulmonary parenchymal) hemorrhage. We are still left with the possibility of a vascular source — specifically, late formation of a fistula at the site of the previous aortic surgery. I would proceed rapidly to aortography or magnetic resonance imaging if the diagnosis was not obvious on the CT scan obtained during the previous admission. Although corticosteroids are frequently used as a nonspecific treatment for many forms of diffuse alveolar hemorrhage, typically to treat the underlying capillaritis that is often responsible for the bleeding, it is generally advisable to confirm a specific diagnosis before such therapy is instituted. I doubt that the corticosteroid treatment in this case had any effect, and I suspect that any temporal relation between the start of corticosteroid therapy and the cessation of bleeding was coincidental.

Repeated CT scanning of the chest revealed a focal irregularity in the posterolateral aortic arch and a small area of consolidation in the adjacent left upper lobe, with central contrast enhancement (Figure 2). Magnetic resonance angiography of the aorta revealed a pseudoaneurysm, 1.7 cm by 1.2 cm, just distal to the origin of the left subclavian artery (Figure 3). No residual coarctation or collateralization was visible. Emergency surgery was performed, and an aortic pseudoaneurysm was found at the site of the coarctation repair. The adjacent left upper lobe of the lung was densely adherent to the aorta, and

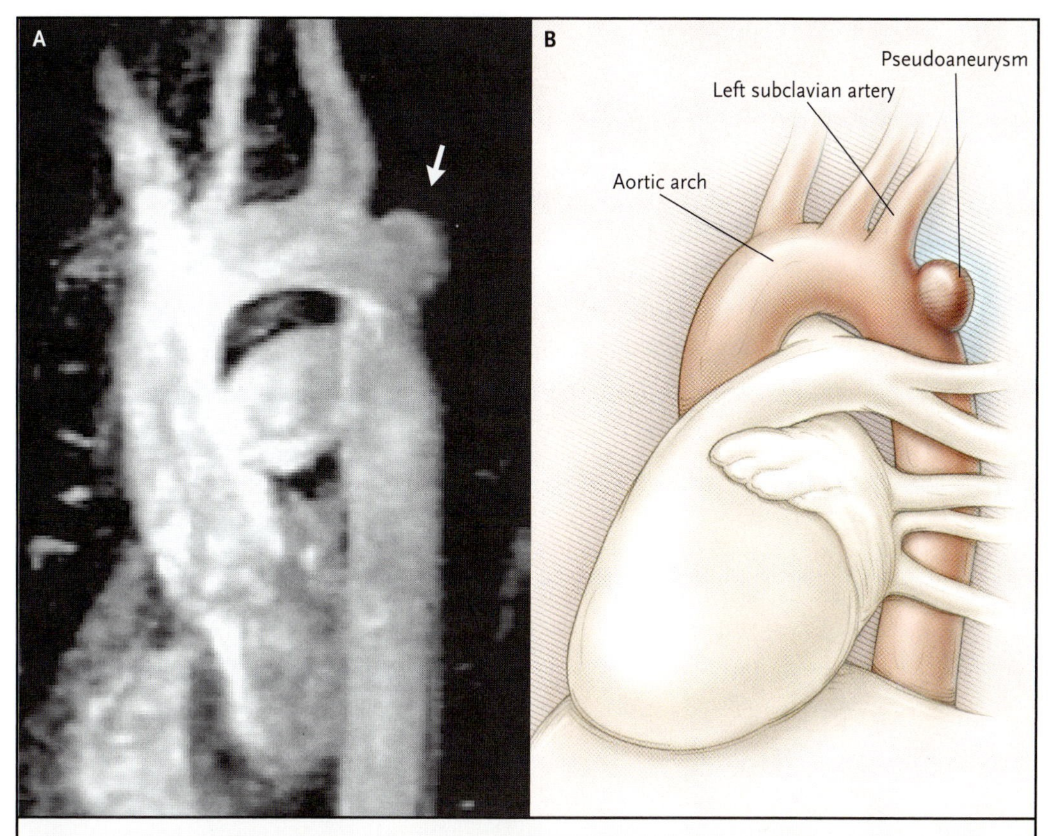

Figure 3. Magnetic Resonance Angiogram (Panel A) and Schematic Diagram (Panel B) of the Aorta.
There is a pseudoaneurysm (arrow in Panel A), 1.7 cm by 1.2 cm, distal to the origin of the left subclavian artery.

exploration revealed a fistulous communication between the pseudoaneurysm and the pulmonary parenchyma. The aortobronchial fistula was repaired by placement of an aortic graft and resection of the involved portion of the lung. The patient did well postoperatively and has not had any recurrence of his hemoptysis.

COMMENTARY

Hemoptysis is a symptom encountered frequently by clinicians. Among patients who present with hemoptysis in the United States, bronchitis, bronchiectasis, and lung cancer each account for about one fifth of the cases, although the proportions vary according to age. Other causes that should be routinely considered include community-acquired pneumonia, congestive heart failure, bleeding diatheses, pulmonary embolism, tuberculosis, aspergillosis, vascular abnormalities, and drugs, including cocaine.[1-3] Patients with recurrent episodes of hemoptysis or massive hemoptysis, defined variably as the expectoration of 1.5 to 3.5 cups (approximately 400 to 800 ml) of blood over a 24-hour period, are important to identify, since they warrant urgent evaluation.

In the majority of patients with hemoptysis, the "textbook" differential diagnosis includes the underlying cause. However, excessive reliance on such a standardized list of conditions may be dangerous, since uncommon causes may be overlooked and a diagnosis may be ascribed prematurely, despite discordant clinical data. The key to a successful diagnosis in this case was threefold: careful attention to the patient's history, expansion of the differential diagnosis according to principles of anatomy and physiology, and continued reassessment of the clinical data to eliminate unlikely causes. This approach allowed conditions such as bronchitis, pneumonia, heart failure, and lung cancer to be ruled out early in the evaluation; permitted reassessment and consideration of aortobronchial fistula as a possible diagnosis as the case progressed; and allowed reevaluation of the possibility of diffuse alveolar hemorrhage, which was considered during the first hospitalization. The decision to treat the patient with corticosteroids in the absence of a definitive diagnosis could have had catastrophic consequences, since fatal hemoptysis could have occurred.

Aortobronchial (or aortopulmonary) fistula is an uncommon but well-established cause of hemoptysis, which in such cases is often massive.[4-6] In 1867, two patients who died from massive hemoptysis were described[7,8]; at autopsy in each case, a fistulous communication between an aortic aneurysm and the left lung was found. Any source of irritation or compression in this region (e.g., an aortic aneurysm or pseudoaneurysm, surgical sutures, an aortic graft, or infection) can lead to inflammation and scarring of the aorta and adjacent lung, with eventual fistula formation.[4,5] Today, most cases are seen in patients who have undergone surgical repair of aortic abnormalities such as an aneurysm, coarctation, or patent ductus arteriosus, in whom hemoptysis may occur months to decades after the operation.[4,9]

Most patients with aortobronchial fistula report episodic massive hemoptysis.[10] Chest radiography generally shows nonspecific abnormalities, whereas CT scanning of the chest may reveal focal consolidation in the region of the left lung that is proximal to the aorta.[4,6,11] Only rarely can the fistulous communication be visualized.[12] Aortography (by means of traditional radiography, CT imaging, or magnetic resonance angiography) is the most sensitive diagnostic test. Untreated, aortobronchial fistula is uniformly fatal. Surgical repair is possible in approximately 80 percent of patients and, when successful, is associated with an excellent rate of survival.[13]

Physicians are often taught that "the diagnosis is in the history." We propose a corollary: that the differential diagnosis is in the careful and continued evaluation of the history and clinical data in the context of anatomy and physiology. This case illustrates the importance of a careful, considered differential diagnosis, even when the interpretation of the patient's initial symptom appears to be straightforward.

Supported by a Career Development Award from the Health Services Research and Development Program of the Department of Veterans Affairs and a Patient Safety Developmental Center Grant from the Agency for Healthcare Research and Quality (P20-HS11540) (both to Dr. Saint).

We are indebted to Dr. David Lynch for providing radiographic images and interpretation of the images and to Dr. Brian Fouty for contributions to the manuscript.

This article first appeared in the September 4, 2003, issue of the New England Journal of Medicine.

REFERENCES

1. Johnston H, Reisz G. Changing spectrum of hemoptysis: underlying causes in 148 patients undergoing diagnostic flexible fiberoptic bronchoscopy. Arch Intern Med 1989;149:1666-8.

2. Santiago S, Tobias J, Williams AJ. A reappraisal of the causes of hemoptysis. Arch Intern Med 1991;151: 2449-51.

3. Hirshberg B, Biran I, Glazer M, Kramer MR. Hemoptysis: etiology, evaluation, and outcome in a tertiary referral hospital. Chest 1997;112:440-4.

4. MacIntosh EL, Parrott JC, Unruh HW. Fistulas between the aorta and tracheobronchial tree. Ann Thorac Surg 1991;51:515-9.

5. Graeber GM, Farrell BG, Neville JF Jr, Parker FB Jr. Successful diagnosis and management of fistulas between the aorta and the tracheobronchial tree. Ann Thorac Surg 1980;29:555-61.

6. Killen DA, Muehlebach GF, Wathanacharoen S. Aortopulmonary fistula. South Med J 2000;93:195-8.

7. Page D. A case of aneurysm of the thoracic aorta bursting into the left bronchus. Lancet 1867;1:43-4.

8. Johnson D. Aneurism of thoracic aorta making its way into the lower lobe of the left lung, which thus formed the sac of the aneurism. Lancet 1867;1:44.

9. Miller JP, Cammarata SK. Massive hemoptysis 17 years after repair of aortic coarctation. Chest 1994;105: 1249-50.

10. Demeter SL, Cordasco EM. Aortobronchial fistula: keys to successful management. Angiology 1980;31:431-5.

11. Posniak HV, Demos TC, Marsan RE. Computed tomography of the normal aorta and thoracic aneurysms. Semin Roentgenol 1989;24:7-21.

12. Higashikawa M, Morikawa J, Nishigaki I, Bamba M. Aortopulmonary fistula detected by CT. AJR Am J Roentgenol 1992;159:673-4.

13. Favre JP, Gournier JP, Adham M, Rosset E, Barral X. Aortobronchial fistula: report of three cases and review of the literature. Surgery 1994;115:264-70.

Occam's Razor versus Saint's Triad

ANTHONY A. HILLIARD, M.D., STEVEN E. WEINBERGER, M.D.,
LAWRENCE M. TIERNEY, JR., M.D., DAVID E. MIDTHUN, M.D.,
AND SANJAY SAINT, M.D., M.P.H.

A 60-year-old woman with a history of radiologically confirmed seronegative rheumatoid arthritis presented to the emergency department with a 10-day history of worsening dyspnea on exertion, nonproductive cough, and subjective fever and a 7-day history of pain in the right leg and buttock, which limited her mobility. There was no sputum production, orthopnea, paroxysmal nocturnal dyspnea, or pleuritic chest pain.

I would start creating my differential diagnosis by taking into account the relatively short time course of the symptoms and the clinical context in which they developed. Given the patient's underlying disease, I am considering several complications of rheumatoid arthritis (although they are unlikely, given her seronegative status), such as parenchymal and distal-airway disease (interstitial pneumonitis, bronchiolitis obliterans with organizing pneumonia, or constrictive bronchiolitis), pleural effusion, or pericardial effusion. Other diseases associated with pulmonary complications and arthritis, such as Wegener's granulomatosis and systemic lupus erythematosus, should also be considered. In addition, she may have a pulmonary infection, particularly if she is receiving immunosuppressive therapy for her underlying rheumatic disease. The leg and buttock pain sounds like sciatica, but other possible explanations include her underlying arthritis, septic arthritis of the hip, or even deep venous thrombosis, which could be complicated by pulmonary embolism.

The patient had been evaluated at her local clinic a few days earlier. A chest radiograph and an ultrasound examination of her right leg showed no abnormalities. An antihistamine for presumed allergic rhinitis was prescribed. Her dyspnea progressed, and on the morning of admission, the patient was seen by her rheumatologist and was found to have a fever, tachypnea, and hypoxemia.

The initially normal chest radiograph was obtained early in the course of her illness and does not dissuade me from considering a process involving the pulmonary parenchyma, which might appear later as radiographic changes. I would focus on four main categories of disease at this point: a primary infectious process within the lungs (particularly if she is receiving immunosuppressive medication); an infection elsewhere (which perhaps would account for her leg and buttock pain) with a secondary process involving the lungs, such as bacteremia or acute respiratory distress syndrome; a noninfectious inflammatory process that may be associated with fever, such as bronchiolitis obliterans with organizing pneumonia, pulmonary embolic disease (despite the absence of abnormalities on the ultrasound examination of the leg), systemic lupus erythematosus, or Wegener's granulomatosis; and drug toxicity, depending on the pharmacologic treatment of her rheumatologic disease. The normal chest radiograph rules out a clinically significant pleural effusion. I do not believe that allergic rhinitis explains her presentation, because this diagnosis should neither cause dyspnea nor be associated with fever.

The patient's history included the CREST syndrome (calcinosis cutis, Raynaud's phenomenon, esophageal dysfunction, sclerodactyly, and telangiectasia), right-knee arthroplasty, right-hip arthroplasty with postoperative deep venous thrombosis five years previously, and hypothyroidism. The patient had been in a monogamous relationship for the past 30 years. She occasionally drank alcohol and reported that she did not use tobacco or illicit drugs. Her inflammatory arthritis was being treated with 5 mg of prednisone taken once a day (for the past 10 years), 25 mg of methotrexate administered subcutaneously once a week (for the past 11 months), and 300 mg of infliximab administered intravenously every 8 weeks (for the past 4 months). Her status with respect to tuberculin skin testing was unknown. Additional medications included levothyroxine, hydrocodone, acetaminophen, and alendronate (to prevent osteoporosis); she also took a folic acid supplement.

The CREST syndrome is associated with pathologic changes in the pulmonary vasculature similar to those in primary pulmonary hypertension, but the fever and the tempo of the presentation in this case argue against that diagnosis. The patient does have prosthetic material from her orthopedic procedures, and the possibility of infection originating in one of these areas remains in the differential diagnosis. Perhaps the most important additional information is that she was receiving drugs that are immunosuppressive, at least one of which (methotrexate) is also associated with inflammatory complications involving the pulmonary parenchyma.

Although her dose of prednisone is relatively low, she is also receiving infliximab in addition to the methotrexate and therefore should be considered immunosuppressed. Immunosuppression places her at risk both for common types of bacterial pneumonia and for infection with a variety of opportunistic pathogens, such as pneumocystis, viruses, fungi, and mycobacteria. A particular concern with the use of infliximab, which is a functional tumor necrosis factor α antagonist, is the development of mycobacterial disease. Since fever accompanies her respiratory symptoms, an opportunistic infection involving the lungs must be considered seriously.

The patient was alert but in moderate respiratory distress. Her temperature was 38.3°C, her heart rate was 82 beats per minute, her blood pressure was 130/72 mm Hg, her respiratory rate was 24 breaths per minute, and her oxygen saturation was 75 percent while she was breathing room air. She was using accessory muscles to breathe. Auscultation revealed crackles in the lower lung fields and dullness to percussion at the bases. There was no pleural friction rub. Cardiovascular examination showed a normal first heart sound but a prominent pulmonic second sound, with no audible murmur of tricuspid insufficiency. The neck veins were not elevated. She had hypertrophic changes of the metacarpal–phalangeal and proximal interphalangeal joints, with bilateral ulnar deviation. There were multiple cutaneous telangiectasias on the face and arms but no rash or nodules. Examination of the right hip showed no acetabular tenderness or edema and revealed a normal range of motion. There was no calf tenderness or edema.

Particularly intriguing in this case is the combination of the dramatically low oxygen saturation and the presence of a prominent pulmonic second sound on cardiac examination. The patient's hypoxemia could contribute to reactive pulmonary vasoconstriction, further complicating the underlying pulmonary vascular disease due to the CREST syndrome. Alternatively, considering her severe hypoxemia along with the prominent second pulmonic sound, I would be concerned about right-to-left intracardiac shunting, perhaps through a patent foramen ovale. Although we generally like to invoke Occam's razor, for some patients we cannot follow the rule of diagnostic parsimony. In this case, I could easily envision an opportunistic pulmonary infection being responsible for the fever, crackles, hypoxemia, and worsening pulmonary hypertension, which is then complicated by right-to-left intracardiac shunting and further deterioration in oxygenation.

The white-cell count was 8000 per cubic millimeter with a normal differential count, the hematocrit was 35 percent, the platelet count was 142,000 per cubic millimeter, the partial-thromboplastin time was 30 seconds (normal range, 19 to 30), and the international normalized ratio for the prothrombin time was 0.9. The serum aspartate aminotransferase level was 107 U per liter, the alanine aminotransferase level was 55 U per liter, the bicarbonate level was 19 mmol per liter, the C-reactive protein level was 12.4 mg per deci-

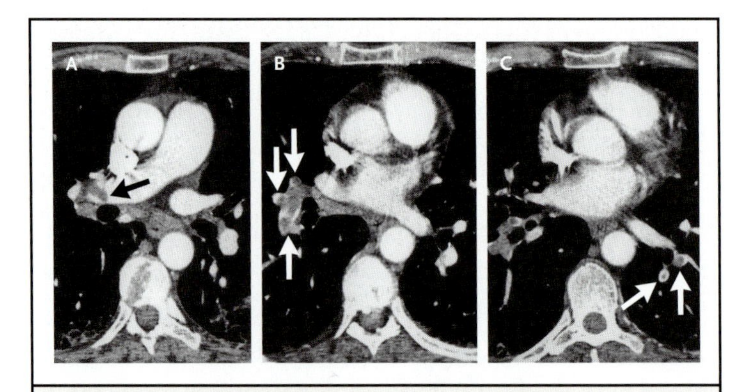

Figure 1. Contrast-Enhanced Spiral CT Scans of the Chest.
The scans show large emboli (arrows) in the right main pulmonary artery (Panel A), right segmental pulmonary arteries (Panel B), and left subsegmental arteries (Panel C).

liter (normal range, 0.020 to 0.800), and the lactate dehydrogenase level was 1142 U per liter (normal range, 104 to 236). The serum levels of alkaline phosphatase, direct and indirect bilirubin, glucose, creatinine, and urea nitrogen were normal. Arterial-blood gas analysis on 15 liters of oxygen delivered by a face mask showed that the partial pressure of oxygen was 230 mm Hg, the partial pressure of carbon dioxide was 29 mm Hg, and the pH was 7.45. The patient's chest radiograph revealed patchy infiltrates scattered throughout both lungs. Her electrocardiogram was normal.

The slightly elevated levels of aminotransferases may reflect an early toxic effect of methotrexate on the liver, although a nonspecific response to a systemic infection is also possible. The patient's acid–base status suggests a mixed metabolic acidosis and respiratory alkalosis. The elevated level of C-reactive protein indicates the presence of inflammation, infection, or both; her underlying rheumatic disease alone might explain this, or there may be an additional contributory process. The pulmonary infiltrates are also nonspecific, reflecting either an inflammatory or an infectious process. I remain most concerned about an opportunistic pulmonary infection (especially tuberculosis, given the treatment with infliximab), an infection complicating a joint prosthesis (with secondary pulmonary manifestations due to septic emboli or the acute respiratory distress syndrome), or a noninfectious inflammatory process, such as methotrexate-associated pneumonitis or bronchiolitis obliterans with organizing pneumonia.

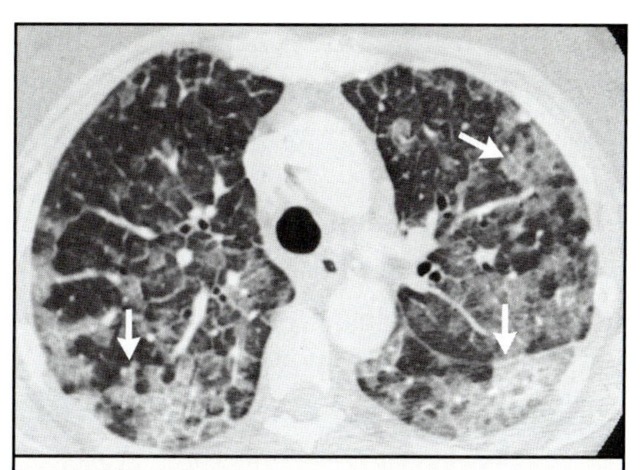

Figure 2. Contrast-Enhanced CT Scan of the Chest Showing Extensive, Peripheral, Patchy Infiltrates (Arrows) Throughout Both Lungs.

Sputum cultures for bacteria were obtained, and empirical antibiotic therapy with levofloxacin, intravenous trimethoprim–sulfamethoxazole, and corticosteroids was begun.

Although empirical antibiotic therapy for pneumocystis pneumonia or community-acquired pneumonia is reasonable, the patient should simultaneously undergo further diagnostic testing, since there are a number of other important possibilities under consideration. I have four key diagnostic questions at this point. Does the patient have an infection involving a prosthetic joint? Does she have thromboembolic disease? Does she have an opportunistic pulmonary infection? Does she have intracardiac right-to-left shunting (presumably through a patent foramen ovale)? Because there may be more than one process present, I favor investigating these diagnostic questions in parallel, beginning with an evaluation for possible thromboembolic disease and opportunistic pulmonary infection.

Spiral computed tomography (CT) of the chest (Figure 1) showed large emboli in the right main pulmonary artery, right segmental pulmonary arteries, and left subsegmental arteries. The CT scan also showed extensive, peripheral, patchy ground-glass infiltrates (Figure 2).

Although I have mentioned deep venous thrombosis as a potential cause of the leg and buttock pain, I am surprised by the diagnosis of extensive pulmonary thromboembolic disease. The additional finding of patchy ground-glass infiltrates is probably not related to the thromboembolic disease, and I remain concerned about another coexisting process, particularly an opportunistic infection. Given the need for anticoagulation and the likelihood of pulmonary hypertension, I would not want to perform a transbronchial biopsy. Rather, I would try to identify an opportunistic pathogen — particularly pneumocystis, given the appearance of the CT scan, or mycobacterium, given the use of infliximab — in induced sputum or bronchoalveolar-lavage fluid.

The patient received an intravenous bolus of unfractionated heparin followed by a continuous infusion of unfractionated heparin. Her clinical status remained stable and unimproved during the several hours between the administration of heparin and bronchoscopy. Bronchoscopy with bronchoalveolar lavage revealed the presence of *Pneumocystis carinii.* Therefore, she continued to receive intravenous trimethoprim–sulfamethoxazole, corticosteroids, and unfractionated heparin, a regimen that constituted treatment for both *P. carinii* pneumonia and pulmonary embolism. She required mechanical ventilation for 24 hours after bronchoscopy, but then her condition improved dramatically. Her trachea was extubated on her second day in the hospital; by the fifth day the supplemental oxygen was discontinued, and she had no further symptoms of dyspnea at rest.

The patient was soon discharged from the hospital while taking an oral corticosteroid (the dose of which was to be tapered), trimethoprim–sulfamethoxazole, and warfarin. After completing treatment for *P. carinii* pneumonia, the patient continued to take trimethoprim–sulfamethoxazole for prophylaxis. She was contacted five months after hospitalization and reported no breathing difficulties.

This case illustrates two important points that come up relatively frequently in puzzling clinical problems. First, diagnostic parsimony is a worthwhile goal, but it is one that cannot always be achieved. Second, pulmonary embolic disease remains one of the most challenging diagnoses to make clinically, and objective confirmation of the presence or absence of thromboembolism is important whenever the diagnosis is considered.

COMMENTARY

Pluralitas non est ponenda sine necessitate.
— William of Occam, 14th century

"What on earth is Saint's Triad?" So asked C.F.M. Saint several decades ago about his own eponym. Saint, a South African surgeon, emphasized the importance of considering the possibility of multiple separate diseases in a patient whenever his or her history and the results of the physical examination were atypical of any single condition.[1] The triad that bears his name is the association of hiatal hernia, gallbladder disease, and diverticulosis. There is no pathophysiological basis for the coexistence of these three diseases; that, perhaps, was his point. Saint emphasized that more than one disease may be responsible for a patient's clinical signs and symptoms. This is, in fact, the same point made by the apocryphal Hickam, credited with Hickam's dictum: "A patient can have as many diagnoses as he darn well pleases."[2] Because physicians are seeing an increasing number of patients with a multitude of acute and chronic illnesses, the views of Saint and Hickam warrant consideration in the practice of modern medicine. Neither name, however, is as well known as that of William Osler, who is credited with applying the teaching of Occam to clinical medicine.[2]

In the 14th century, William of Occam stated, "Plurality must not be posited without necessity." A subsequent version of this statement was expressed as "Among competing hypotheses, favor the simplest one" — hence the term "Occam's razor."[3] As the discussant points out, parsimony of diagnosis is an important standard in modern medicine; however, this principle can fail us. As the population continues to age — and as diagnostic studies increase in number and sophistication — the dulling of Occam's razor is certain to continue. Indeed, this patient's dyspnea had two distinct causes: pulmonary embolism and *P. carinii* pneumonia.

Why Hickam's dictum in this particular case? This patient's inflammatory arthritis required that she receive immunosuppressive therapy to control her symptoms. Chronic immunosuppression then placed her at increased risk for an opportunistic infection. *P. carinii* pneumonia then led to shortness of breath, fever, and lethargy that may have prompted her to reduce her physical activity, a change that, in turn, may have predisposed her to the development of venous thromboembolism. Though only a hypothesis, this line of reasoning provides one explanation for her risks of multiple, seemingly unrelated diseases.

How should we balance the competing philosophies of Occam and Saint in the modern era? As people live longer and as the prevalence of disease increases, physicians must anticipate the greater likelihood of multiple diagnoses. A recent population-based study concluded that in patients 65 years of age or older who have chronic medical diseases and receive prescription medications free of charge, additional unrelated disorders are undertreated, as compared with the same disorders in patients who do not have another underlying medical condition.[4] An accompanying editorial suggested that this finding may be related to the application of Occam's principle of parsimony by the health care providers.[5] If physicians consider the tenets of Saint and Hickam as well, patients may receive better care.

Although the view of Saint is useful for complicated medical cases, can the diagnostic parsimony that medicine has adhered to for so many years be abandoned? Will physicians err by assigning, for example, separate diagnoses of arthritis, dermatitis, and kidney disease to a patient who has systemic lupus erythematosus? It is clear that in patient care we cannot embrace either principle exclusively; rather, we should keep the views of both Occam and Saint in mind.

Supported by a Career Development Award from the Health Services Research and Development Program of the Department of Veterans Affairs and a Patient Safety Developmental Center Grant (P20-HS11540) from the Agency for Healthcare Research and Quality (both to Dr. Saint).

This article first appeared in the February 5, 2004, issue of the New England Journal of Medicine.

REFERENCES

1.
Firkin BG, Whitworth JA. Dictionary of medical eponyms. 2nd ed. Pearl River, N.Y.: Parthenon Publishing Group, 1996:354.

2.
Miller WT. Occam versus Hickam. Semin Roentgenol 1998;33:213.

3.
Drachman DA. Occam's razor, geriatric syndromes, and the dizzy patient. Ann Intern Med 2000;132:403-4.

4.
Redelmeier DA, Tan SH, Booth GL. The treatment of unrelated disorders in patients with chronic medical diseases. N Engl J Med 1998;338:1516-20.

5.
Steinbrook R. Patients with multiple chronic conditions — how many medications are enough? N Engl J Med 1998;338:1541-2.

A Pain in the Neck

SANDRA J. BLISS, M.D., SCOTT A. FLANDERS, M.D.,
AND SANJAY SAINT, M.D., M.P.H.

A previously healthy 16-year-old girl presented to her physician because of a two-day history of sore throat, fatigue, fever, headache, and vomiting; she had not had rhinorrhea or a cough. On examination, her temperature was 36.7°C, and she appeared fatigued. She had mild erythema and white plaques on her tonsillar pillars and mild tenderness of the anterior neck, without lymphadenopathy.

The signs and symptoms on presentation are consistent with the presence of acute pharyngitis. Infections with rhinovirus, adenovirus, influenzavirus, and parainfluenzavirus are among its most common causes. Infection with mycoplasma or Epstein–Barr virus (EBV) is also possible, but diagnostic efforts should initially focus on the identification of group A streptococcal infection, if present, since treatment can prevent serious sequelae. The tonsillar exudates, fever, anterior cervical adenopathy, and absence of cough in this case are highly suggestive of streptococcal pharyngitis. The vomiting, however, is more commonly seen in younger children with group A streptococcal pharyngitis.

I would obtain a swab from her pharynx for a rapid streptococcal-antigen test and treat the patient with antibiotics if the test result was positive. Rapid streptococcal-antigen tests are, at best, 80 to 90 percent sensitive, so if the result was negative I would send the throat swab for culture and await the results before prescribing antibiotics.

The result of a rapid streptococcal-antigen assay was negative. Viral pharyngitis was diagnosed. Treatment with analgesics and adequate fluid intake were advised.

Four days later, the patient returned to her physician with a worsening sore throat. She was having difficulty swallowing and reported dizziness while standing. She continued to feel fatigued, chilled, and achy but stated that she had not had further fever. She described a bifrontal headache and some mild stiffness of the neck. She stated that she had not vomited since the previous visit and that she did not have abdominal pain or diarrhea. The streptococcal culture obtained during the previous visit was sterile.

Although group A streptococcal infection is still possible, the sterile culture, combined with the new and worsening symptoms, leads me to broaden my differential diagnosis. Most symptoms due to viral or streptococcal pharyngitis should be improving or resolved by the sixth day of illness. The patient's throat pain and difficulty swallowing may be due to a complication such as a peritonsillar abscess or to a less common cause of pharyngitis, such as acute human immunodeficiency virus (HIV) infection, EBV infection, or gonococcal infection. Her headache and neck stiffness raise the possibility of meningitis. Bacterial meningitis would be unlikely without fever and severe clinical deterioration, although viral or aseptic meningitis remains a possibility.

The patient had a history of depression and childhood asthma. She was taking paroxetine and trazodone, as well as ibuprofen for her sore throat; she had no allergies to medication. She was a junior in high school and did not smoke, consume alcohol, or use illicit drugs. She stated that she had never been sexually active.

On examination, she was thin and pale and appeared ill. Her temperature was 36.3°C, her blood pressure 93/64 mm Hg, her pulse 120 beats per minute, her respiratory rate 22 breaths per minute, and her oxygen saturation 98 percent while she was breathing room air. She had some difficulty fully opening her mouth and protruding her tongue, but there was no anatomical distortion. Her oropharynx was dry, and there was right tonsillar erythema. Her anterior cervical lymph nodes were tender, especially on the right side; otherwise, her neck was supple. The findings on a cardiovascular examination were normal except for tachycardia, and her lungs were clear. The findings on an abdominal examination were normal, and she had no rash.

Her appearance and vital signs are alarming. Her blood pressure alone would not be cause for concern in an adolescent, but in this case it is associated with tachycardia and orthostatic symptoms. She also has trismus, as well as some asymmetric tonsillar erythema and cervical adenopathy, which may explain her neck stiffness. I am concerned that this patient has an undiagnosed bacterial infection, in particular a deep-tissue infection. Ludwig's angina could explain the findings, but this disorder is usually associated with gingivitis, dental infection, and foul-smelling breath. Peritonsillar abscesses are often visualized on examination of the throat, but a parapharyngeal or submandibular infection might be harder to diagnose.

The white-cell count was 9000 per cubic millimeter, the hemoglobin level 11.6 g per deciliter, and the platelet count 10,000 per cubic millimeter. Examination of a peripheral-

blood smear confirmed the thrombocytopenia and showed that the white-cell differential count included 89 percent segmented neutrophils and 10 percent band forms. No schistocytes were seen. The urea nitrogen level was 125 mg per deciliter (44.6 mmol per liter), the creatinine level 2.1 mg per deciliter (185.6 μmol per liter), the serum aspartate aminotransferase level 153 U per liter, the serum alanine aminotransferase level 90 U per liter, the alkaline phosphatase level 270 U per liter, the total bilirubin level 1.7 mg per deciliter (29.1 μmol per liter), and the lactate dehydrogenase level 451 U per liter. Urinalysis revealed three to five nondysmorphic red cells per high-power field and occasional hyaline casts.

Given these laboratory findings, I would search for a soft-tissue infection; streptococcal toxic shock syndrome could cause any of these abnormalities. The patient's thrombocytopenia is profound, and given the relative preservation of her other cell lines, I would focus on platelet-specific destruction rather than on sequestration or a bone marrow process. In the setting of bacterial infection, destruction would most likely be a result of disseminated intravascular coagulation. Thrombocytopenia and elevated aminotransferase levels may have a viral cause, such as infection with EBV, cytomegalovirus, parvovirus, coxsackievirus, acute HIV, or acute hepatitis. Many of these infections, however, are associated with a rash and with lymphocytosis or the presence of atypical lymphocytes. This patient's renal failure probably represents a preglomerular process, since the ratio of urea nitrogen to creatinine is high in the setting of orthostasis and ibuprofen use. On urinalysis, there are no dysmorphic red cells or cellular casts, which would suggest glomerulonephritis.

I would stop the ibuprofen and begin aggressive rehydration. Given the possibility of meningitis, a lumbar puncture should be performed, but not before the thrombocytopenia is corrected, preferably to a level above 50,000 platelets per cubic millimeter. Although infection is the most likely explanation for the illness in this case, lymphoma is a remote possibility in an ill-appearing adolescent with adenopathy, unexplained thrombocytopenia, and an elevated lactate dehydrogenase level.

Chest radiographs showed several ill-defined nodular opacities within the right lower lobe and retrocardiac region (Figure 1). Posteroanterior and lateral plain-film radiographs of the neck showed a normal tracheal air column and no evidence of retropharyngeal abscess. An abdominal ultrasound study showed sludge in the gallbladder but otherwise no abnormalities. Computed tomography (CT) of the head, performed without the use of intravenous contrast material, showed no abnormalities.

Aggressive rehydration was begun, and the patient's tachycardia and hypotension resolved. Lumbar puncture was deferred because of her thrombocytopenia. Adminis-

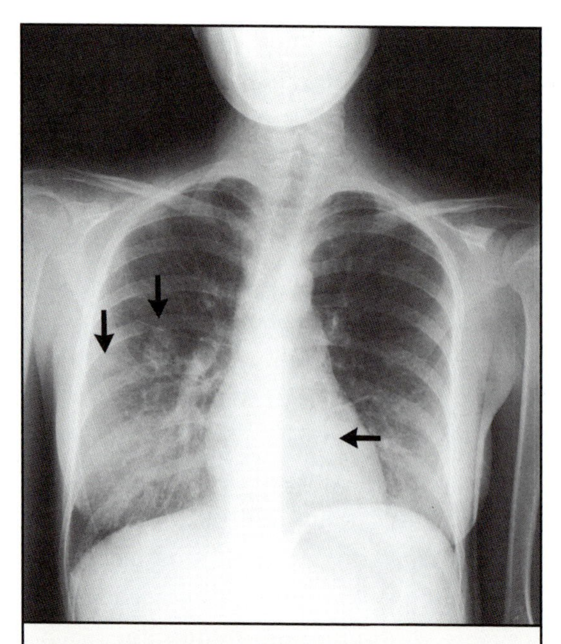

Figure 1. Posteroanterior Chest Radiograph Showing Nodular Opacities (Arrows) within the Right Lower Lobe and Retrocardiac Region.

tration of vancomycin, gentamicin, and piperacillin–tazobactam was begun after blood cultures were obtained.

Nodular opacities on chest radiography are found in a variety of disorders, but most commonly they are associated with septic emboli, disseminated fungal infection, and cancer — primarily lymphoma or metastatic disease. In a patient with a history of pharyngitis and findings signaling a possible deep-tissue infection of the neck, Lemierre's syndrome — septic thrombophlebitis of the jugular vein — should be considered. The absence of abnormalities on plain films of the patient's neck argues against the presence of a large obstructing abscess but would not rule out a smaller, parapharyngeal infection complicated by extension to the jugular veins. I would carefully palpate the tender areas of her neck for an affected vein and would request CT studies of her neck with the use of contrast material. Like endocarditis, this syndrome can be associated with multiorgan involvement, which might explain the abnormalities on her liver-function tests and her hematuria and which would put her at risk for meningitis.

Over the next 12-hour period, the patient reported that her headache and neck pain were becoming increasingly severe. Her renal function improved with rehydration; however, she became progressively acidemic and hypoxemic.

The erythrocyte sedimentation rate was 60 mm per hour. The prothrombin and partial-thromboplastin times were normal. The fibrinogen level was elevated, at 1027 mg per deciliter (normal range, 150 to 450); the D-dimer level was 0.2 to 0.4 μg per milliliter (normal range, <0.2). Serologic studies for hepatitis viruses A, B, and C were negative, as were antibody tests for EBV (tests for IgG and IgM antibodies to viral capsid antigen and for antibodies against early antigen and Epstein–Barr nuclear antigen). There was no detectable antinuclear antibody, and the levels of complements C3 and C4 were normal. Tests for urinary histoplasma antigen, HIV antibody, and antineutrophil cytoplasmic antibody and measurement of von Willebrand factor antigen were ordered. The streptococcal-antibody screen was positive, at a titer of 1:400.

These laboratory results, combined with the absence of a microangiopathic process on the blood smear, argue against disseminated intravascular coagulation as the sole cause of the patient's thrombocytopenia. At present, she has no evidence of splenic sequestration (since no splenomegaly was detected on examination or on abdominal imaging) and no evidence of bone marrow failure or of a nonspecific consumptive process, such as thrombotic thrombocytopenic purpura; thus, her thrombocytopenia is most likely an immune-mediated process. In the absence of potential offending drugs, I would continue to look for an infection that might be associated with the production of antiplatelet antibodies. Examination of a bone marrow biopsy specimen would probably show large megakaryocytes; this procedure may be indicated if an infectious source is not identified soon.

The elevated erythrocyte sedimentation rate is nonspecific; the streptococcal-antibody screen, however, shows that the patient has recently had a streptococcal infection and suggests a causative role for this organism in her pharyngeal process. The HIV antibody test, if negative, would not rule out the presence of acute HIV disease; a viral-load assay would be more helpful. The patient's worsening acidemia and oxygenation are reasons for concern because they may indicate that she has sepsis or the acute respiratory distress syndrome. The patient should be monitored closely in an intensive care unit. Given her worsening headache and neck pain, a lumbar puncture should be performed after platelet transfusion, in addition to CT study of her neck.

CT scans of the patient's neck, chest, abdomen, and pelvis were obtained to evaluate the possibility of lymphoma. Multiple ill-defined pulmonary masses, small bilateral pleural

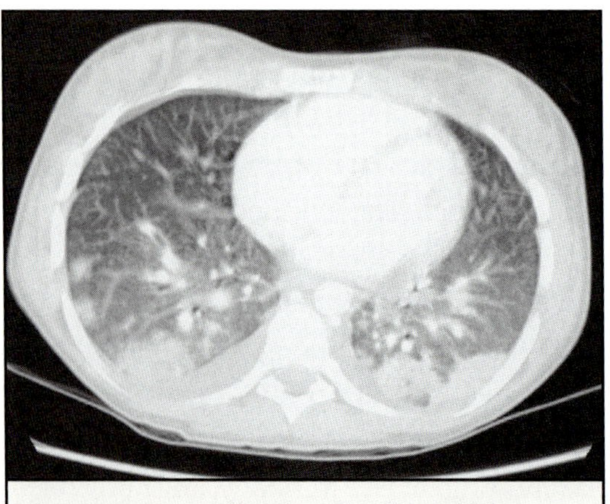

Figure 2. CT Scan of the Chest Showing Multiple Ill-Defined Pulmonary Opacities, Bilateral Pleural Effusions, and Air-Space Disease.

effusions, and widespread air-space disease were seen (Figure 2). There was asymmetric thickening of the right pharyngeal soft tissues, and the right internal jugular vein was occluded to the level of the thoracic inlet (Figure 3). The rest of the vasculature was normal, and there was no lymph-node enlargement. The abdomen and pelvis were unremarkable. Blood cultures grew gram-negative rods and gram-positive cocci in chains.

These findings are consistent with a diagnosis of septic thrombophlebitis of the internal jugular vein, or Lemierre's syndrome. The gram-negative rods, if anaerobic, are likely to be a fusobacterium species; I expect that a beta-hemolytic streptococcal species will also be identified. Polymicrobial causes are not unusual in deep-tissue pharyngeal infections. The antibiotics that the patient is currently receiving provide appropriately broad coverage, but at this time I would stop the vancomycin, since infection with methicillin-resistant *Staphylococcus aureus* or highly penicillin-resistant *Streptococcus pneumoniae* is unlikely. She does not appear to have an organized abscess that requires drainage, but she does need antibiotic therapy of at least four weeks' duration. The role of anticoagulation is controversial, but in this case, given the patient's thrombocytopenia, I would reserve it for use if there is clot progression or perhaps for use later in her clinical course, as the acute embolic phase resolves. She will need careful monitoring and evaluation for septic complications of the disease, including meningitis, empyema, and septic arthritis.

Because her illness was rapidly progressing, the patient was urgently taken to the operating room for exploration of the right side of the neck. Extensive thrombosis of the right

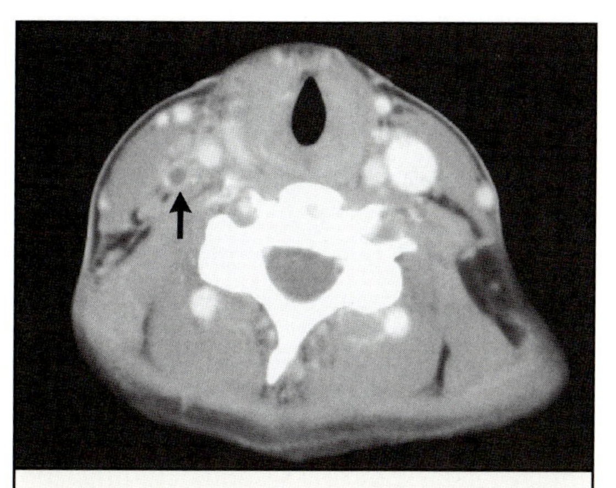

Figure 3. CT Scan of the Neck Showing Occlusion of the Right Jugular Vein (Arrow) with Adjacent Swelling of the Right Pharyngeal Soft Tissues.

jugular vein extended from the base of the skull to the clavicle. Surrounding phlegmon adhered to but did not invade the carotid artery or the deep muscles of the cervical neck. No frank abscess was identified. The internal jugular vein was ligated.

Postoperatively, vasopressor support was required because of the development of the acute respiratory distress syndrome and hypotension. Organisms from the blood were identified as *Eikenella corrodens, S. milleri,* and *Fusobacterium necrophorum.* Anticoagulation was initiated when magnetic resonance imaging with venography showed propagation of thrombosis into the intracranial venous sinuses. The patient recovered with supportive care, including intravenous antibiotics for six weeks and anticoagulant therapy for six months. At follow-up one year later, she had moderate rightward deviation of the tongue as a result of hypoglossal-nerve weakness but no other stigmata of her infection.

COMMENTARY

A sore throat is one of the most common symptoms for which patients seek medical care and accounts for at least 12 million ambulatory visits annually.[1] In the majority of cases, the sore throat is caused by a common viral pathogen; approximately 15 to 30 percent of sore throats in children and 5 to 10 percent in adults are caused by group A beta-hemolytic streptococci.[2] The growing use of antibiotics for upper respiratory infections has fostered increasing antimicrobial resistance,[3] and efforts to promote the judicious use of these drugs have meant that fewer patients with pharyngitis have been receiving them.[1]

Most episodes of pharyngitis are benign and self-limited. However, when symptoms do not remit, the clinician must consider other causes of the illness, such as infectious mononucleosis, acute HIV infection, or a suppurative complication such as cervical adenitis or a peritonsillar or retropharyngeal infection. Symptoms suggesting the presence of a deep pharyngeal infection include neck pain and limited mobility of the jaw, neck, or tongue.[4] Trismus develops when the muscles of mastication are inflamed or reflexively irritated[5] as a result of infectious spread to the lateral pharyngeal space.

Despite this patient's clinically significant oropharyngeal findings, her physicians did not initially attribute her systemic symptoms to an underlying, deep pharyngeal infection. As her care shifted from an outpatient to an inpatient setting, her presenting symptom — pharyngitis — became secondary, and her systemic findings took priority. The multiple pulmonary nodules, acute renal failure, liver-enzyme abnormalities, and thrombocytopenia framed the differential diagnosis and led to such discordant possibilities as thrombotic thrombocytopenic purpura, vasculitis, and lymphoma. The context in which physicians frame a diagnostic question helps to generate the differential diagnosis and guides the subsequent evaluation.[6] In this case, the inpatient clinicians initially marginalized the neck-related symptoms, whereas the discussant in this article placed the systemic findings into the context of an antecedent pharyngitis and arrived relatively easily at the correct diagnosis.

In 1936, André Lemierre, a Parisian bacteriologist, described 20 cases of anaerobic thrombophlebitis of the internal jugular vein with metastatic infection.[7] Most cases of Lemierre's syndrome occur in adolescents and young adults with tonsillopharyngitis, or less commonly, those with an odontogenic infection, mastoiditis, or sinusitis.[8] Oral anaerobes invade the peritonsillar tissue, and infection spreads to the adjacent lateral pharyngeal space, which contains the internal jugular vein. *F. necrophorum*, an anaerobic, gram-negative rod that commensally inhabits the oral cavity and gastrointestinal and female genital tracts, is identified in 82 percent of the cases.[8] It is not known why fusobacterium species invade the mucosa; antecedent EBV infection may promote the invasion, possibly by inducing immunosuppression.[9,10] From the neck, the infection spreads hematogenously, most commonly to the lungs, but also to the joints, liver, spleen, bones, kidneys, and meninges.[10]

Patients with Lemierre's syndrome usually present with systemic findings within one week after the onset of the inciting oropharyngeal infection.[8,9] Ipsilateral neck pain and swelling occur in only half the patients; a minority will have trismus or evidence of a thrombosed jugular vein on examination.[8] Signs of metastatic infection include pulmonary infiltrates, hepatosplenomegaly, hyperbilirubinemia, elevation in liver-enzyme levels, hematuria, and disseminated intravascular coagulation with thrombocytopenia.[8-11] Thrombocytopenia in the absence of disseminated intravascular coagulation has been reported,[12,13] although the exact pathogenic mechanism of thrombocytopenia in the current case is not entirely clear.

The diagnosis of Lemierre's syndrome is usually made after a variety of infectious and noninfectious illnesses have been considered. The diagnosis may first be suggested when *F. necrophorum* grows in blood culture[8,10,11]; contrast-enhanced CT studies of the neck can confirm the diagnosis. Although the optimal treatment is unknown, antimicrobial therapy effective against anaerobic pathogens is critical. Penicillin, cephalosporins, clindamycin, metronidazole, chloramphenicol, and tetracyclines all have efficacy against fusobacterium species.[9] Since anticoagulation may facilitate embolic spread, it is usually reserved for cases of retrograde propagation of thrombus.[9] Ligation of the internal jugular vein is rarely required, although it may help to prevent further embolism if the infection spreads despite appropriate medical therapy. Before antibiotics became available, the mortality rate approached 90 percent[7]; even with systemic antibiotic therapy, up to 18 percent of patients may die.[8,9,14]

In the era before antibiotics, Lemierre's syndrome was common, but reports declined in the 1960s and 1970s as the use of antimicrobial agents for pharyngitis became increasingly common.[9] In the past decade, the frequency of Lemierre's syndrome has again increased,[11,15] and some have attributed this change to the increasingly judicious use of antibiotics.[9,11,14] Because the number of physicians familiar with its dramatic signs and symptoms is diminishing, Lemierre's syndrome has been referred to as the "forgotten disease."[8,9,11] Changes affecting the neck may be subtle or absent at the time of a patient's presentation with metastatic infection, and the diagnosis may be overlooked. In their search for a unifying diagnosis, the clinicians caring for the patient in the current case would have been well served to remember her chief symptom: a pain in the neck.

Supported by a Career Development Award from the Health Services Research and Development Program of the Department of Veterans Affairs and a Patient Safety Developmental Center Grant (P20-HS11540) from the Agency for Healthcare Research and Quality (both to Dr. Saint).

We are indebted to Peter Strouse, M.D., for assistance with the radiographic images and their interpretation.

This article first appeared in the March 4, 2004, issue of the New England Journal of Medicine.

REFERENCES

1.
Steinman MA, Gonzales R, Linder JA, Landefeld CS. Changing use of antibiotics in community-based outpatient practice, 1991-1999. Ann Intern Med 2003;138:525-33.

2.
Bisno AL, Gerber MA, Gwaltney JM Jr, Kaplan EL, Schwartz RH. Practice guidelines for the diagnosis and management of group A streptococcal pharyngitis. Clin Infect Dis 2002;35:113-25.

3.
Jacobs RF. Judicious use of antibiotics for common pediatric respiratory infections. Pediatr Infect Dis J 2000;19:938-43.

4.
Ortiz JA, Hudkins C, Kornblut A. Adenitis, adenopathy, and abscesses of the head and neck. Emerg Med Clin North Am 1987;5:359-70.

5.
Tveterås K, Kristensen S. The aetiology and pathogenesis of trismus. Clin Otolaryngol 1986;11:383-7.

6.
Kassirer JP, Kopelman RI. Cognitive errors in diagnosis: instantiation, classification, and consequences. Am J Med 1989;86:433-41.

7.
Lemierre A. On certain septicæmias due to anaerobic organisms. Lancet 1936;1:701-3.

8.
Chirinos JA, Lichtstein DM, Garcia J, Tamariz LJ. The evolution of Lemierre syndrome: report of 2 cases and review of the literature. Medicine (Baltimore) 2002;81:458-65.

9.
Hagelskjaer Kristensen L, Prag J. Human necrobacillosis, with emphasis on Lemierre's syndrome. Clin Infect Dis 2000;31:524-32.

10.
Golpe R, Marin B, Alonso M. Lemierre's syndrome (necrobacillosis). Postgrad Med J 1999;75:141-4.

11.
Hagelskjær LH, Prag J, Malczynski J, Kristensen JH. Incidence and clinical epidemiology of necrobacillosis, including Lemierre's syndrome, in Denmark 1990-1995. Eur J Clin Microbiol Infect Dis 1998;17:561-5.

12.
Ellis GR, Gozzard DI, Looker DN, Green GJ. Postanginal septicaemia (Lemmiere's disease) complicated by haemophagocytosis. J Infect 1998;36:340-1.

13.
Ghosh TK, Khan N, Malik A. Platelet auto-antibodies in septicaemic patients. Indian J Pathol Microbiol 1999;42:31-5.

14.
Liu ACY, Argent JD. Necrobacillosis — a resurgence? Clin Radiol 2002;57:332-8.

15.
Jones JW, Riordan T, Morgan MS. Investigation of postanginal sepsis and Lemierre's syndrome in the south west peninsula. Commun Dis Public Health 2001;4:278-81.

Red Snapper or Crab?

PAUL B. CORNIA, M.D., BENJAMIN A. LIPSKY, M.D.,
GURPREET DHALIWAL, M.D., AND SANJAY SAINT, M.D., M.P.H.

A 68-year-old man originally from the Philippines presented with a three-month history of increasing dyspnea on exertion and orthopnea. He also reported an unintentional weight loss of 7 kg (15 lb), night sweats, and abdominal bloating. He stated that he had not had fever, chills, cough, vomiting, chest pain, or swelling of the legs.

The patient's dyspnea could be due to congestive heart failure, pulmonary disease, anemia, or deconditioning associated with a cachexia-inducing illness. The absence of upper and lower gastrointestinal symptoms, even in the presence of abdominal bloating, points me away from further consideration of luminal gastrointestinal disorders. Ascites could account for the increasing abdominal girth, and in a patient who has lost weight, it may indicate a chronic infection, cancer, or cirrhosis.

Because tuberculosis is endemic in the Philippines, tuberculous peritonitis is a consideration. Patients with extrapulmonary tuberculosis often present without associated pulmonary infection, so the absence of a cough is not inconsistent with this diagnosis. Any intraabdominal cancer can lead to abdominal distention as a result of a mass effect or malignant ascites, which may occur by way of widespread hepatic metastasis or peritoneal carcinomatosis.

The patient's medical history included prostate cancer with bony metastasis (stage D2), which had been diagnosed 15 years previously and treated by radical prostatectomy, followed by radiation therapy and bilateral orchiectomy. The patient had had a positive tuberculin skin test with purified protein derivative, without prior active tuberculosis or antituberculosis therapy, and had a history of gastroesophageal reflux and hypercholesterolemia. His medications were rabeprazole and simvastatin. He had last traveled to the Philippines two years previously and had never used tobacco or illicit substances. He had served in the Navy for 20 years and had then worked as a custodian.

The positive tuberculin skin test is not surprising, but his history of service in the Navy is intriguing. He may have worked in shipyards where asbestos is abundant, raising the pos-

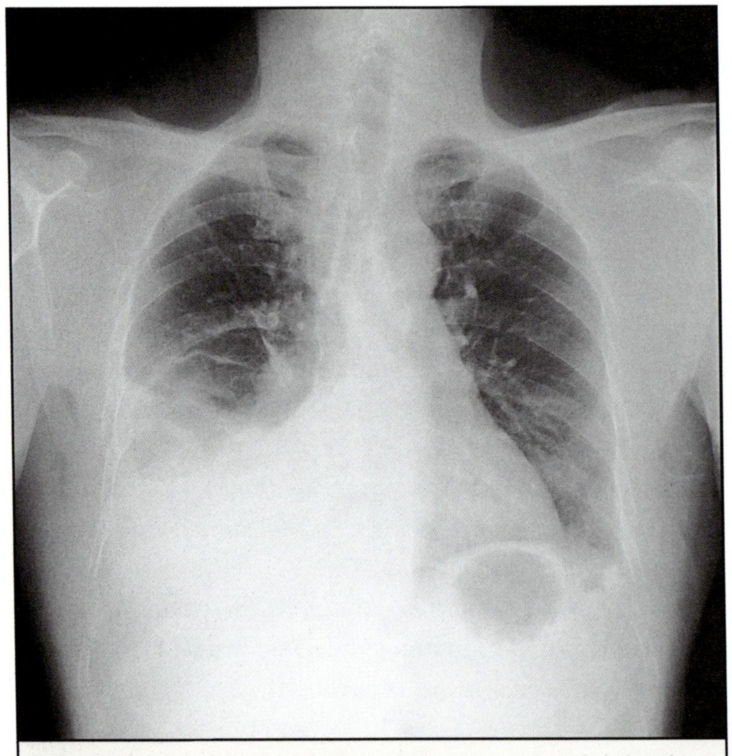

Figure 1. Posteroanterior Chest Radiograph Showing a Right-Sided Pleural Effusion.

sibility of malignant peritoneal mesothelioma. Pleural mesothelioma, which is more common, could also explain his dyspnea. If gastroesophageal reflux was diagnosed without endoscopic confirmation, gastric carcinoma is possible. I am still considering ascites to be the cause of his abdominal bloating and weight loss. The only identifiable risk factor for liver disease is his country of origin, where hepatitis B infection is common. Tuberculosis, gastrointestinal cancer, and malignant mesothelioma can all cause ascites. Metastatic prostate cancer could account for the weight loss, but cardiopulmonary and gastrointestinal manifestations are uncommon in that form of cancer.

The patient was afebrile, and his pulse, respiratory rate, and blood pressure were normal. Examination of the chest revealed dullness to percussion and an absence of breath sounds posteriorly over three quarters of the right hemithorax. The heart sounds and jugular venous pulses were normal, and there was no peripheral edema. The abdomen was distended, but there was no tenderness, organomegaly, or fluid wave.

The hematocrit was 34 percent, with a normal mean corpuscular volume. The platelet count was 439,000 per cubic millimeter, and the white-cell count 9800 per cubic millimeter; the differential count was normal. Serum electrolyte levels, renal function, and the results of liver function tests were normal. The serum albumin level was 3.6 g per deciliter, and the international normalized ratio was 1.0. Prostate-specific antigen was undetectable. Chest radiography revealed no abnormalities except for a right-sided pleural effusion (Figure 1), which appeared to be freely mobile in the lateral decubitus view. The electrocardiogram was unremarkable. The patient was admitted to the hospital.

The normal results on the cardiovascular examination and the absence of edema make congestive heart failure, the most common cause of pleural effusion, unlikely. I remain suspicious of tuberculosis as a possible diagnosis. The fact that prostate-specific antigen was undetectable essentially rules out metastatic prostate cancer, with rare exceptions; pleural effusion would be unusual in metastatic prostate cancer. A malignant pleural effusion is plausible, but a primary cancer is not evident. Cirrhosis is unlikely without the characteristic findings on physical examination or laboratory evidence of chronic liver disease. An ultrasound study would be useful to confirm the presence of ascites in the absence of known liver disease or marked abdominal distention. If ascites due to cirrhosis were unexpectedly found, hepatic hydrothorax would be a consideration. Pleural effusion and abdominal bloating could be explained by an abdominal tumor with metastases to the lung or by a bronchogenic carcinoma with an associated paraneoplastic autonomic neuropathy.

Infection (particularly tuberculosis) and cancer remain my primary considerations. The tests that will guide my decision making are analysis of the pleural fluid and computed tomography (CT) of the abdomen.

CT scanning of the chest showed the right-sided pleural effusion, but no pulmonary parenchymal nodules, enlarged lymph nodes, or pleural plaques were visible. On CT scanning of the abdomen, all the organs were normal, but there were multiple enhancing omental nodules (Figure 2), along with minimal ascites confined to the pelvis. Thoracentesis was performed, and 1 liter of bloody fluid was removed. Findings on analysis of the fluid were as follows: total protein level, 7.2 mg per deciliter; lactate dehydrogenase level, 745 U per liter; red-cell count, 220,000 per cubic millimeter; and white-cell count, 11,000 per cubic millimeter (35 percent neutrophils, 32 percent lymphocytes, 25 percent monocytes, and 8 percent mesothelial cells). The total protein level in the serum was 8.2 mg per deciliter, and the serum lactate dehydrogenase level was 192 U per liter. Cultures of the

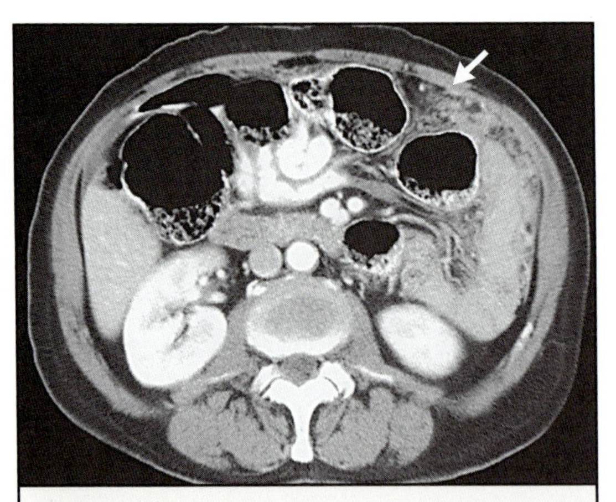

Figure 2. CT Scan of the Abdomen, Showing Omental Nodules (Arrow) in the Anterior Aspect of the Left Upper Abdomen.

pleural fluid grew no bacteria, and stains of the pleural fluid for acid-fast bacilli were negative. Cytologic examination revealed mesothelial cells without malignant features. The patient's dyspnea resolved after thoracentesis, and he asked to be discharged.

The patient has a bloody, exudative effusion according to Light's criteria (which indicate that the effusion is exudative when at least one of the following is true: when the ratio of pleural-fluid protein to serum protein is greater than 0.5, the ratio of pleural-fluid lactate dehydrogenase to serum lactate dehydrogenase is greater than 0.6, or the pleural-fluid lactate dehydrogenase level is greater than two thirds the upper limit of the normal range for serum lactate dehydrogenase). He also has a diseased omentum with a small amount of ascites. Bloody pleural fluid usually signifies one of three processes: trauma, cancer, or pulmonary embolism.

The pleura and the peritoneum may be affected simultaneously in a number of diseases, including primary tumors (e.g., mesothelioma), infections (e.g., tuberculosis), metastatic carcinoma (usually adenocarcinoma), and systemic lupus erythematosus. Each would cause an exudative effusion, and the results in this case are not sufficiently characteristic to narrow the differential diagnosis further.

The patient's positive tuberculin skin test, night sweats, and pleural-fluid pleocytosis with an elevated protein level suggest tuberculosis. The negative stain for acid-fast bacilli is not surprising, since a tuberculous pleural effusion is a hypersensitivity reaction to a small number of bacilli in the pleural space. However, fever often accompanies tuberculous pleuritis, the effusion is typically lymphocytic, and rarely are there numerous mesothelial cells. Mesothelioma remains a serious concern because of the possible asbestos exposure (a long latency period would be typical) and because of the aggressive disease that affects two serosal surfaces. The absence of pleural thickening or irregularity on the CT scan of the chest would be uncharacteristic, but malignant mesothelial cells are often absent in the pleural fluid. Finally, I must consider the possibility that another tumor has metastasized to the pleura and peritoneum. Cytologic studies may be negative for malignant cells in a patient with a malignant pleural effusion, but this patient's history, laboratory data, and images do not suggest another primary cancer.

Two weeks after hospital discharge, the patient presented with fever and with pain and swelling of the left side of the neck. He otherwise felt well and stated that he had not had dyspnea since his discharge. He had not sustained trauma to the neck or undergone surgical procedures involving the neck. On examination, the left side of the neck was indurated, with overlying erythema, and was exquisitely tender; the oropharynx was unremarkable. The white-cell count was 16,000 per cubic millimeter.

Is this acute inflammatory mass a lymph node? The differential diagnosis of cervical lymphadenopathy is primarily one of infection versus cancer. The fever, tenderness, erythema, and leukocytosis favor the former, particularly a bacterial lymphadenitis. Tuberculous lymphadenitis deserves consideration, although intense pain and inflammation are not typical of that disease. If this new finding is not lymphadenopathy, bacterial infections such as cellulitis, infection of the branchial-cleft cyst, submandibular abscess, or suppurative thrombosis of the internal jugular vein are possible.

This finding is perplexing. The neck abnormality sounds like an acute bacterial infection, but the pleural–peritoneal disease seems chronic in nature, and I cannot easily link the two. If inflammatory soft tissue cannot be distinguished from lymphadenopathy on physical examination, I would obtain a neck CT scan.

CT scanning revealed thrombosis of the left internal jugular vein with extensive surrounding inflammation, but no mass or lymphadenopathy. Chest radiography revealed reaccumulation of the right-sided pleural effusion. The patient was readmitted for anticoagulant therapy.

Spontaneous thrombosis of a neck vein is very uncommon and leads me to suspect a hypercoagulable state, perhaps from an underlying cancer. Could a pulmonary embolus be responsible for the pleural effusion in this case? Pulmonary embolism is usually an acute condition and is out of step with the tempo of this patient's illness. Am I missing some other cause of his exudative pleural effusion?

Because the patient had previously undergone abdominal surgery and pelvic irradiation, pleuroscopy (rather than laparoscopy) was performed. The findings included an area of abnormal-appearing tissue deep in the posterior inferior pleural space on the right side. Intraoperative frozen sections of this tissue were examined, and the findings were interpreted as indicative of metastatic carcinoma, consistent with a primary focus in the prostate. Talc pleurodesis was performed to prevent reaccumulation of pleural fluid, and the patient was discharged.

I am fairly convinced that the patient does not have tuberculosis, since it would be difficult to confuse carcinoma with a tuberculous granuloma. I also doubt that he has metastatic prostate cancer, because recurrence would be extremely unusual in a patient who has been free of disease for 15 years since treatment and in whom prostate-specific antigen is undetectable. Because mesothelioma could be misinterpreted as adenocarcinoma, I would await further review of the tissue by a pathologist. If the diagnosis remains in question, I would obtain another biopsy specimen. Since the pleural surface would be inaccessible after pleurodesis, I would further investigate the omental nodules. I am increasingly interested in knowing what the patient did while in the Navy.

At a clinic visit one week later, the patient reported anorexia and persistent abdominal distention. Repeated abdominal CT scanning showed an increase in the number and size of the omental nodules and in the amount of ascitic fluid. Ultrasound-guided paracentesis yielded 20 ml of clear yellow fluid with a serum–ascitic fluid albumin gradient of 0.7 g per deciliter. The ascitic fluid contained 15,400 white cells per cubic millimeter (30 percent neutrophils, 5 percent lymphocytes, 35 percent monocytes, and 30 percent mesothelial cells) and 1900 red cells per cubic milliliter. Bacterial and mycobacterial cultures were sterile. Cytologic examination showed inflammatory cells and normal-appearing mesothelial cells. The final interpretation of the biopsy specimens obtained during pleuroscopy was hemorrhagic fibrin clot with a small, benign-appearing overgrowth of mesothelial cells, a finding not consistent with the presence of metastatic prostate carcinoma.

Since the ascites originates from the peritoneum, the low serum–ascitic fluid albumin gradient (less than 1.1 g per deciliter) was expected. (In contrast, processes that result in portal hypertension are associated with an elevated serum–ascitic fluid albumin gradient [1.1 g per deciliter or higher].) The cell counts and the white-cell differential count are not diagnostic and again raise the question of tuberculosis as opposed to cancer. The white-cell count is substantially elevated, and the neutrophil count is greater than 250 per cubic millimeter, but I doubt that he has spontaneous bacterial peritonitis. That condition almost always occurs in the setting of liver disease and is usually accompanied by a predominance of neutrophils.

This patient has two diseased serosal surfaces with exudative effusions, complicated by hypercoagulability, and there is no strong evidence of tuberculosis, which is the competing diagnosis. I think that he has malignant pleural and peritoneal mesothelioma and would thus proceed with laparoscopic peritoneal biopsy.

Exploratory laparoscopy revealed a peritoneal surface with diffuse plaques and an omentum caked with soft, nodular plaques. Pathological evaluation of the biopsy specimens by immunocytochemistry and electron microscopy revealed malignant mesothelioma. On further questioning, the patient reported that while serving in the Navy he had been continually exposed to asbestos-covered pipes, both while scraping and repainting them and while working below deck as a cook.

COMMENTARY

The venerable adage that careful history taking and physical examination usually lead to the correct diagnosis is especially true in perplexing cases. Unfortunately, because of advances in medical technology and specialized diagnostic tests, physicians have begun to place less emphasis on these skills. Despite the methodical evaluation of this patient by his physicians, the diagnosis remained elusive. The discussant, however, zeroed in on two key aspects of the history: the patient's country of origin (an area where tuberculosis is endemic) and his service in the Navy (a clue to potential asbestos exposure). The discussant was then able to place infection with *Mycobacterium tuberculosis* (sometimes called the "red snapper" because of its characteristic appearance on acid-fast staining) and cancer (Latin for crab) at the top of his differential diagnosis for this patient with diseased pleural and peritoneal surfaces. As additional information was presented, he interpreted it in the context of these two historical linchpins.

Disseminated tuberculosis (with pleuritis and peritonitis) was appropriately considered because of the patient's positive tuberculin skin test. The likelihood of tuberculous pleuritis was lessened by the absence of typical clinical findings (e.g., fever, cough, and pleuritic chest pain)[1] and the atypical findings in the pleural fluid (more than 5 percent mesothelial cells and an absence of a lymphocytic predominance).[1,2] The patient's history of metastatic prostate cancer was also considered and briefly led to an incorrect diagnosis. Despite the initial misreading of the pleural biopsy specimen, the discussant recognized that metastatic prostate cancer was unlikely because prostate-specific antigen was undetectable.[3] Mesothelioma can be mistaken for adenocarcinoma histologically.[4] The distinction can be, and was in this case, made by immunocytochemical staining and electron microscopy. Although the findings described made disseminated tuberculosis or prostate cancer unlikely, several features suggested mesothelioma as a potential diagnosis. The combination of several factors — the possibility of heavy asbestos exposure (not recognized until late in the workup), the involvement of both the pleural and the peritoneal surfaces, the long latency period between the exposure and the onset of symptoms, and hypercoagulability — led the discussant to the correct diagnosis: malignant mesothelioma.

Asbestos was used extensively in World War II–era ships. Its use did not decline until the mid-1970s, when the adverse health consequences of prolonged exposure became widely known. Exposure to asbestos can cause the fibrotic interstitial lung disease called asbestosis; it has also been linked to lung cancer (and the risk appears to increase synergistically with tobacco use), malignant mesothelioma, and benign pleural disorders (pleural plaques and effusions). Although asbestosis has been recognized since the early 1900s, asbestos exposure was not linked to malignant mesothelioma until the 1960s.[5]

The incidence of mesothelioma in the United States rose during the 1970s and early 1980s, primarily as a result of occupational exposure during the preceding decades, and was projected to peak in 2000.[6] Malignant mesothelioma may arise from the pleural or peritoneal surfaces or, less commonly, the pericardium or tunica vaginalis. Pleural involvement is more common than peritoneal involvement, which usually occurs in persons with the heaviest asbestos exposure. After inhalation, the lung's mucociliary system attempts to clear the asbestos fibers. Fibers that are coughed up and swallowed may lead to peritoneal mesothelioma. A latency period of 20 to 40 years between asbestos exposure and the onset of symptoms of mesothelioma is typical.

Peritoneal mesothelioma tends to progress locally, resulting in vague abdominal symptoms, including pain, increased girth (due to malignant ascites), and weight loss.[7,8] Examination of the abdomen usually reveals evidence of ascites but little else.[8] As the tumor advances locally, it may cause bowel obstruction. Surgical debulking followed by intraperitoneal chemotherapy may be attempted in selected patients with localized disease. Palliative systemic chemotherapy is an option for those with advanced disease.

Because of the rarity of peritoneal mesothelioma and its frequently nonspecific features at the time of presentation, the diagnosis is often delayed. Five months elapsed between this patient's initial presentation and the correct diagnosis. Because the prognosis is poor and treatment options are limited, this delay probably did not alter the outcome, but it may have been avoidable. Two main factors contributed to the delay. First, the patient was discharged from the hospital twice (once at his request) before his evaluation had been completed. Although rapid discharge may help constrain costs, it may not be optimal for patients who require certain diagnostic tests or evaluations by multiple subspecialists. Second, there was an initial reluctance to perform exploratory abdominal surgery (to obtain biopsy specimens of the omental nodules) because of the patient's prior abdominal surgery and pelvic irradiation. This initial decision not to obtain specimens of the omental nodules was not revisited for several months. Had the patient's extensive asbestos exposure been recognized earlier, the primary and consulting physicians would probably have pursued exploratory abdominal surgery soon after the nondiagnostic pleuroscopy.

More than half a century ago, Platt asserted that most diagnoses could be made on the basis of the history alone.[9] Subsequent studies have confirmed that the history is the key to the final diagnosis in 56 to 82 percent of cases.[10-12] The commonly passed-on clinical aphorism, "What you do not ask, you will not find out," remains true.

Supported by a Career Development Award from the Health Services Research and Development Program of the Department of Veterans Affairs and a Patient Safety Developmental Center Grant (P20-HS11540) from the Agency for Healthcare Research and Quality (both to Dr. Saint).

This article first appeared in the April 1, 2004, issue of the New England Journal of Medicine.

REFERENCES

1.
Light RW. Pleural diseases. 3rd ed. Baltimore: Williams & Wilkins, 1995.
2.
Valdés L, Alvarez D, San José E, et al. Tuberculous pleurisy: a study of 254 patients. Arch Intern Med 1998;158:2017-21.
3.
Ruckle HC, Klee GG, Oesterling JE. Prostate-specific antigen: concepts for staging prostate cancer and monitoring response to therapy. Mayo Clin Proc 1994;69:69-79.
4.
Antman KH. Natural history and epidemiology of malignant mesothelioma. Chest 1993;103:Suppl:373S-376S.
5.
Wagner JC, Sleggs CA, Marchand P. Diffuse pleural mesothelioma and asbestos in the North Western Cape Province. Br J Ind Med 1960;17:260-71.
6.
Price B. Analysis of current trends in United States mesothelioma incidence. Am J Epidemiol 1997;145:211-8.
7.
Mohamed F, Sugarbaker PH. Peritoneal mesothelioma. Curr Treat Options Oncol 2002;3:375-86.
8.
Asenio JA, Goldblatt P, Thomford NR. Primary malignant peritoneal mesothelioma: a report of seven cases and a review of the literature. Arch Surg 1990;125:1477-81.
9.
Platt R. Two essays on the practice of medicine. Manch Univ Med Sch Gaz 1947;26:139-45.
10.
Hampton JR, Harrison MJG, Mitchell JRA, Prichard JS, Seymour C. Relative contributions of history-taking, physical examination, and laboratory investigation to diagnosis and management of medical outpatients. Br Med J 1975;2:486-9.
11.
Sandler G. Importance of the history in the medical clinic and the cost of unnecessary tests. Am Heart J 1980;100:928-31.
12.
Peterson MC, Holbrook JH, Von Hales D, Smith NL, Staker LV. Contributions of the history, physical examination, and laboratory investigation in making medical diagnoses. West J Med 1992;156:163-5.

Index of Suspicion

UPTAL D. PATEL, M.D., HARRY HOLLANDER, M.D.,
AND SANJAY SAINT, M.D., M.P.H.

A 26-year-old woman with end-stage renal disease from primary membranoproliferative glomerulonephritis presented with a two-week history of intermittent fever, with temperatures as high as 39°C. She had received her second cadaveric renal transplant 11 months previously.

Disease categories to consider in a febrile patient who has received a transplanted organ include infection, rejection, a post-transplantation lymphoproliferative disorder, and the reappearance of an underlying inflammatory disease that resulted in previous organ failure and transplantation. In this patient, both routine community-acquired infections and opportunistic infections associated with immunosuppression deserve consideration; the differential diagnosis of the latter would be shaped by the patient's epidemiologic characteristics (e.g., her travel history) and additional clinical and laboratory data. Fever caused by cellular rejection is often accompanied by allograft dysfunction, so a new elevation in the level of serum creatinine in conjunction with fever would raise this possibility. Post-transplantation lymphoproliferative disorder, which may occur six weeks or more after transplantation, is also possible. If this patient had received treatment for prior episodes of rejection it would place her at increased risk for this complication.

The patient had received her first transplant 10 years before presentation; she had received the second transplant as a result of allograft failure due to chronic rejection. Two weeks before presentation, she had a fever almost daily; the fevers were associated with diffuse myalgias and drenching sweats and chills. She was evaluated by her local physician, who was unable to identify an obvious infectious cause; no new treatment was prescribed. She reported generalized malaise, anorexia, and a weight loss of 1.4 kg (3 lb) since the onset of the fevers. In addition, she noted slight swelling and nontender erythema of her left index finger, which had started one week before presentation. She reported that she had not had any other symptoms or recent contact with sick persons and that she had not traveled out of Michigan, her state of residence.

Whereas myalgias are nonspecific, a new, localized change involving a swollen finger and erythema is highly clinically significant and frames the differential diagnosis. If the abnormalities appear to be confined to the skin, the morphologic features become important; well-demarcated erythema implies cellulitis, whereas a nonblanching lesion increases the likelihood of an embolic infection (e.g., endocarditis or fungal disease) or a vasculitis. The tempo of this presentation and the appearance of erythema after one week of fever argue strongly against one of the usual gram-positive causes of cellulitis. Certain opportunistic infections — such as nocardial or mycobacterial infection — may cause an indolent soft-tissue infection that mimics cellulitis.

The medications she took were cyclosporine, mycophenolate mofetil, prednisone (10 mg per day), propranolol, amlodipine, and valacyclovir (prescribed by an emergency department physician five days before presentation for presumed herpetic whitlow, without confirmatory tests). Approximately six weeks before presentation, the patient received bolus doses of corticosteroids (250 mg of intravenous methylprednisolone daily for three days) as treatment for moderate acute cellular rejection. She was married and did not have children or pets. She worked as a veterinary assistant and had recently had contact with various domestic animals, mostly cats and dogs.

Despite the low current dose of corticosteroids, the patient must be considered to have clinically significant cellular immunodeficiency in the light of her treatment with two other agents that inhibit T-cell function and the recent bolus doses of methylprednisolone for rejection. Patients who have received a solid-organ transplant remain at increased risk for herpesvirus infection; a diagnosis of herpetic whitlow is possible, although the finger is not a common site of herpesvirus reappearance.

The patient's occupational history is intriguing. Several zoonotic infections that can be worrisome in immunocompromised hosts are transmitted from cats. Toxoplasmosis is most often acquired through inadvertent ingestion of feline feces and may be manifested with atypical symptoms in a transplant recipient. Enteric pathogens include salmonella and campylobacter species; the latter especially should be considered, since infection with any of several campylobacter-like organisms may manifest as bacteremia and migratory cellulitis, rather than enteritis, in immunocompromised patients. Another cat-borne illness that is heralded by fever and new cutaneous findings is infection with *Bartonella henselae*. The lesions of bacillary angiomatosis are typically nonblanching and vascular, which may lead to their confusion with Kaposi's sarcoma, another opportunistic complication of

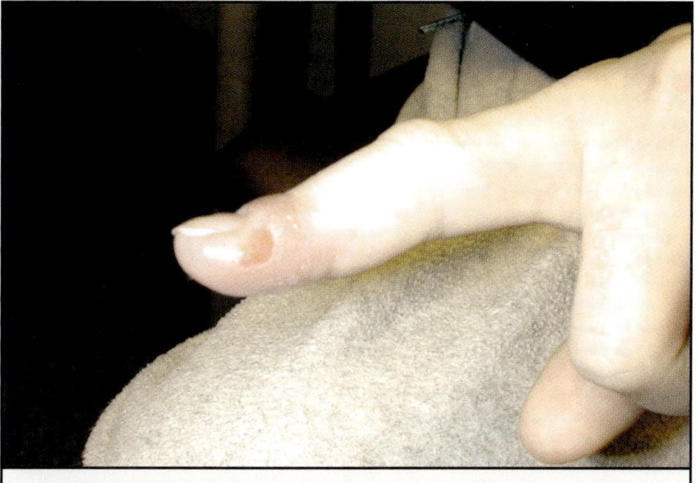

Figure 1. Photograph Showing a Nodular, Erythematous Lesion on the Medial Aspect of the Distal Phalanx of the Left Index Finger.

transplantation in persons previously exposed to human herpesvirus 8. The physical examination would help distinguish among these possibilities.

The patient's temperature was 37.2°C, her heart rate was 74 beats per minute, her respiratory rate was 14 breaths per minute, and her blood pressure was 96/50 mm Hg. She was a thin, pale woman in no distress. The oropharynx was free of exudates, and the neck was supple. The chest was clear on auscultation; heart sounds were regular, and a grade 3 systolic ejection murmur was heard throughout the precordium. Abdominal examination revealed no abnormalities; in the region of the bilateral renal allografts, no audible bruits or palpable tenderness was detected. There were multiple enlarged, soft, rubbery, mobile left axillary lymph nodes, with the largest measuring approximately 2 cm in diameter. No epitrochlear or clavicular lymph nodes were palpable. The skin was normal except for a slightly nodular, soft, erythematous lesion, 8 mm in diameter, on the medial aspect of the distal phalanx of the left index finger (Figure 1).

The patient's white-cell count was 4000 per cubic millimeter, with a differential count of 81 percent neutrophils, 12 percent lymphocytes, 3 percent monocytes, and 4 percent eosinophils. The hematocrit was 22 percent, and the platelet count was 125,000 per cubic millimeter. The results of liver-function tests were normal, and the lactate dehydrogenase level was 156 U per liter. The creatinine level was 2.0 mg per deciliter (176.8 μmol per liter), similar to previously observed levels, and the results of urinalysis were normal.

The patient's low blood pressure raises the possibility of sepsis syndrome due to an underlying infection. The cardiac murmur probably represents a flow murmur due to her anemia, but with a distal digital lesion, endocarditis must be considered. The morphologic features and position of the digital lesion do not support the possibility of herpetic whitlow. Hematogenously spread bacterial, fungal, or mycobacterial infections could have this appearance. The tempo of the illness suggests the presence of indolent organisms such as bartonella and nocardia. If the lesion were caused by direct inoculation, I would think primarily of certain mycobacteria (e.g., *Mycobacterium marinum*) and environmental fungi, such as aspergillus or cryptococcus. Several of these organisms are relevant to her occupation, assuming the appropriate contact with animals such as fish, birds, cats, or dogs.

Given the hematologic abnormalities, I must also consider bone marrow involvement with a disseminated infection. Granulomatous infections such as fungal diseases (especially histoplasmosis and cryptococcosis) and mycobacterial diseases are the most common marrow-infiltrative infections. The presence of adenopathy may also indicate disseminated infection or cancer (e.g., lymphoma).

Cultures of blood and urine obtained on admission revealed no growth. The results of serologic tests for Epstein–Barr virus (EBV), cytomegalovirus (CMV), parvovirus B19, and bartonella were all negative for acute infection; serum polymerase-chain-reaction (PCR) assays for EBV and CMV were also negative. Transthoracic echocardiography revealed a bicuspid aortic valve but no evidence of endocarditis. Computed tomography of the chest, abdomen, and pelvis revealed left axillary lymph-node enlargement but no other remarkable findings. The patient was presumed to have an unspecified viral illness. The mycophenolate mofetil was discontinued, and she was discharged home, with close outpatient observation anticipated.

Clinicians must be cautious in the interpretation of the results of serologic tests in immunosuppressed patients. These patients may have a component of humoral immunodeficiency that impairs the ability to mount typical antibody responses to acute or recrudescent infection. Thus, the absence of IgM antibodies to EBV or CMV, for example, would have limited negative predictive value. Genomic or antigen-based studies are generally more reliable in this setting. Parvovirus B19 infection was a consideration because of the hematologic cytopenias, but it would not fully explain the skin findings. The absence of detectable parvovirus B19 in a PCR study of the blood provides strong evidence against this infection.

At this point, I am uncomfortable ascribing the fever to an undefined viral illness. The clinical setting, duration of illness, and associated physical findings warrant additional evaluation for specific treatable causes. Since less invasive tests have been unrevealing, histologic evaluation of the skin lesion, enlarged lymph nodes, or bone marrow should be considered next.

Two days after discharge from the hospital, the patient was readmitted because of persistent fever, malaise, and anorexia. The small erythematous lesion on her left index finger had persisted without change. While she was hospitalized, the patient continued to have a fever, with temperatures up to 40.5°C. Blood cultures from the previous admission remained sterile after a one-week incubation period. The results of all the following investigations were negative: repeated blood and urine cultures; PCR assays for human herpesvirus 6, CMV, EBV, hepatitis C virus, ehrlichia, and babesia; serologic tests for human immunodeficiency virus, hepatitis B virus, and toxoplasma; a test for urinary histoplasma; and tests for rheumatoid factor and antinuclear antibody. The erythrocyte sedimentation rate and the C-reactive protein level were normal, and the results of a serum PCR assay for polyomavirus type BK (BK virus) was positive, at 5200 copies per milliliter.

Reactivation of BK virus occurs commonly in transplant recipients who are infected with this agent; the most common associated clinical syndrome is hemorrhagic interstitial cystitis. I doubt that BK virus infection explains the entire picture here. A general principle in the evaluation of a patient with fever of unknown origin is to focus on and pursue any focal abnormalities. Biopsy of the involved tissue may have been a more efficient approach in this case.

At this point, I still favor a diagnosis of disseminated infection with lymphatic and bone marrow involvement; infection with bartonella is an intriguing possibility because of the patient's occupation and the presence of a skin lesion. Mycobacteria and fungi have not yet been ruled out as possible causes; post-transplantation lymphoproliferative disorder would be lower on my differential diagnosis.

The patient's white-cell count decreased to 900 per cubic millimeter (with an absolute neutrophil count of 200 per cubic millimeter), the hematocrit decreased to 20 percent, and the platelet count decreased to 75,000 per cubic millimeter. A bone marrow biopsy revealed normocellular marrow, which was negative for signs of cancer, infection with acid-fast bacilli, fungal infection, or other, atypical infections.

Bone marrow examination has value in establishing the diagnosis of an infection such as histoplasmosis or tuberculosis when there are abnormalities in the peripheral-blood count. The results must be interpreted cautiously in this situation, since immunosuppres-

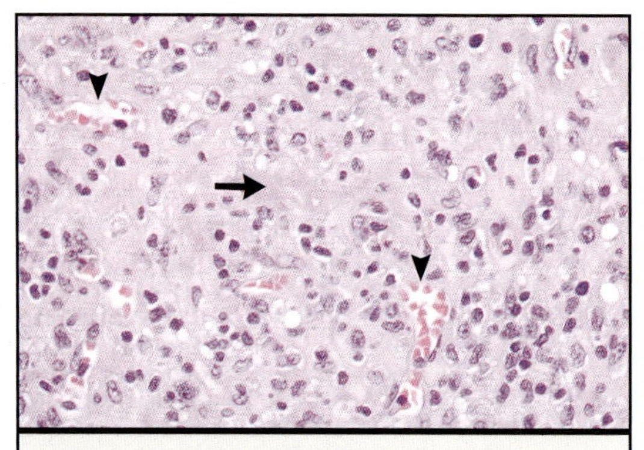

Figure 2. Biopsy Specimen of the Left Axillary Lymph Node, Showing Multiple Amorphous, Granular Deposits (Arrow) between and around Proliferated Blood Vessels (Arrowheads) (Hematoxylin and Eosin, ×40).

sive therapy may mask important histopathologic clues, particularly granulomas and lymphoid aggregates suggestive of lymphoproliferative disease.

Examination of a specimen obtained by core biopsy of the left axillary lymph node revealed vascular proliferation that appeared to be morphologically benign. However, the possibility of cancer could not be definitively ruled out because there was insufficient tissue for analysis.

The vascular proliferation seen in the lymph-node aspirate from the core-biopsy specimen must be pursued with an excisional lymph-node biopsy. The diagnoses suggested by the vascular proliferation are Kaposi's sarcoma, angioimmunoblastic lymphadenopathy, and bartonellosis. A larger specimen would be needed to demonstrate the typical findings in Kaposi's sarcoma, which would be slit-like vascular proliferation with extravasation of erythrocytes. When Kaposi's sarcoma involves the lymph nodes or other visceral organs, fever may be a prominent feature. In angioimmunoblastic lymphadenopathy, one of the atypical lymphoproliferative disorders that are often associated with viral oncogenesis, systemic symptoms are common. Finally, lymphatic involvement with bartonella should be easily demonstrable on examination of a lymph-node biopsy specimen if proper staining is done for the causative organism. Bartonellosis and disseminated Kaposi's sarcoma may be very difficult to distinguish without a biopsy, but I favor the former, given the patient's occupation and the relatively low probability of previous infection with human herpesvirus 8.

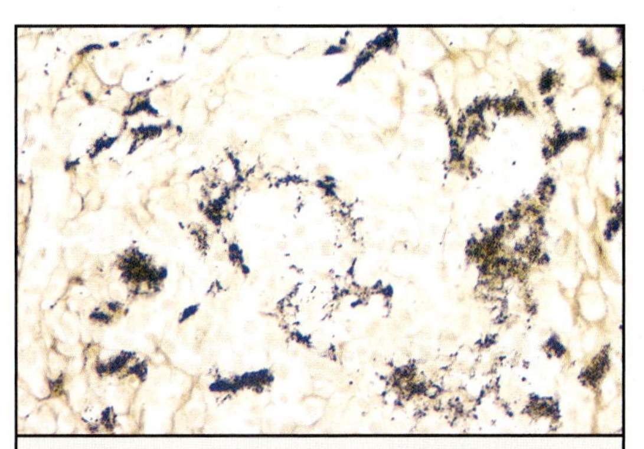

Figure 3. Biopsy Specimen of the Left Axillary Lymph Node Showing Dark, Granular Deposits (Warthin–Starry, x40).

The deposits are aggregates of rod-shaped bacteria.

An excisional biopsy of the patient's left axillary lymph node was performed. Pathological examination showed multiple coalescent nodules of proliferated blood vessels surrounded by amorphous, granular, eosinophilic deposits (Figure 2). A Warthin–Starry stain revealed the amorphous deposits to be aggregates of small, rod-shaped bacteria (Figure 3); the results of further study with special stains for acid-fast bacilli and fungi were negative. These findings were diagnostic of bacillary angiomatosis.

The patient remained persistently febrile until treatment with oral levofloxacin was initiated for bartonella infection. Repeated serologic testing for bartonella was performed, three weeks after the previous (negative) titers had been obtained. Whereas the IgM titers for both *B. henselae* and *B. quintana* remained normal (range, less than 1:20), the IgG titers for both species were now positive, at greater than 1:1024. Two weeks after antibiotic therapy was initiated, the patient reported that her symptoms had dissipated, and the lesion on her finger and the lymphadenopathy had almost resolved.

This case highlights the potential limitations of some diagnostic tests for opportunistic infections, particularly in immunosuppressed patients. Not only were the genomic and serologic evaluations extremely expensive, the PCR assay yielded a positive result (for polyomavirus) that was unrelated to the final diagnosis, and the initial serologic tests yielded a false negative result (for bartonella). Histologic and microbiologic examinations of clinically involved tissues may be warranted even when the results of serologic testing are negative.

COMMENTARY

Fever of unknown origin is defined as a temperature of 38.3°C or greater on several occasions over a period of more than three weeks, accompanied by an uncertain diagnosis after three days of inpatient investigation or three outpatient visits.[1] The majority of cases are caused by infections, tumors, and various noninfectious inflammatory diseases.[1,2] However, the spectrum of disease in immunocompromised patients who present with fever of unknown origin tends to include infections more often than other illnesses.[1] The increased risk of rapid clinical deterioration in immunocompromised patients underscores the importance of prompt diagnosis.[3] Errors in the processing of available information during the diagnostic evaluation can result in delays and missed diagnoses,[2,4] as occurred in the case under discussion.

The primary impediment to a more timely diagnosis in this case was the excessive reliance on noninvasive diagnostic tests rather than tissue biopsy for direct examination early in the presentation. As the discussant notes, the findings of an erythematous lesion on the left index finger and of ipsilateral axillary lymphadenopathy warranted directed evaluation. The negative results on the serologic tests markedly reduced the treating physicians' suspicion of bartonella infection and thus delayed biopsy and appropriate therapy.

Several aspects of the diagnostic challenge merit review. Undirected serologic and immunologic tests have poor predictive value for evaluating fever of unknown origin because of the low prevalence of the disorders for which they screen. Even with tests with high specificity, the rate of false positive results remains unacceptably high.[1] The positive PCR assay for BK virus provides an example of this general principle. Conversely, an example of the opposite phenomenon occurred in the search for bartonella infection (since there was a high pretest probability of the infection and a false negative test result).

Although they are commonly used to evaluate the possibility of bartonella infection,[5] serologic tests have variable sensitivities and specificities.[6,7] These discrepancies are probably related to differences in the available tests and to spectrum bias, which can occur when a diagnostic test is used in a patient who has characteristics different from those of the reference population in which the test characteristics were defined.[8] The discussant correctly emphasizes the low predictive value of serologic testing given that the patient's antibody response was probably blunted because of impaired T-cell function.[3,9] Although the results of blood cultures were also negative, the yield of this test is generally low.[10]

A PCR test is available for bartonella,[11] but it requires examination of tissue samples. In this case, PCR examination of the specimen from the core biopsy might have provided an earlier diagnosis. Repeated serologic testing after a reduction in the level of immunosuppression revealed a delayed antibody response, with elevated IgG titers. The diagnosis of bacillary angiomatosis often requires a biopsy of lesions and the subsequent detection of characteristic histopathological features or identification of the bacillus by Warthin–Starry staining or electron microscopy.[5]

Both *B. henselae* and *B. quintana* have been associated with cat scratch disease, bacillary angiomatosis, bacillary peliosis, splenitis, osteomyelitis, bacteremia, and endocarditis.[10,12,13] Whereas cat scratch disease most often affects healthy people, bacillary angiomatosis occurs predominantly in patients with the acquired immunodeficiency syndrome. Cases also have been described in organ-transplant recipients as well as in immunocompetent patients.[5,14] Exposure usually occurs through the scratch or bite of a cat.[13,15] This patient was probably exposed while working as a veterinary assistant.

Patients with bacillary angiomatosis often present with cutaneous or subcutaneous vascular proliferative lesions at the site of inoculation, as did this patient. These lesions can be difficult to distinguish clinically from those associated with Kaposi's sarcoma.[16] Extracutaneous lesions may involve bone, mucosal surfaces, the central nervous system, and even bone marrow,[5] providing a potential explanation for this patient's pancytopenia.[17] Although the blood cultures were sterile, a bacteremic syndrome probably accounts for this patient's insidious, prolonged constellation of symptoms.[5] In general, prompt treatment of bacillary angiomatosis may prevent the illness and death associated with progressive disease.[18]

Despite their early recognition of bartonella infection as a potential cause of this patient's fever of unknown origin, the physicians pursued a noninvasive investigation. Appropriate interpretation of negative serologic tests in an immunosuppressed patient requires that a high index of suspicion for probable causes be maintained.

Supported by a Career Development Award from the Health Services Research and Development Program of the Department of Veterans Affairs and a Patient Safety Developmental Center Grant from the Agency for Healthcare Research and Quality (P20-HS11540, to Dr. Saint).

We are indebted to Camilla Payne, R.N., for her careful review of an earlier draft of this manuscript; to Kamal Amin, M.D., for his generous provision of the photograph used in Figure 1; and to Riccardo Valdez, M.D., for his assistance with photomicrographs and pathologic interpretation.

This article first appeared in the May 6, 2004, issue of the New England Journal of Medicine.

REFERENCES

1.
Knockaert DC, Vanderschueren S, Blockmans D. Fever of unknown origin in adults: 40 years on. J Intern Med 2003;253:263-75.

2.
Arnow PM, Flaherty JP. Fever of unknown origin. Lancet 1997;350:575-80.

3.
Pizzo PA. Fever in immunocompromised patients. N Engl J Med 1999;341: 893-900.

4.
Kassirer JP, Kopelman RI. Cognitive errors in diagnosis: instantiation, classification, and consequences. Am J Med 1989;86:433-41.

5.
Adal KA, Cockerell CJ, Petri WA. Cat scratch disease, bacillary angiomatosis, and other infections due to Rochalimaea. N Engl J Med 1994;330:1509-15.

6.
Sander A, Posselt M, Oberle K, Bredt W. Seroprevalence of antibodies to Bartonella henselae in patients with cat scratch disease and in healthy controls: evaluation and comparison of two commercial serological tests. Clin Diagn Lab Immunol 1998;5:486-90.

7.
Bergmans AM, Peeters MF, Schellekens JF, et al. Pitfalls and fallacies of cat scratch disease serology: evaluation of Bartonella henselae-based indirect fluorescence assay and enzyme-linked immunoassay. J Clin Microbiol 1997;35:1931-7.

8.
Ransohoff DF, Feinstein AR. Problems of spectrum and bias in evaluating the efficacy of diagnostic tests. N Engl J Med 1978;299: 926-30.

9.
Denton MD, Magee CC, Sayegh MH. Immunosuppressive strategies in transplantation. Lancet 1999;353:1083-91.

10.
Cotell SL, Noskin GA. Bacillary angiomatosis: clinical and histologic features, diagnosis, and treatment. Arch Intern Med 1994;154: 524-8.

11.
Relman DA, Loutit JS, Schmidt TM, Falkow S, Tompkins LS. The agent of bacillary angiomatosis: an approach to the identification of uncultured pathogens. N Engl J Med 1990; 323:1573-80.

12.
Koehler JE, Quinn FD, Berger TG, LeBoit PE, Tappero JW. Isolation of Rochalimaea species from cutaneous and osseous lesions of bacillary angiomatosis. N Engl J Med 1992;327: 1625-31.

13.
Zangwill KM, Hamilton DH, Perkins BA, et al. Cat scratch disease in Connecticut: epidemiology, risk factors, and evaluation of a new diagnostic test. N Engl J Med 1993; 329:8-13.

14.
Cline MS, Cummings OW, Goldman M, Filo RS, Pescovitz MD. Bacillary angiomatosis in a renal transplant recipient. Transplantation 1999;67:296-8.

15.
Tappero JW, Mohle-Boetani J, Koehler JE, et al. The epidemiology of bacillary angiomatosis and bacillary peliosis. JAMA 1993;269: 770-5.

16.
Tappero JW, Koehler JE. Bacillary angiomatosis or Kaposi's sarcoma? N Engl J Med 1997;337:1888.

17.
Kiriakos J, Ranchin B, Gillet Y, et al. Systemic bacillary angiomatosis after kidney transplantation. Pediatr Nephrol 2003;18:C46. abstract.

18.
van der Wouw PA, Hadderingh RJ, Reiss P, Hulsebosch HJ, Walford N, Lange JM. Disseminated cat-scratch disease in a patient with AIDS. AIDS 1989;3:751-3.

Forgotten but Not Gone

ASHISH K. JHA, M.D., KAVEH G. SHOJANIA, M.D.,
AND SANJAY SAINT, M.D., M.P.H.

A 74-year-old man was brought to the emergency department after being found confused and incapacitated at home. The patient lived in a residential hotel and had previously been healthy and socially active. Having not seen him for three days, his friends entered his room and found him on the floor, covered in stool. The patient was conversant but confused, recalling only a recent fall and his inability to get up.

Causes of acute alteration in mental status fall primarily into four categories: infectious, neurologic, drug-related, and metabolic. In elderly patients, infections are the most common cause, although the other causes remain frequent enough to be pursued just as assiduously. Neurologic causes include hemorrhagic and nonhemorrhagic stroke, seizures, and subdural hematoma. Medications such as sedatives and opiates commonly cause confusion. Metabolic disturbances include alcohol withdrawal, sodium disorders, hyperosmolar coma, and uremia. Other conditions, such as acute myocardial infarction or an intraabdominal infection, can develop atypically in the elderly, predominantly with confusion as the main finding.

The patient's conversation was tangential. He reported fatigue, diffuse weakness, and a minimally productive cough of four days' duration. He reported that he had no previous medical problems and had not sought medical care for many years; that he took no regular medications; and that he had not traveled outside the United States in more than 30 years. He had quit smoking 15 years earlier and reported no serious alcohol or illicit-drug use.

Pneumonia is now my leading diagnosis. Elements of the clinical assessment do not indicate which type of pneumonia, although *Streptococcus pneumoniae* is probably the leading cause of severe community-acquired pneumonia. Pneumococcal pneumonia could certainly account for the patient's confusion, even without overt bacteremia. Lung cancer presenting as postobstructive pneumonia is possible, given his smoking history, as is cancer-induced hypercalcemia. An acute exacerbation of chronic bronchitis is unlikely to present in this manner.

On physical examination, the patient was disheveled but in no acute distress. He was afebrile with a heart rate of 103, a respiratory rate of 16 breaths per minute, a blood pressure of 145/72 mm Hg, and an oxygen saturation of 95 percent breathing room air. He had mildly icteric sclera and several missing front teeth; the remainder of the examination of his head was normal. His neck was supple without evidence of meningeal irritation. He had occasional inspiratory crackles in the lower left lung field, and the cardiac examination revealed a 2/6 early systolic murmur at the lower left sternal border that did not change with inspiration. His abdomen was soft without tenderness or hepatosplenomegaly. Bowel sounds were present. The rectal examination revealed guaiac-positive brown stool. Motor strength was 4/5 in the upper and lower extremities bilaterally. The sensory examination was normal, with symmetric reflexes in the upper and lower extremities. The patient could recall his name and where he lived but did not know the name of the hospital, the date, or the year. He was able to recall only one of three objects mentioned.

The patient's vital signs and lung findings are consistent with the presence of pneumonia, but the icterus adds additional possibilities. Though the patient reported that he did not drink heavily, his appearance obliges us to consider the possibility of alcoholic liver disease, complicated by pneumonia and hepatic encephalopathy. We should also consider other causes of jaundice. Acute viral hepatitis seems unlikely without recent exposure risks. Cholecystitis or gallstone pancreatitis could cause icterus, but he reported no abdominal pain. Hemolytic causes of jaundice, including unrecognized chronic lymphocytic leukemia, should be considered. Given the presence of a heart murmur, endocarditis is possible. Nevertheless, community-acquired pneumonia remains the most likely diagnosis.

Laboratory tests revealed a white-cell count of 8300 per cubic millimeter, a hematocrit of 43 percent with a mean corpuscular volume of 89.5 μm3, and a platelet count of 69,000 per cubic millimeter. The serum sodium concentration was 132 mmol per liter, and the serum calcium concentration was 8.1 mg per deciliter (2.0 mmol per liter); other serum electrolyte levels were normal. The results of other laboratory tests were as follows: blood urea nitrogen, 31 mg per deciliter (11.1 mmol per liter); aspartate aminotransferase, 256 U per liter; alanine aminotransferase, 77 U per liter; alkaline phosphatase, 214 U per liter; total bilirubin, 6.2 mg per deciliter (106.0 μmol per liter); direct bilirubin, 3.5 mg per deciliter (59.8 μmol per liter); and creatine kinase, 26 U per liter. His albumin level was 1.9 g per deciliter, and the prothrombin time was 13.4 seconds (international normalized ratio, 1.2). The partial-thromboplastin time was elevated, at 37.9 seconds. Other than revealing

tachycardia, his electrocardiogram was normal. A chest radiograph obtained with portable equipment revealed slight haziness in the left lower lobe with clearly visible borders of the left heart and diaphragm — findings that are most consistent with the presence of atelectasis. Radiographs of his hips and lower extremities revealed no fractures. Two sets of blood cultures were performed.

Despite the patient's denial of excessive alcohol use, it is increasingly difficult to discount the possibility of cirrhosis. The levels of aspartate aminotransferase and alanine aminotransferase in combination with thrombocytopenia (not to mention the several missing teeth) all suggest the possibility of alcoholic cirrhosis. Acute causes of liver injury seem less likely, as they would leave unexplained the low albumin level, and the history was not consistent with chronic malnutrition. Given the hyperbilirubinemia, I would also consider cholestatic processes, especially cancer of the gallbladder or pancreas. Intrahepatic causes of cholestasis are possible, including infiltrative disorders (e.g., sarcoidosis or amyloidosis), infections (e.g., abscess or tuberculosis), and metastatic carcinoma.

Regardless of the underlying problem, an acute event has also occurred. Given the patient's age, the absence of fever does not diminish my concern about infection; this remains the most likely cause. Although the findings on the chest radiograph appear to be consistent with atelectasis, pneumonia is a reasonable diagnosis. At this point, I would err on the side of administering empirical antibiotics to provide coverage for common bacterial causes of pneumonia and for an abdominal infection such as cholangitis. I would obtain a measurement of the serum ammonia level to see whether hepatic encephalopathy may account for the patient's delirium.

The patient was admitted with a diagnosis of dehydration and possible community-acquired pneumonia and was treated with intravenous saline, intravenous cefuroxime, and oral doxycycline. He was given thiamine and folate. On the second hospital day, the patient's clinical condition improved. He was conversant, interactive, and lucid. He could identify the month and year and stated that he felt better. On the third hospital day, the patient became tachypneic, and his mental status worsened. By the end of the third hospital day, he was unresponsive and required supplemental oxygen to maintain the blood oxygen saturation above 92 percent. A second chest radiograph revealed bilateral patchy opacities (Figure 1). Arterial-blood gas analysis revealed a partial pressure of oxygen of 70 mm Hg, a partial pressure of carbon dioxide of 32 mm Hg, and a pH of 7.38 while the patient was breathing 6 liters of oxygen through a nasal cannula. A computed tomographic (CT) scan of the head, obtained without the administration of contrast material, was nor-

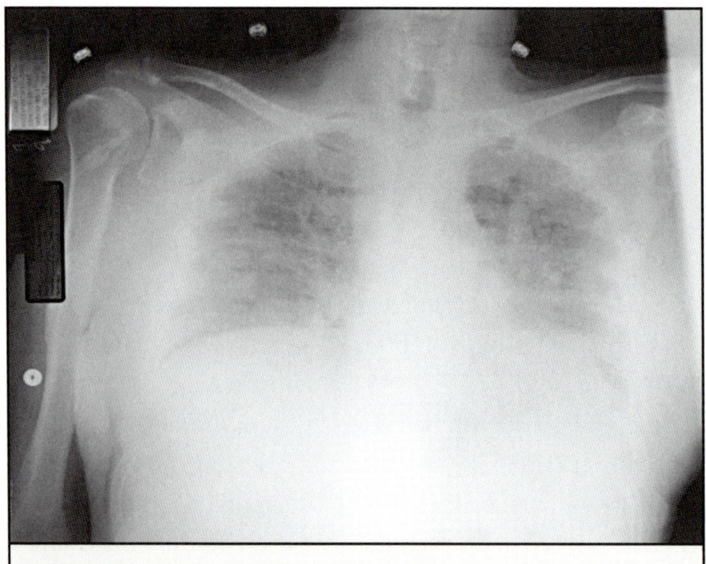

Figure 1. Chest Radiograph Obtained on the Third Hospital Day, Showing Bilateral Patchy Opacities.

mal except for the finding of multiple small old infarcts that were consistent with hypertensive disease. Blood cultures showed no growth of any organisms. Intravenous fluids were stopped, and the patient was given intravenous furosemide for presumed pulmonary edema. His mental status worsened.

Although empirical treatment for pneumonia was reasonable, the possible hepatobiliary problem seems to have been largely ignored. Abdominal imaging to evaluate the liver, biliary tract, portal vein, and pancreas remains important. What about the lungs? Lack of improvement for 24 to 48 hours is possible with uncomplicated community-acquired pneumonia, but improvement followed by worsening is a reason for concern. One possibility is that though he has pneumonia, the organism is resistant to the antibiotics administered. Another possibility is that the primary problem is delirium and that he has aspirated and now has chemical pneumonitis or a new pneumonia. Finally, one must consider the possibility that the patient mistakenly did not receive his antibiotics.

Instead of pneumonia, the patient may have cardiogenic or noncardiogenic pulmonary edema. Given his murmur, it is possible that he has valvular heart disease or alcoholic cardiomyopathy. Right-sided endocarditis with septic emboli to the lungs is unlikely unless he uses injection drugs. Also, the murmur's characteristics are not suggestive of tricuspid regurgitation, and the negative blood cultures to date are reassuring. The patchy infiltrates on his chest radiograph may represent acute respiratory distress syndrome due to worsening sepsis rather than pneumonia. The cause of the sepsis may be an intraabdominal infection (e.g., cholangitis) that responded partially to the treatment for community-acquired pneumonia but has now progressed.

On the fourth hospital day, the patient's condition worsened, with a body temperature of 35.4°C, a respiratory rate of 24 breaths per minute, a pulse of 120 beats per minute, and a blood pressure of 85/50 mm Hg. Worsening hypoxemia necessitated intubation and transfer to the intensive care unit, where a third chest radiograph showed increased patchy infiltrates bilaterally. Multiple cultures of blood and urine were performed, and a test for the human immunodeficiency virus (HIV) was obtained. His antibiotic regimen was changed to include piperacillin–tazobactam and gentamicin. Pulmonary-artery catheterization revealed a cardiac index of more than 5 liters per minute per square meter of body-surface area, a systemic vascular resistance of less than 300 dyn • sec • cm^{-5}, and a pulmonary-capillary wedge pressure of 15 mm Hg.

Although hepatic dysfunction can cause hypotension, we must assume that the patient has sepsis on the basis of his hemodynamic measurements and hypothermia. The patient either has pneumonia as the cause of these infiltrates with sepsis secondary to pneumonia or has some other cause of sepsis (probably an intraabdominal cause) with pulmonary edema. Pneumonia has been the leading diagnosis from the start and remains so, with an increasing likelihood of a resistant organism. Thus, while I agree with broadening the antibiotic coverage, vancomycin is also indicated for penicillin-resistant pneumococcal infection. I am also concerned about legionella infection, given his nonproductive cough, hyponatremia, and poor response to β-lactam antibiotics and aminoglycosides. Tuberculosis or a fungal infection seems unlikely, given the acute presentation and brief improvement with cefuroxime and doxycycline.

To look for other possible sources of sepsis, I would order an abdominal CT scan and an echocardiogram. One additional possibility is adrenal insufficiency, which may complicate critical illness. In this patient with hypotension, hypothermia, and hyponatremia, I would perform a corticotropin stimulation test or consider measuring the cortisol level in a random serum specimen, but would initiate empirical treatment with corticosteroids while awaiting the result.

The patient remained hypotensive, despite the use of dopamine and phenylephrine hydrochloride, and hypoxemic, despite 100 percent inspired oxygen delivered by a ventilator. All

blood and urine cultures and the HIV test were negative. An echocardiogram was notable only for hyperdynamic left ventricular function, without wall-motion abnormalities. Abdominal ultrasonography revealed a thickened gallbladder wall with pericholecystic fluid but no stones and normal hepatic and biliary ducts. Further radiographic studies or bronchoscopy was not performed, because of the patient's unstable clinical condition. His hemoglobin level decreased to 6 g per deciliter. He passed large amounts of black stool that were guaiac-positive. His blood pressure continued to drop, despite aggressive fluid support and use of vasopressor medications. The patient died on the sixth hospital day. An autopsy was performed.

The patient's subsequent deterioration did not undermine the initial diagnosis of pneumonia but shifted concern to a resistant organism — penicillin-resistant *Streptococcus pneumoniae,* multidrug-resistant *Haemophilus influenzae, Pseudomonas aeruginosa,* or legionella. The tempo of the illness still seemed quick for tuberculosis or fungal infection. I expect the autopsy to reveal pneumonia and hope that tissue cultures identify the organism.

The autopsy revealed a normal gallbladder and bile ducts and a slightly enlarged liver with micronodular cirrhosis. Evidence of a previous myocardial infarction, congestive hepatopathy, and diffuse alveolar damage with pulmonary edema and hyaline membranes were present. There was blood in the stomach and small bowel. Pathological specimens from the lungs (Figure 2A), mediastinal lymph nodes (Figure 2B), liver, and kidney showed necrotizing granulomas, with acid-fast bacilli appreciable in some specimens, a finding that is diagnostic of systemic tuberculosis infection. Both adrenal glands had extensive involvement of necrotizing granulomas as well (Figure 2C). Examination of the brain and spinal cord revealed no acute abnormalities. Two physicians involved in the patient's care subsequently had positive tests with purified protein derivative for mycobacterium exposure. Their chest radiographs were normal, and they received six months of prophylactic therapy.

COMMENTARY

Although the severe acute respiratory syndrome (SARS), West Nile virus infection, anthrax, and infections with various poxviruses are claiming the attention of patients and physicians, tuberculosis remains a major cause of morbidity throughout the world. In 2002, tuberculosis was responsible for more than 2 million deaths worldwide[1] and, in 2001, more than 15,000 infections in the United States.[2] However, if tuberculosis is not consid-

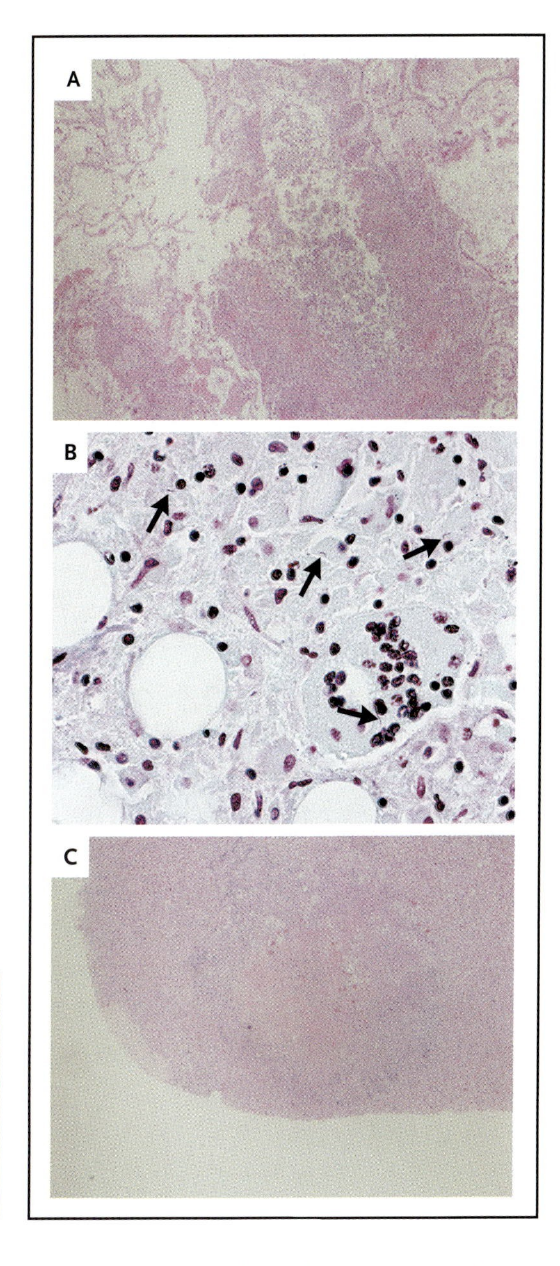

Figure 2. Tissue Specimens Obtained at Autopsy from the Patient.

Specimens from the lung (Panel A, hematoxylin and eosin, ×40) and adrenal gland (Panel C, hematoxylin and eosin, ×40) contain multiple caseating granulomas. A specimen from a mediastinal lymph node (Panel B, acid-fast stain, ×400) contains acid-fast bacilli (arrows).

ered, it will not be diagnosed. In retrospect, the diagnosis of tuberculosis warranted consideration in a marginally housed, elderly man with probable chronic liver disease. As the discussant points out, the lack of response to the initial antibacterial therapy also indicated the need for further consideration of atypical infections, among them tuberculosis.

This diagnosis, however, was far from straightforward. The original presentation did not obviously indicate tuberculosis. Clinicians often try to find simple explanations to expedite the evaluation and care of elderly patients found incapacitated.[3] Here, the clinicians considered common causes, such as urinary tract infection, pneumonia, electrolyte abnormalities, and cardiovascular events, and treated the patient empirically for a bacterial pneumonia. In one study of patients who were found helpless or dead in their homes, one out of three patients had an infection.[3] Neurologic events and cardiac disorders were the next most likely causes of being found in this state. Unless the cause is obvious, all these possibilities should be evaluated. Aside from pneumonia, other causes, including a neurologic event, warranted greater attention in this case. Early evaluation of hepatic encephalopathy, stroke, or a central nervous system infection (due to subacute meningitis, for example) would have been appropriate though unlikely to lead to the correct antemortem diagnosis.

Initially, the patient's condition seemed to improve. Dehydration and malnutrition can complicate many disease processes, especially infections, and correction of these problems can result in apparent improvement, while the underlying cause remains untreated. Such improvements should not curtail the evaluation of other diagnoses. As noted by the discussant, adrenal insufficiency warranted consideration when the patient remained hypotensive. The threshold for evaluating and empirically treating adrenal insufficiency in critically ill patients should be low, given an incidence as high as 40 percent in this population.[4] Although cortisol levels were not measured, the diffuse involvement of the adrenal glands that was apparent at autopsy suggests that adrenal insufficiency due to tuberculosis probably complicated the patient's illness. Tuberculosis remains an important cause of primary adrenal insufficiency.[5]

This case highlights the value of autopsy. Unfortunately, the autopsy rate continues to decline in the United States; in 1994, the most recent year for which figures are available, autopsies were performed after only 6 percent of deaths in nonforensic cases.[6] Yet there continues to be a large discrepancy between clinical diagnoses and autopsy findings, with a median major-error rate of 24 percent.[6] Without an autopsy, the patient's clinicians would have neither recognized their exposure to tuberculosis nor had the opportunity to learn in order to improve the care of future patients. The possibility that an autopsy will unearth important clinical information is sufficiently high that initiatives to improve autopsy rates are needed.

Finally, it is important to remember that tuberculosis has varying clinical manifestations, especially when infection is widely disseminated. The discussant considered but rejected tuberculosis as a diagnosis, because the clinical course was too quick. Although miliary tuberculosis commonly has a subacute presentation,[7,8] it may be manifested as a syndrome of rapidly progressing multiorgan dysfunction with sepsis[9,10] or as the acute respiratory distress syndrome.[11,12] Miliary tuberculosis is more common among immunocompromised patients, including those with the acquired immunodeficiency syndrome, children under the age of five years, and the elderly. The mortality associated with miliary tuberculosis approaches 50 percent. Because miliary tuberculosis reflects hematogenous spread of the mycobacterium, it typically affects multiple organs (e.g., the liver, spleen, and adrenal glands), with central nervous system involvement in up to 20 percent of patients.[7,8] Though miliary tuberculosis derives its name from the tiny, discrete granulomas resembling millet seeds seen on chest radiography, the chest radiograph is interpreted as normal in approximately 40 percent of cases.[13] Transmission to others is uncommon but may have occurred in this case.

Although not as headline-grabbing as SARS or West Nile virus infection, tuberculosis remains a major cause of morbidity and mortality throughout the world and in the United States. With rising numbers of elderly people and the increasing rate of chronic immunosuppression, clinicians should consider the possibility of tuberculosis even if the clinical manifestations and presentation are atypical.

Supported by a National Research Service Award from the Agency for Healthcare Research and Quality (to Dr. Jha) and a Career Development Award from the Health Services Research and Development Program of the Department of Veterans Affairs and a Patient Safety Developmental Center Grant (P20HS11540) from the Agency for Healthcare Research and Quality (both to Dr. Saint).

We are indebted to Henry Holdt for his critical aid in obtaining pathological and radiologic data.

This article first appeared in the June 3, 2004, issue of the New England Journal of Medicine.

REFERENCES

1. Tuberculosis. Fact sheet no. 104. Rev. Geneva: World Health Organization, August 2002.

2. Reported tuberculosis in the United States, 2001. Atlanta: Centers for Disease Control and Prevention, September 2002.

3. Gurley RJ, Lum N, Sande M, Lo B, Katz MH. Persons found in their homes helpless or dead. N Engl J Med 1996;334:1710-6.

4. Marik PE, Zaloga GP. Adrenal insufficiency during septic shock. Crit Care Med 2003;31:141-5.

5. Oelkers W. Adrenal insufficiency. N Engl J Med 1996; 335:1206-12.

6. Shojania KG, Burton EC, McDonald KM, Goldman L. Changes in rates of autopsy-detected diagnostic errors over time: a systematic review. JAMA 2003;289: 2849-56.

7. Maartens G, Willcox PA, Benatar SR. Miliary tuberculosis: rapid diagnosis, hematologic abnormalities, and outcome in 109 treated adults. Am J Med 1990;89: 291-6.

8. Kim JH, Langston AA, Gallis HA. Miliary tuberculosis: epidemiology, clinical manifestations, diagnosis, and outcome. Rev Infect Dis 1990;12:583-90.

9. Ahuja SS, Ahuja SK, Phelps KR, Thelmo W, Hill AR. Hemodynamic confirmation of septic shock in disseminated tuberculosis. Crit Care Med 1992;20: 901-3.

10. George S, Papa L, Sheils L, Magnussen CR. Septic shock due to disseminated tuberculosis. Clin Infect Dis 1996; 22:188-9.

11. Dyer RA, Chappell WA, Potgieter PD. Adult respiratory distress syndrome associated with miliary tuberculosis. Crit Care Med 1985;13:12-5.

12. Heffner JE, Strange C, Sahn SA. The impact of respiratory failure on the diagnosis of tuberculosis. Arch Intern Med 1988;148: 1103-8.

13. Kwong JS, Carignan S, Kang EY, Muller NL, FitzGerald JM. Miliary tuberculosis: diagnostic accuracy of chest radiography. Chest 1996;110:339-42.

A Twist of Fate?

MICHAEL D. CHRISTIAN, M.D., AND ALLAN S. DETSKY, M.D., PH.D.

A 39-year-old Sri Lankan male physiotherapist presented to an emergency department in Toronto with a three-day history of headache, chills, diarrhea, nausea, vomiting, and neck stiffness. He reported having had vertigo, left-sided facial paresthesia, incoordination, and dysarthria, which had lasted for several minutes at the onset of his illness. These symptoms disappeared and were followed by the other symptoms noted above. His history was significant only for type 2 diabetes mellitus and chronic neck symptoms following a motor vehicle collision seven years earlier.

The patient reported that his symptoms had begun shortly after he had eaten a dorado fish that was freshly caught and imported from the Dominican Republic by his brother. He was worried about possible poisoning due to "red tide," a contamination of water by toxic algae.

The dorado fish, along with other species of fish from the Caribbean, has been associated with ciguatera poisoning. Although at first glance this may seem unlikely in an urban center in North America, such poisoning is possible outside of regions where ciguatera is endemic if fish that have been contaminated with ciguatoxin are exported or are eaten locally by travelers who then return home. During the past decade, we have seen several cases of this disorder per year at the hospital where the patient presented. The hospital is situated near a large fresh-food market.

The patient has some symptoms that are consistent with ciguatera poisoning, including paresthesia beginning in the face, headache, vertigo, incoordination, diarrhea, nausea, and vomiting. However, other findings make this diagnosis unlikely. Among those findings is the transient nature of the paresthesia. Although the gastrointestinal manifestations of ciguatera may resolve within hours, the neurologic manifestations tend to last for a minimum of several days. The lateralization of the neurologic symptoms is also inconsistent with ciguatera poisoning and raises concern about a focal lesion in the central nervous system that could have been caused by a stroke, a tumor, or an abscess.

The patient's brother was contacted. He confirmed that the fish had been caught the day before its consumption. He had transported it on ice by airplane to Toronto, where he was

visiting family. A physician who was contacted in the Dominican Republic reported that the algae containing ciguatoxin were not in bloom at that time.

While the report that algae were not in bloom does not complately rule out ciguatera poisoning (large fish can accumulate the toxin over time), the constellation of signs and symptoms (and their duration) make this diagnosis unlikely. (See addendum.)

On examination, the patient appeared acutely ill, with a dazed appearance, a heart rate of 96 beats per minute, a respiratory rate of 14 breaths per minute, a blood pressure of 124/80 mm Hg, and a temperature of 35.8°C. The neurologic examination was normal except that the patient was drowsy and had a sustained horizontal nystagmus on leftward gaze. His neck was supple and was negative for Kernig's and Brudzinski's signs. The remainder of the physical examination was normal. The results of initial laboratory tests were as follows: hemoglobin level, 15.2 g per deciliter; white-cell count, 13,100 per cubic millimeter (neutrophilia); platelet count, 267,000 per cubic millimeter; and normal levels of electrolytes, creatinine, glucose, and prothrombin and a normal partial-thromboplastin time.

The combination of acute headache and neck pain with focal neurologic symptoms initially suggests a primary neurologic disorder. The diagnoses that come to mind first are the stroke syndrome, migraine headache, and infections of the central nervous system.

While the patient was in the emergency department, his temperature increased to 38.0°C.

The presence of fever, headache, and drowsiness arouses concern about the possibility of meningoencephalitis. Although I would want to evaluate the patient for infection as quickly as possible, the history of paresthesia, dysarthria, and incoordination at the onset of the illness, plus nystagmus when the patient was examined, calls for neuroimaging studies to rule out a mass lesion before a lumbar puncture is performed. Computed tomographic (CT) scanning would be reasonable to rule out a mass lesion; if no mass effect is found, a lumbar puncture should be performed. The presence of transient focal neurologic deficits provides a rationale for ordering magnetic resonance imaging (MRI) of the brain if the CT scan and lumbar puncture fail to explain the symptoms and signs. MRI is more sensitive than CT for detecting strokes and abnormalities associated with infectious meningoencephalitis.

CT scanning of the head showed no evidence of a space-occupying lesion or an intracranial hemorrhage. An emergency room physician then performed a lumbar puncture, which was uncomplicated and successful on the first attempt. Analysis of the clear and colorless cerebrospinal fluid revealed the following values: in the first tube, 197 leukocytes per cubic millimeter and 7690 erythrocytes per cubic millimeter; in the fourth tube, 237 leukocytes per cubic millimeter (90 percent of which were neutrophils), 4700 erythrocytes per cubic millimeter, 181 mg of protein per deciliter, and 124 mg of glucose per deciliter (6.9 mmol per liter); the serum glucose level was 162 mg per deciliter (9.0 mmol per liter). Staining was negative for bacteria, acid-fast bacilli, and yeast. A rapid latex-agglutination test for cryptococcal antigen was negative.

The elevated red-cell count in the cerebrospinal fluid is probably not an indication of a subarachnoid hemorrhage, given the marked fall in the erythrocyte count between the first and fourth tubes and the absence of xanthochromia. Even though the lumbar puncture was reported as uncomplicated, it was most likely traumatic. The leukocyte count can be elevated with traumatic lumbar puncture, but the ratio of the white-cell count to the red-cell count should be no more than 1:500 in this setting. In the fourth tube, the ratio of the white-cell count to the red-cell count was 1:20, suggesting there is a true leukocytosis. Faced with a fever and leukocytosis in the cerebrospinal fluid, with a high proportion of neutrophils, the first consideration is always bacterial meningitis. However, that diagnosis is unlikely in this case since I would expect the white-cell count in the cerebrospinal fluid to be higher and the glucose level lower, and that, after 72 hours of illness, the patient would be more severely ill. The negative results of Gram's staining are not particularly helpful, given its low sensitivity. Although bacterial meningitis is unlikely, a negative culture is required to exclude the possibility in this case. Viral meningoencephalitis can also cause fever and an elevated white-cell count in the cerebrospinal fluid, but again that diagnosis does not fit well with the findings in this case. Typically, the leukocytosis in the cerebrospinal fluid will have a lymphocytic predominance in viral infections. A final consideration with respect to infectious agents is mycobacterial meningitis, which can also cause focal neurologic symptoms. In the small proportion of patients who present with acute tuberculous meningitis, the findings in the cerebrospinal fluid may include a neutrophil-predominant leukocytosis, often with a count above 1000 per cubic millimeter. However, most patients with tuberculous meningitis present with a longer duration of symptoms and a leukocytosis with a lymphocytic predominance.

While awaiting the results of the cerebrospinal fluid cultures, I would administer broad-spectrum antibiotics to cover meningococcus, pneumococcus, *Haemophilus influen-*

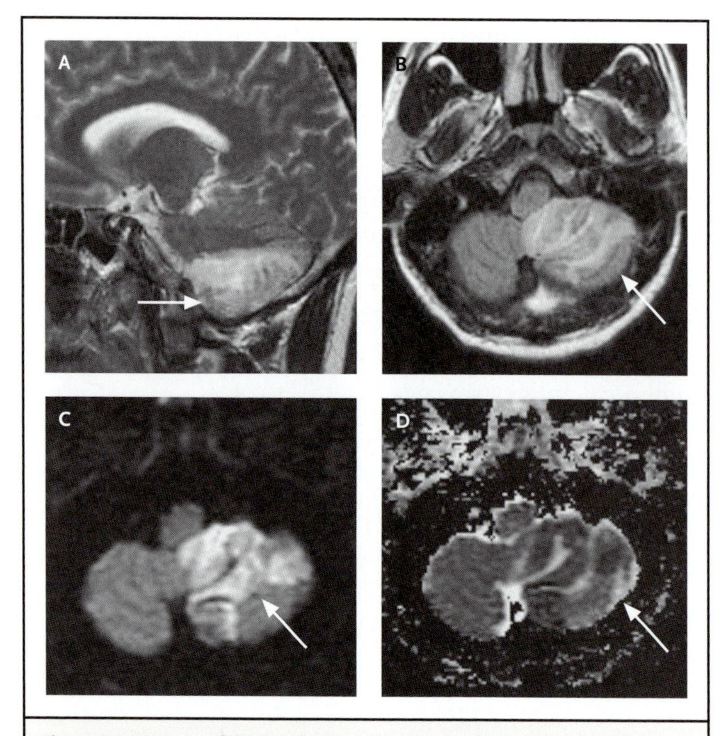

Figure 1. MRI Scan of the Cerebellum Showing Increased Signal Intensity in the Left Cerebellar Hemisphere.

Acute infarction in the territory of the left posteroinferior cerebellar artery is evident in the sagittal T_2-weighted view (Panel A, arrow), the axial view obtained with a fluid-attenuated inversion recovery (FLAIR) sequence (Panel B, arrow), an axial diffusion-weighted image (Panel C, arrow), and an apparent-diffusion-coefficient image (Panel D, arrow).

zae, and listeria. I would also administer acyclovir to cover meningoencephalitis caused by herpes simplex virus.

Treatment was started with cefotaxime (2 g given intravenously every 6 hours), vancomycin (1 g given intravenously every 12 hours), and acyclovir (700 mg given intravenously every 8 hours).

When questioned further about other antecedent events, the patient reported that several hours before the onset of his symptoms, one of his patients (who may have been a retired chiropractor) had manipulated his neck in an attempt to alleviate his chronic neck pain. On the basis of his description, the manipulation appeared to involve a high-velocity rotary movement.

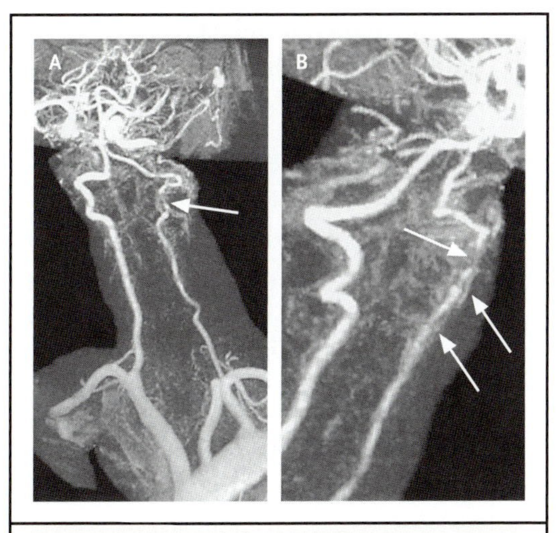

Figure 2. Magnetic Resonance Angiogram Showing Vertebral-Artery Dissection.

Irregular stenotic segments — a finding consistent with the diagnosis of arterial dissection — can be seen within the distal left vertebral artery in the left anterior oblique view (Panel A, arrow) and the magnified right anterior oblique view (Panel B, arrows). Both images were obtained with the use of an autotriggered gadolinium-enhanced technique. The cervical carotid arteries have been eliminated from the image.

This new information makes me consider the possibility of a vertebral-artery dissection that resulted in a stroke (either ischemic or hemorrhagic). If the stroke occurred in the cerebellum or brain stem, it could explain the patient's nausea and vomiting on presentation. Ischemic events may also cause fever and abnormalities in the cerebrospinal fluid. The increase in both the neutrophil count and the protein level and the normal glucose level are consistent with the inflammatory and repair processes that have been reported after a stroke. Even though the CT scan did not show a hemorrhage or an infarct, MRI (and possibly magnetic resonance angiography) is warranted, since it is more sensitive than CT is for revealing small strokes and dissection. MRI will also be useful in evaluating the patient for the possibility of certain infections, such as herpes simplex virus, in which inflammation and hemorrhage of the temporal lobe can be found, or meningitis, in which MRI shows enhancement and thickening of the leptomeninges (especially around the cranial nerves), increased fluid in the subarachnoid space, local venous thrombi, or edema of the adjacent brain. These findings associated with meningoencephalitis may be seen on a CT scan but are usually more evident on an MRI scan.

MRI of the brain showed an abnormality in the left cerebellar hemisphere. However, the study was considered nondiagnostic since the images were of poor quality due to movement artifact. Another scan was obtained (Figure 1) in conjunction with three-dimensional magnetic resonance angiography (Figure 2). This study showed increased signal intensity on T_2-weighted images, with enhancement after the administration of contrast material, in the posteroinferior arterial territory of the left cerebellar hemisphere. The magnetic resonance angiogram showed irregularities in the left vertebral artery at the C1–2 level, which is consistent with vertebral-artery dissection; there was no evidence of hemorrhage. All the cultures were negative, as were polymerase-chain-reaction assays of the cerebrospinal fluid for herpes simplex virus, cytomegalovirus, and *Mycobacterium tuberculosis*; a test for serum antibodies against human immunodeficiency virus types 1 and 2; and serologic Venereal Disease Research Laboratory tests for syphilis.

Given the MRI results showing vertebral-artery dissection and the negative results on investigations for infection, I would discontinue all antimicrobial agents and initiate anticoagulation.

Warfarin was administered, and the patient's condition improved, with complete resolution of his fever, nausea, vomiting, and diarrhea. He was discharged with a plan for warfarin to be discontinued after three months if repeated magnetic resonance angiography showed a normal vertebral artery and reestablishment of normal blood flow.

COMMENTARY

In this case, the patient's initial presentation included nausea, vomiting, and transient neurologic symptoms. His rapidly increasing fever and the cerebrospinal fluid abnormalities confused the clinical picture. Since the patient had recently eaten a dorado fish, he was concerned about ciguatera poisoning,[1-4] but this proved to be a red herring. When considering diagnostic possibilities, clinicians must first consider those that have serious consequences if left untreated. However, clinicians must also attend to the patient's concerns. In this case, the pattern and time course of signs and symptoms ruled out the diagnosis that was his primary concern. (See addendum.)

The diagnosis of vertebral-artery dissection could have been made earlier if MRI had been performed initially instead of CT. However, the decision regarding which neuroimaging technique to use is neither easy nor without controversy. The American College of Emergency Physicians recently considered the question about choice of neuroimaging when it was developing its guidelines for the management of acute headaches.[5] After carefully considering the evidence, the group recommended CT without the administration of contrast material for patients with acute headaches and neurologic symptoms. In addition, CT is more sensitive than MRI for detecting hemorrhage in the central nervous system. On a practical level, in many emergency departments such as ours, CT is more readily available and faster to perform than MRI is, and unlike MRI, CT can be used in patients who have metal or implantable devices in their bodies and can be performed more easily in patients who have claustrophobia. These are important considerations, given that time is of the essence when considering a diagnosis of bacterial meningitis. Whereas CT is more sensitive for the detection of acute hemorrhage, MRI provides more detailed images of the brain and may detect strokes and other conditions that are missed by CT, including signs of meningoencephalitis, which was a serious concern in this case. In the end, it seems reasonable to start with CT in order to rule out contraindications for lumbar puncture and then move to MRI if further information is required to explain the focal neurologic deficits.[5]

Several aspects of this case made it difficult to arrive at a diagnosis immediately. The first was the patient's concern about the possibility of ciguatera poisoning. Although a diagnosis of vertebral-artery dissection would account for fever, nausea, and vomiting, it would not account for diarrhea and chills.

Once the history of neck manipulation came to light, stroke caused by vertebral-artery dissection became an important consideration. Since the CT scan was negative, there was an urgent indication for MRI followed by magnetic resonance angiography, with its increased sensitivity for detecting infarcts and vertebral-artery dissection.[6,7]

Because of their anatomy, the vertebral arteries are particularly susceptible to injury resulting from head or neck torsion. When dissection occurs, the initial symptoms of neck pain and headache are caused by the direct trauma to the arteries. Subsequently, focal neurologic symptoms may develop as a result of ischemic injury to the cerebellum or brain stem from arterial occlusion by the intimal flap or artery-to-artery thromboembolism.[6] The hallmark symptoms are neck pain and headache, which occur in 47 to 79 percent of cases.[8,9] Patients tend to describe the headache as very severe, sharp, one-sided, and radiating from the neck,[6] and as being different from any other pain they have experienced. The onset of neck pain or headache typically precedes the development of neurologic symptoms. The delay before the neurologic symptoms and signs develop is usually less than 24 hours[6,8,9] but may range from several minutes to two months. Symptoms and signs reflect the territory of the brain involved, such as a lateral medullary stroke (i.e., Wallenberg's syndrome) or cerebellar stroke, and include vertigo, nausea, vomiting, diplopia, tinnitus, dysarthria, dysphagia, and hemiparesthesia. In the present case, nausea, vomiting, and nystagmus were consistent with infarction of the cerebellum.

In this case, the neck manipulation may have caused the dissection. Twisting of the neck from a wide variety of activities (including coughing, sports, lifting, ceiling painting, yoga, archery, and falls) has been associated with vertebral-artery dissection. Several recent reports have described an association of the condition with chiropractic neck manipulation.[7,10-13] When patients, especially those under 60 years of age, present with an acute onset of a focal neurologic deficit (i.e., a stroke syndrome) involving a part of the brain that is supplied by the posterior circulation, they should be routinely questioned about neck manipulation or other activities that cause rapid neck movements.

The management of vertebral-artery dissection remains controversial and has not been examined in any randomized, controlled trials. Anticoagulant therapy is the current standard of care in the absence of apparent hemorrhage on imaging and is typically continued for three to six months,[14] followed by long-term antiplatelet therapy. The rationale is to prevent thromboembolism from the vertebral artery to the brain, which is the most frequent complication of vertebral-artery dissection.[6] The main exception is intradural vertebral-artery dissection, in which anticoagulation is contraindicated because of the high incidence of associated subarachnoid hemorrhage. In such cases, antiplatelet agents are sometimes used instead. The optimal time to begin anticoagulation remains uncertain. Recently, interest has been growing in the use of angioplasty and stenting to treat vertebral-artery dissection. However, there is evidence that anticoagulant therapy alone often results in the resolution of neurologic symptoms and may prevent recurrence.[15]

We are indebted to Dr. Richard Farb for interpretation of the neuroimaging studies and preparation of the images, and to Dr. Hillar Vellend for his insights into the case and years of mentorship.

This article first appeared in the July 1, 2004, issue of the New England Journal of Medicine.

REFERENCES

1.
Angibaud G, Rambaud S. Serious neurological manifestations of ciguatera: is the delay unusually long? J Neurol Neurosurg Psychiatry 1998;64:688-9.

2.
Lange WR, Snyder FR, Fudala PJ. Travel and ciguatera fish poisoning. Arch Intern Med 1992;152: 2049-53.

3.
Pearn J. Neurology of ciguatera. J Neurol Neurosurg Psychiatry 2001;70:4-8.

4.
Poli MA, Lewis RJ, Dickey RW, Musser SM, Buckner CA, Carpenter LG. Identification of Caribbean ciguatoxins as the cause of an outbreak of fish poisoning among U.S. soldiers in Haiti. Toxicon 1997;35:733-41.

5.
American College of Emergency Physicians. Clinical policy: critical issues in the evaluation and management of patients presenting to the emergency department with acute headache. Ann Emerg Med 2002;39:108-22.

6.
Sturzenegger M. Headache and neck pain: the warning symptoms of vertebral artery dissection. Headache 1994; 34:187-93.

7.
Ernst E. Life-threatening complications of spinal manipulation. Stroke 2001;32: 809-10.

8.
Frisoni GB, Anzola GP. Vertebrobasilar ischemia after neck motion. Stroke 1991;22:1452-60.

9.
Norris JW, Beletsky V, Nadareishvili ZG. Sudden neck movement and cervical artery dissection. CMAJ 2000;163:38-40.

10.
Kapral MK, Bondy SJ. Cervical manipulation and risk of stroke. Can Med Assoc J 2001;165:907-8.

11.
Phillips SJ, Maloney WJ, Gray J. Pure motor stroke due to vertebral artery dissection. Can J Neurol Sci 1989;16:348-51.

12.
Rothwell DM, Bondy SJ, Williams JI. Chiropractic manipulation and stroke: a population-based case-control study. Stroke 2001; 32:1054-60.

13.
Sherman DG, Hart RG, Easton JD. Abrupt change in head position and cerebral infarction. Stroke 1981; 12:2-6.

14.
Schievink WI. The treatment of spontaneous carotid and vertebral artery dissections. Curr Opin Cardiol 2000;15: 316-21.

15.
Kitanaka C, Tanaka J, Kuwahara M, et al. Nonsurgical treatment of unruptured intracranial vertebral artery dissection with serial follow-up angiography. J Neurosurg 1994;80:667-74. [Erratum, J Neurosurg 1994; 80:1132.]

ADDENDUM

The fifth paragraph of our article states that "A physician who was contacted in the Dominican Republic reported that the algae containing ciguatoxin were not in bloom at that time." In the original article, the subsequent statement (removed in this compilation) suggested that the information was useful in ruling out the possibility of ciguatera poisoning. In a letter to the editor, Dr. Selcer pointed out that the seasonality of the toxin-containing algae blooms is not sufficient to rule out ciguatera poisoning.[1]

Although some investigators have noted a seasonality in the incidence of ciguatera poisoning,[2,3] others have not.[4] Ciguatera most often results when humans consume reef-eating fish, which in turn have consumed herbivorous fish, which in their turn have ingested the original toxin in marine algae. The marine algae carrying the toxin do bloom in a seasonal pattern during periods with warmer seawater temperatures. However, despite this seasonal variation, because humans eat fish from the higher end of the food chain in which biomagnification of the toxin has occurred, the seasonality is not as distinct, nor is it sufficient in itself to rule out ciguatera poisoning.

The patient's presentation, in particular the duration of symptoms and their unilateral distribution, most convincingly argue against the diagnosis of ciguatera poisoning.

1. Selcer UM. Ciguatera poisoning N Engl J Med 2004;351:2020.

2. Hales S, Weinstein P, Woodward A. Ciguatera (fish poisoning), El Nino, and Pacific sea surface temperatures. Ecosystem Health 1999;5(1):20-5.

3. Lawrence DN, Enriquez MB, Lumish RM, Maceo A. Ciguatera fish poisoning in Miami. JAMA 1980;244:254-8.

4. Morris JG Jr, Lewin P, Smith CW, Blake PA, Schneider R. Ciguatera fish poisoning: epidemiology of the disease on St. Thomas, U.S. Virgin Islands. Am J Trop Med Hyg 1982;31:574-8.

A Bitter Tale

LORI S. NEWMAN, M.D., PH.D., MARK W. FEINBERG, M.D.,
AND HOWARD E. LEWINE, M.D.

A 53-year-old woman presented to an outpatient urgent care clinic with persistent nausea and vomiting. On the previous evening, she had had an acute onset of nausea that was followed by vomiting and light-headedness. The vomiting had occurred approximately every hour for 18 hours. She had mild discomfort in the chest and abdomen but reported no headache, fever, chills, diarrhea, shortness of breath, or diaphoresis.

These symptoms are nonspecific. The most likely cause is gastroenteritis or gastritis. Other gastrointestinal disorders — including hepatitis, cholecystitis, and pancreatitis — are possible, especially if she is febrile. The persistence of nausea and vomiting also raises the possibility of gastrointestinal obstruction. Knowledge of the quantity and quality of the emesis might help in differentiating the level, if obstruction is indeed the cause. A central nervous system process may cause nausea and vomiting; however, the patient did not have a headache or report other neurologic symptoms. I am concerned about an atypical presentation of an acute coronary syndrome. Women are more likely than men to present without classic chest pain; nausea and abdominal discomfort may be the primary presenting symptoms.

The patient had a history of the irritable bowel syndrome, attention-deficit disorder, hypercholesterolemia, and allergic rhinitis. Her medications included atorvastatin and methylphenidate. She had gone through menopause one year earlier and had been taking estrogen and medroxyprogesterone since that time. A brother had coronary artery disease with an onset before the age of 50 years. The patient had stopped smoking at the age of 40. She reported drinking a glass of wine occasionally, with no recent increase in alcohol consumption, and exercising for three hours per week.

A prescription medication, over-the-counter drug, herb, or supplement can induce gastritis or acute hepatitis or have a neurotoxic effect that might cause her symptoms. Of her medications, statins are associated with a mild increase in the aminotransferase level, but they very rarely induce symptomatic hepatitis. The patient should be asked specifically about the use of aspirin and nonsteroidal antiinflammatory drugs, which have gastric toxicity, and acetaminophen, in view of its hepatic toxicity. The patient's postmenopausal status, her use of hormone-replacement medications for the previous year, and her brother's premature coronary disease add to my concern about an acute ischemic event.

On physical examination, the patient had a heart rate of 36 beats per minute, with a regular rhythm, and a supine blood pressure of 110/60 mm Hg. When sitting up, she had a heart rate of 38 beats per minute and a blood pressure of 90/50 mm Hg. She was afebrile and had an oxygen saturation of 98 percent while breathing room air. She had minimal tenderness in the right upper quadrant of the abdomen without guarding or rebound. The cardiac examination revealed no murmurs, gallops, or rubs. The patient's lungs were clear on auscultation. Her extremities were warm, with intact pulses and no edema. She had no impairment of cognition or memory and no focal neurologic abnormalities.

With the patient's history of vomiting and orthostasis, I am surprised she does not have tachycardia. Perhaps she has a gastrointestinal illness with an exaggerated vagal response. However, this would be an unusual cause of persistent bradycardia. I would wonder about an underlying conduction defect that predisposed her to an exaggerated vagal response. Although she engages in regular physical activity, it is unlikely that the amount of exercise she reports could account for this degree of bradycardia. Hypothyroidism might cause a sinus bradycardia, but even with increased vagal tone, her heart rate is extremely slow. It is possible that she has the sick sinus syndrome, but she is rather young for this disorder.

The patient might have an underlying infiltrative cardiomyopathy with a conduction defect, such as Lyme disease, sarcoid, or amyloidosis. Undiagnosed congenital heart disease or muscular dystrophy with heart block would be expected to present at a younger age.

I am still very concerned about an acute coronary syndrome, particularly an inferior-wall myocardial infarction with heart block. If this is not an exaggerated vagal response or active ischemia, then ingestion of a drug (such as a beta-blocker, a calcium-channel blocker, or digoxin) or other toxin that causes bradycardia needs to be considered, although the patient reports no such history. At this time, I would order an electrocardiogram, establish intravenous access, give her an aspirin, and call for an ambulance to transport her to the hospital.

The patient was transferred to the emergency department. On arrival, she continued to have bradycardia, with a blood pressure of 100/50 mm Hg. An electrocardiogram revealed a marked sinus bradycardia at a rate of 36 beats per minute with nonspecific ST–T wave abnormalities (Figure 1). Her initial creatine kinase level was 247 U per liter (normal

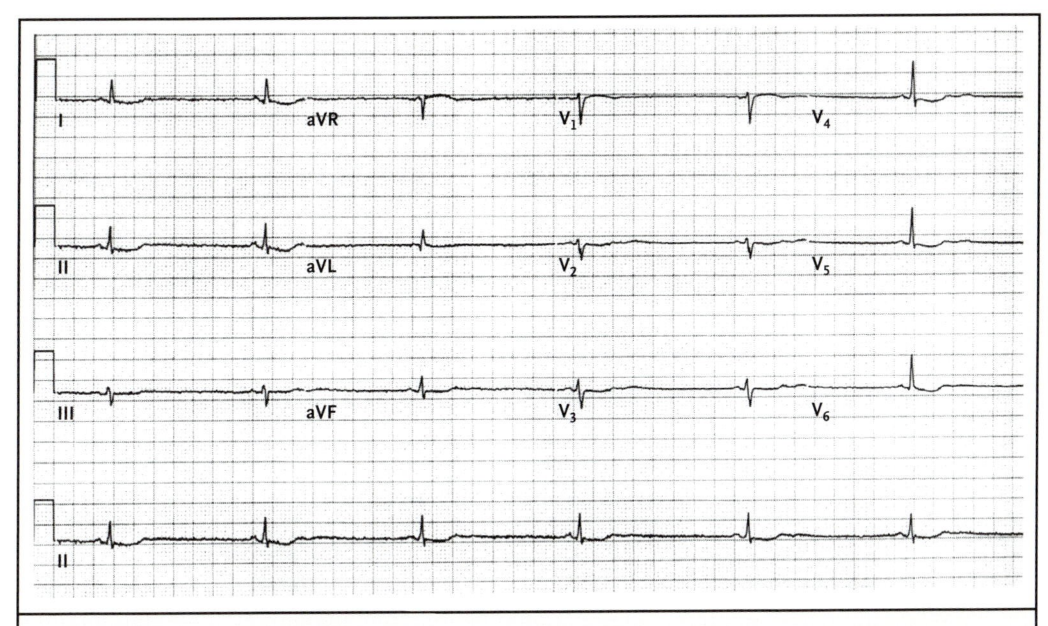

Figure 1. Electrocardiogram from the Patient.
The 12-lead electrocardiogram shows sinus bradycardia and diffuse, "scooping" ST–T wave abnormalities.

range, 27 to 218) with an MB fraction of 5.8 ng per milliliter (normal range, 0.0 to 5.0); troponin was 0.0 ng per milliliter. The serum potassium level was 5.2 mmol per liter, and the magnesium level was 1.6 mg per deciliter (0.7 mmol per liter); other electrolyte values were normal, as was the complete blood count. The serum urea nitrogen level was 12 mg per deciliter (4.3 mmol per liter), and the creatinine level was 0.9 mg per deciliter (79.6 μmol per liter). The calcium level was 8.6 mg per deciliter (2.2 mmol per liter), with a normal albumin level. The results of liver-function tests and measurements of amylase and lipase were within normal limits. Toxicologic screening of serum and urine was performed. The findings on a chest radiograph and an ultrasound of the right upper quadrant were normal. The patient was admitted to the hospital.

The electrocardiogram shows profound sinus bradycardia, diffuse ST-segment depressions in a "scooping" or "coving" pattern, and the presence of U waves. There are no Q waves to suggest prior myocardial infarction, and there is normal R-wave progression across the precordial leads.

The diffuse nature of the ST-segment depressions suggests a drug or electrolyte imbalance rather than ischemia. Also, the cardiac enzyme measurements obtained 12 to 24 hours after the onset of the patient's symptoms are somewhat reassuring. Since she is symptomatic, serial electrocardiography, measurement of cardiac enzyme levels, and cardiac monitoring are still appropriate, but attention should be focused on diagnoses other than cardiac ischemia.

I am surprised that the serum potassium level is slightly elevated in the setting of vomiting and normal renal function. However, the presence of U waves suggests that either intracellular potassium levels may be reduced or the initial laboratory value was an error. U waves can also be a toxic effect of medication (e.g., quinidine). The sinus bradycardia in conjunction with the concave pattern of the ST depressions also raises the suspicion of a toxic effect of digoxin; however, other drugs can have this effect as well.

The patient continued to have a heart rate in the 30s, with persistent nausea and occasional vomiting. She was given 0.5 mg of atropine intravenously, which was followed by a prompt increase in the heart rate to 70 beats per minute. Additional details of her history confirmed that she had not taken any unusual medications and that her most recent refills of medications did not appear to differ from her usual pills. She reported no recent travel, hiking, or tick bites. She said that she had consumed a salad with dandelion leaves from her partner's inner-city garden two days before admission and again one day before admission.

With this additional information, a toxic ingestion seems most likely. Eating dandelion leaves is relatively safe, especially when they are eaten as part of a salad. The two most commonly reported side effects of ingesting dandelions are diuresis and an elevation in the blood glucose level.

What else might the patient have consumed or been exposed to that could cause this clinical picture? Her nausea, abdominal discomfort, and bradycardia might indicate organophosphate poisoning. However, the onset of symptoms from excessive acetylcholine activity can occur within 4 hours after pesticide exposure and routinely occurs within 12 hours, whereas this patient's symptoms started more than a day after she first ate the salad. Also, she did not have some of the other classic symptoms of organophosphate poisoning, such as headache, abdominal cramping, diarrhea, blurred vision with small pupils, excessive sweating, and increased salivation.

Since her bradycardia responded to a small dose of atropine, there is no urgent indication for placement of a temporary pacemaker. If her hemodynamic status became compromised, advanced heart block developed, or she did not have a response to atropine, she then would be a candidate for a pacemaker.

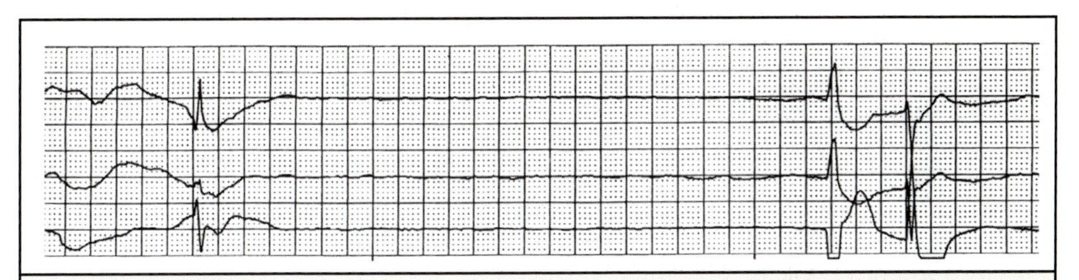

Figure 2. Rhythm Strip Obtained during Telemetric Monitoring on the Second Night of the Patient's Hospitalization.
The single-lead rhythm strip shows a five-second sinus pause with ventricular escape beats.

The bradycardia and nonspecific electrocardiographic changes persisted for two days after admission. On the night of the second day, she had a syncopal episode with a five-second pause on telemetry after having a bowel movement (Figure 2). Serial cardiac enzyme measurements remained normal. Repeated tests of potassium and magnesium levels were normal. Toxicologic screening was negative. The level of thyrotropin was normal, and a serologic test for Lyme disease was negative. An echocardiogram showed normal left and right ventricular size and function, without wall-motion abnormalities and with structurally normal valves. An exercise stress test with perfusion imaging revealed no evidence of ischemia. Although the patient said that she had not taken digoxin, the persistent electrocardiographic findings and the absence of a clear cause of her condition prompted a test for serum digoxin on the third hospital day, which showed a level of 1.3 ng per milliliter.

Why does the patient have digoxin in her serum? Possibilities include surreptitious digoxin use by the patient, poisoning by someone else, or accidental ingestion of a cardiac glycoside from consumption of plants containing the compound. Other possibilities include laboratory error and a false positive test result due to the presence of endogenous digoxin-like immunoreactive factors, as has been described, for example, in patients with renal or hepatic disease or in those taking aldosterone inhibitors, such as spironolactone. However, the symptoms and signs that are consistent with digoxin toxicity argue strongly against a false positive test result.

Given the marked bradycardia and electrocardiographic changes with a serum digoxin concentration of only 1.3 ng per milliliter and normal renal function, other sources of glycoside-containing substances should be explored, including plants and herbal medications. Such glycosides may only partly cross-react or may not be detected at all in a standard digoxin serum assay. The serum digoxin level is only a rough indication of possible toxicity. A serum digitoxin level may correlate more closely with symptoms and cardiac manifestations of toxicity.

The patient and her partner reaffirmed that the patient had not taken digoxin. However, the patient's partner reported that he was growing foxglove in his garden. The patient described where she had picked dandelion leaves for her salad, and he confirmed that this was the location where he was growing foxglove. The digitoxin level, measured on the third hospital day, was 43 ng per milliliter (therapeutic range, 10 to 32).

Digitoxin is the principal active agent in the foxglove leaf. Therefore, the patient's digitoxin level is consistent with recent ingestion of foxglove. Digitoxin differs from digoxin in that digitoxin has a much higher gastrointestinal absorption, has a longer half-life (four to six days rather than two), is more protein-bound, and is cleared less by the kidneys and metabolized more in the liver. Because the effects of digitoxin are likely to persist longer than those of digoxin, the patient should be monitored in the hospital until her symptoms and bradycardia resolve.

Should the patient be treated with digoxin-specific–antibody Fab fragments? The generally accepted indications for this therapy are persistent hyperkalemia, life-threatening ventricular or supraventricular arrhythmias, hemodynamically significant bradycardia, high-degree heart block that is unresponsive to atropine, and cardiac arrest.

The patient's nausea and light-headedness began to improve, but her heart rate remained slow, at an average of 40 beats per minute. By the seventh hospital day, her heart rate had increased to the high 40s. The patient's partner brought in a sample of the foxglove, and the patient immediately recognized it as the plant she had eaten. Analysis of the plant confirmed the presence of digitoxin. The patient was well enough to go home on the ninth hospital day, with a resting heart rate in the 50s.

COMMENTARY

Accidental digitalis toxicity associated with consumption of plants that contain cardiac glycosides is rare.[1] Although foxglove is indigenous to temperate climatic zones, few people consume it because of its bitter taste.[2] Exposure is more common among infants and children under six years of age than among adults.[1] Ingestion may also

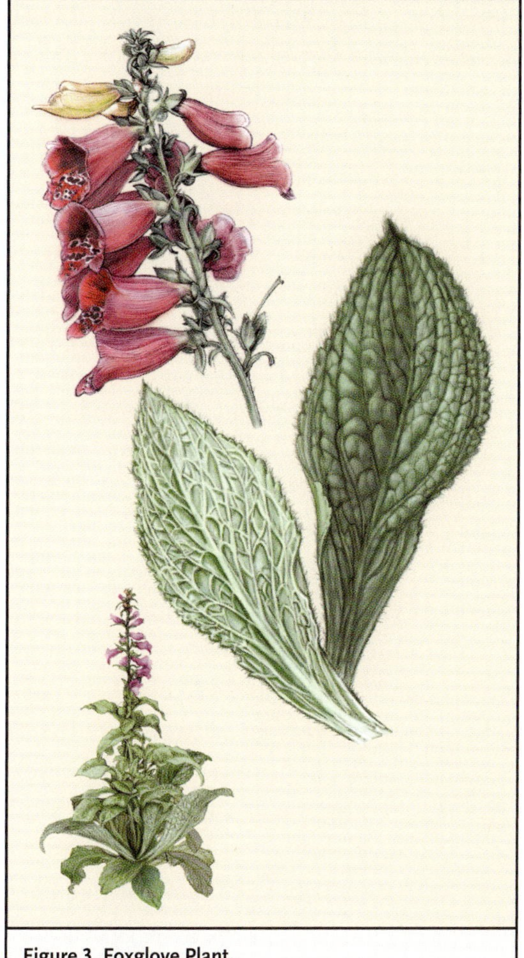

Figure 3. Foxglove Plant.

occur from consumption of contaminated field water near places where these plants grow, from homemade herbal preparations, and from homegrown gardens, as occurred in this case.

Toxicity due to consumption of leaves from the foxglove plant (*Digitalis purpurea*) produces clinical findings that are similar to those associated with an overdose of digoxin. Although some patients may present with typical side effects, such as gastrointestinal symptoms (nausea, vomiting, anorexia, or diarrhea), others may have central nervous system effects (fatigue, confusion, insomnia, or psychosis), visual effects (seeing yellow "halos" around lights, blurred or double vision, or photophobia), and cardiac effects (palpitations, light-headedness, or chest pain). Such diverse manifestations can mislead the clinician and delay the diagnosis, as occurred with this patient. It should be noted that symptoms associated with digitalis toxicity do not necessarily correspond to the serum digoxin concentration, and a person may have toxic effects at a level that is considered to be normal or therapeutic.[2]

In general, plant-derived cardiac glycosides have properties that affect the myocardium in a manner that is similar to that of digoxin. Cardiac glycosides enhance cardiac inotropy by inhibiting the cellular membrane Na^+/K^+–ATPase and ultimately increasing intracellular calcium within cardiomyocytes.[3,4] In addition, cardiac glycosides promote parasympathetic activity, thereby slowing the basal resting heart rate or the ventricular response to supraventricular tachycardia. This patient's syncopal episode probably occurred because of the higher vagal state associated with having a bowel movement, coupled with the increased parasympathetic activity from foxglove-derived digitalis toxicity.

In addition to foxglove (Figure 3), several other plant and herbal sources of cardiac glycosides may be detected by serum immunoassays for digoxin or digitoxin (as in this case), including woolly foxglove (*D. lanata*), ornamental oleander (*Nerium oleander*), yellow oleander (*Thevetia peruviana*), squill or sea onion (*Uriginea maritima*), lily of the valley (*Convallaria majalis*), and ouabain (*Strophanthus gratus*).[2] Another source of cardiac glycosides is venom extracted from skin glands in certain species of toads (*Bufo marinus* and *B. alvarius*). This compound has turned up in some aphrodisiacs and Chinese medications (e.g., chan su).[5,6] Ingestion may cause symptoms and clinical findings similar to those of digitalis overdose, and deaths have been reported.[6]

Patients with cardiac-glycoside toxicity from plant or herbal sources, like those with pharmaceutical digitalis toxicity, can be treated initially with activated charcoal. If toxicity is life-threatening, administration of digoxin-specific–antibody Fab fragments should be considered for rapid reversal of the cardiac complications. Because of the large volume of distribution of cardiac glycosides, dialysis is ineffective for treating this type of digitalis toxicity.[2] Early consultation with a medical toxicologist or poison control center may help the clinician to identify the toxic source and guide decisions about treatment.

Could the diagnosis have been made sooner in this case? Several clues to the diagnosis were not initially recognized. The potassium level was elevated, which is unusual in the setting of nausea and vomiting. In addition, the combination of persistent bradycardia and the patient's other electrocardiographic findings should have raised the suspicion of digitalis intoxication. Had the diagnosis been established earlier, the administration of digoxin-specific–antibody Fab fragments might have been useful. In contrast to the well-established efficacy of Fab fragments for treating pharmaceutical digitalis toxicity,[2,3,7,8] there is less experience with Fab fragments for treating toxicity associated with plant-containing cardiac glycosides.[9,10] Nevertheless, Fab treatment is generally benign and might have reversed the patient's symptoms and shortened her hospital course.

We are indebted to Joseph L. Dorsey, M.D., and Michael E. Hurwitz, M.D., Ph.D., for their critical review of the manuscript.

This article first appeared in the August 5, 2004, issue of the New England Journal of Medicine.

REFERENCES

1.
Watson WA, Litovitz TL, Rodgers GC Jr, et al. 2002 Annual report of the American Association of Poison Control Centers Toxic Exposure Surveillance System. Am J Emerg Med 2002;21:353-421.

2.
Hoffman BF, Bigger TJ. Digitalis and allied cardiac glycosides. In: Gilman AG, Rall TW, Nies AS, Taylor P, eds. Goodman and Gilman's the pharmacological basis of therapeutics. 8th ed. New York: Pergamon Press, 1990:814-39.

3.
Smith TW, Haber E. Digitalis. N Engl J Med 1973;289:1125-9.

4.
Hauptman PJ, Kelly RA. Digitalis. Circulation 1999;99:1265-70.

5.
Kwan T, Paiusco AD, Kohl L. Digitalis toxicity caused by toad venom. Chest 1992;102:949-50.

6.
Gowda RM, Cohen RA, Khan IA. Toad venom poisoning: resemblance to digoxin toxicity and therapeutic implications. Heart 2003;89:e14. (Accessed July 12, 2004, at http://heart.bmjjournals.com/cgi/content/full/89/4/e14.)

7.
Kelly RA, Smith TW. Recognition and management of digitalis toxicity. Am J Cardiol 1992;69:108G-118G.

8.
Antman EM, Wenger TL, Butler VP Jr, Haber E, Smith TW. Treatment of 150 cases of life-threatening digitalis intoxication with digoxin-specific Fab antibody fragments: final report of a multicenter study. Circulation 1990;81:1744-52.

9.
Rich SA, Libera JM, Locke RJ. Treatment of foxglove extract poisoning with digoxin-specific Fab fragments. Ann Emerg Med 1993;22:1904-7.

10.
Thierry S, Blot F, Lacherade J-C, Lefort Y, Franzon P, Brun-Buisson C. Poisoning with foxglove extract: favorable evolution without Fab fragments. Intensive Care Med 2000;26:1586.

Undercover and Overlooked

ANDREW WANG, M.D., AND THOMAS M. BASHORE, M.D.

A 67-year-old overweight man was seen by his physician because of a two-month history of shortness of breath, a nonproductive cough, and bilateral swelling of the lower extremities. He also reported a tight sensation in the neck, occasional wheezing, and an increase in dyspnea after meals. The patient noted the onset of symptoms soon after a hunting trip in November. He had no other constitutional symptoms and had not ingested or had contact with anything unusual during his trip. His history was notable for gastroesophageal reflux and a remote pneumonia. He had no history of lung or heart disease, occupational exposure, allergies, or tobacco use.

The onset of symptoms after the patient's hunting trip raises the possibility of a relationship between this event and the illness. However, he reports no unusual exposures. Given his history of gastroesophageal reflux and increased dyspnea after meals, bronchospasm due to reflux may be a contributing factor. However, bilateral edema of the lower extremities is suggestive of a cardiac cause of his dyspnea. The patient's history suggests broadly either a pulmonary or cardiac disorder, so the differential diagnosis at this point is extensive, including pulmonary infection, pulmonary emboli, obstructive airway disease, hypersensitivity pneumonitis, pulmonary hypertension, and heart failure.

Because of worsening respiratory symptoms, the patient was admitted to a local medical center. At the time of his admission, he had a nonproductive cough and was able to walk only a short distance without stopping, because of dyspnea. He reported orthopnea but not paroxysmal nocturnal dyspnea. On examination, he was afebrile, his blood pressure was 150/86 mm Hg, his heart rate was 110 beats per minute, and his respiratory rate was 28 breaths per minute. His weight was 109 kg, with a body-mass index (the weight in kilograms divided by the square of the height in meters) of 34.4 kg. The lung examination demonstrated scattered, brief expiratory wheezes in both lungs. The jugular venous pressure could not be visualized. The heart sounds were distant, with no audible murmur, rub, or gallop. The lower extremities had symmetric, pitting edema (2+).

The results of blood tests were as follows: hemoglobin, 13.1 g per deciliter; hematocrit, 40 percent; platelet count, 182,000 per cubic millimeter; white-cell count, 6000 per cubic

millimeter, with a normal differential count; sodium, 136 mmol per liter; potassium, 5.0 mmol per liter; chloride, 105 mmol per liter; bicarbonate, 24 mmol per liter; blood urea nitrogen, 13 mg per deciliter (4.6 mmol per liter); serum creatinine, 1.1 mg per deciliter (97.2 μmol per liter); blood glucose, 128 mg per deciliter (7.1 mmol per liter); total protein, 6.9 g per deciliter; albumin, 3.5 g per deciliter; total bilirubin, 1.0 mg per deciliter (17.1 μmol per liter); aspartate aminotransferase, 33 U per liter; alanine aminotransferase, 33 U per liter; and alkaline phosphatase, 160 U per liter. Urinalysis and liver-function tests showed no abnormalities. Initial arterial-blood gas analysis (with the patient breathing room air) revealed the following values: pH 7.47; partial pressure of carbon dioxide, 34 mm Hg; partial pressure of oxygen, 62 mm Hg; and bicarbonate concentration, 25 mmol per liter. A chest radiograph showed cardiomegaly and mildly increased pulmonary vasculature. An electrocardiogram showed sinus tachycardia at a rate of 110 beats per minute with diffuse T-wave inversions and low voltage. The values for creatine kinase and the MB fractions, measured serially, were normal.

Although cough and dyspnea may reflect either cardiac or pulmonary disease, the presence of orthopnea suggests elevated left ventricular filling pressure in the setting of increased venous return and points to a cardiac cause. Physical examination is often helpful in distinguishing the cause of these symptoms but provides little guidance in the present case. It is unfortunate that the jugular venous pressure could not be adequately evaluated, since an elevated pressure would point to possible heart failure. The findings on the chest radiograph are consistent with a cardiac condition. I would also want to know the level of B-type natriuretic peptide, since an elevated level would also support heart failure as the cause of dyspnea, particularly in the setting of left ventricular systolic dysfunction.

A transthoracic echocardiogram showed normal left ventricular size and function. The right ventricle was mildly thickened but not enlarged or hypocontractile. The aortic valve was thickened, with no stenosis or regurgitation. There was no other valvular abnormality. A perfusion imaging study was performed with the use of dobutamine and single-photon-emission computed tomography (CT). During infusion of dobutamine (30 μg per kilogram per minute intravenously), the patient's heart rate increased to 132 beats per minute (85 percent of the predicted heart rate, 130 beats per minute). Perfusion imaging of the left ventricle was normal at the peak heart rate and at rest.

The echocardiographic finding of right ventricular thickening without evidence of dilation suggests that the pulmonary-artery pressure is elevated, but the absence of tricuspid regurgitation precludes estimation of the right ventricular (and thus, pulmonary-artery) systolic pressure. There was no apparent left ventricular systolic dysfunction or valvular abnormality. It would be useful to know whether there was echocardiographic evidence of diastolic dysfunction. The results of myocardial perfusion imaging suggest that myocardial ischemia is not the cause of the patient's dyspnea.

Spiral CT scanning of the chest, which was performed with the intravenous administration of contrast material, showed no evidence of pulmonary embolus or infiltrate. Hilar, subcarinal, and pretracheal lymph nodes that were small and calcified and a small right-sided pleural effusion were noted. An ultrasound study of the bilateral lower extremities showed no evidence of deep venous thrombosis.

The patient sought a second opinion at another regional medical center. Pulmonary-function testing there showed a forced vital capacity (FVC) of 2.5 liters (59 percent of the predicted value), a forced expiratory volume in one second (FEV_1) of 1.9 liters (65 percent of the predicted value), a ratio of FEV_1 to FVC of 76 percent, a forced expiratory flow (between 25 percent and 75 percent of FVC) of 1.5 liters per second (54 percent of the predicted value), a total lung capacity of 5.4 liters (85 percent of the predicted value), and a residual volume of 1.9 liters (77 percent of the predicted value). There was no response to bronchodilator testing. A sleep study showed 21 apneic and 12 hypopneic episodes per hour of sleep, with a minimal oxygen saturation of 83 percent. Treatment with nasal continuous positive airway pressure (CPAP) of 17 cm of water resulted in a reduction in apneic and hypopneic episodes to 20 per hour and a minimal oxygen saturation of 90 percent. Nocturnal CPAP and empirical therapy with oral diuretics were started.

Pulmonary thromboembolism, a possible cause of dyspnea and hypoxemia, is probably not the cause of the patient's symptoms on the basis of the chest CT scan. The results of pulmonary-function testing indicate a mixed restrictive and obstructive process. The patient's obesity may contribute to restrictive lung disease. Presumably, sleep apnea was suspected on the basis of the patient's obesity, hypertension, and significant edema. However, dyspnea is not a common symptom of sleep apnea. A minority of patients with obstructive sleep apnea have pulmonary hypertension, a condition that has been associated with an elevation of left ventricular filling pressure and the duration of oxygen desaturation. Sleep apnea is associated with left ventricular systolic and diastolic dysfunction, which may improve with CPAP therapy.

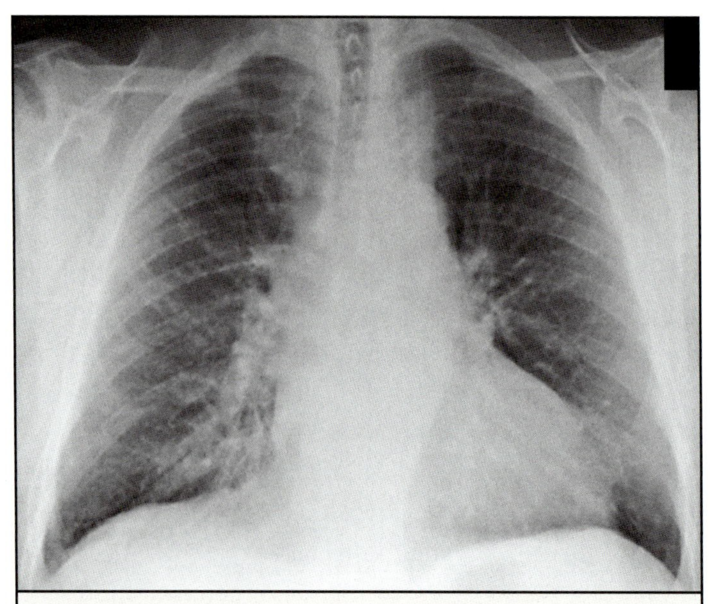

Figure 1. Radiograph of the Chest Showing Cardiomegaly and Increased Interstitial Markings.

Despite these interventions, the patient had worsening dyspnea and edema. His weight increased to 130 kg. He presented to our institution for evaluation nine months after his initial symptoms developed. A chest radiograph showed mild cardiomegaly and increased interstitial markings with possible septal lines (Figure 1). To evaluate for possible interstitial lung disease, a high-resolution CT scan of the chest was ordered; it showed no evidence of pulmonary disease but did show a thickened pericardium (Figure 2).

The focus of attention has shifted from the pulmonary system to the cardiovascular system. A repeated CT scan of the chest showed a thickened pericardium, which raises the possibility of constrictive pericarditis. Although radiographic evidence of pericardial thickening is the anatomical hallmark of constrictive pericarditis, this finding is not specific for constrictive pericarditis and may occur in patients without physiological constriction. Conversely, patients with constrictive pericarditis may not have pericardial thickening on imaging studies. Hemodynamic measurements during cardiac catheterization may be necessary to diagnose constrictive pericarditis if noninvasive methods, such as echocardiography or pericardial imaging, are not conclusive.

The patient underwent right- and left-heart catheterization, which showed the following hemodynamic values: mean right atrial pressure, 20 mm Hg; right ventricular pressure,

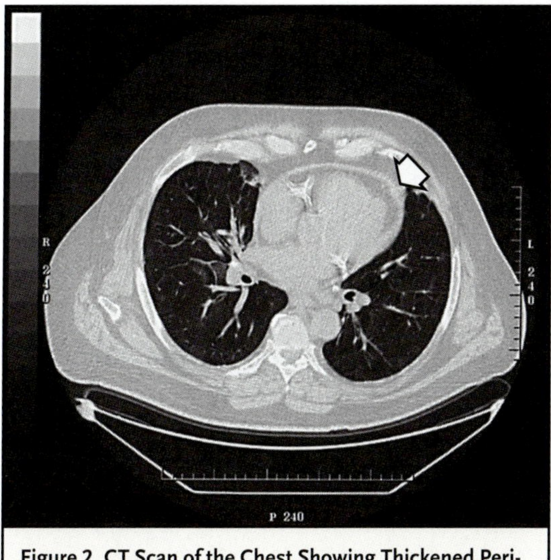

Figure 2. CT Scan of the Chest Showing Thickened Pericardium (Arrow) and a Small Pericardial Effusion.

48/20 mm Hg; pulmonary-artery pressure, 48/22 mm Hg (mean pressure, 30 mm Hg); mean pulmonary-capillary wedge pressure, 20 mm Hg; left ventricular pressure, 130/20 mm Hg; and aortic pressure, 130/80 mm Hg. Simultaneous right and left ventricular diastolic pressures showed equalization and a dip-and-plateau waveform pattern; simultaneous measurements of ventricular systolic pressure showed discordance, a finding that is consistent with increased ventricular interaction (Figure 3). Cardiac output, as measured by the Fick method, was 5.3 liters per minute, and the cardiac index was 2.2 liters per minute per square meter of body-surface area. The left ventricular ejection fraction was normal. There were no clinically significant coronary-artery stenoses present.

The hemodynamic findings of equalized diastolic pressures and rapid early filling of the ventricles (a dip-and-plateau waveform pattern) is suggestive of constrictive pericarditis. However, these findings are not specific for constrictive pericarditis and may be present in other causes of heart failure, particularly restrictive cardiomyopathy. A number of hemodynamic criteria have been used to differentiate constrictive pericarditis from restrictive cardiomyopathy, since the two conditions are similar with respect to the clinical presentation, findings on physical examination, and catheterization results. However, the diagnosis of constrictive pericarditis should be based on two physiological findings: a dissociation of intrathoracic and intracardiac pressures and an increased ventricular interaction.

In normal persons, changes in intrathoracic pressure during respiration are transmitted to the heart through the pericardium, resulting in decreased intracardiac pressure

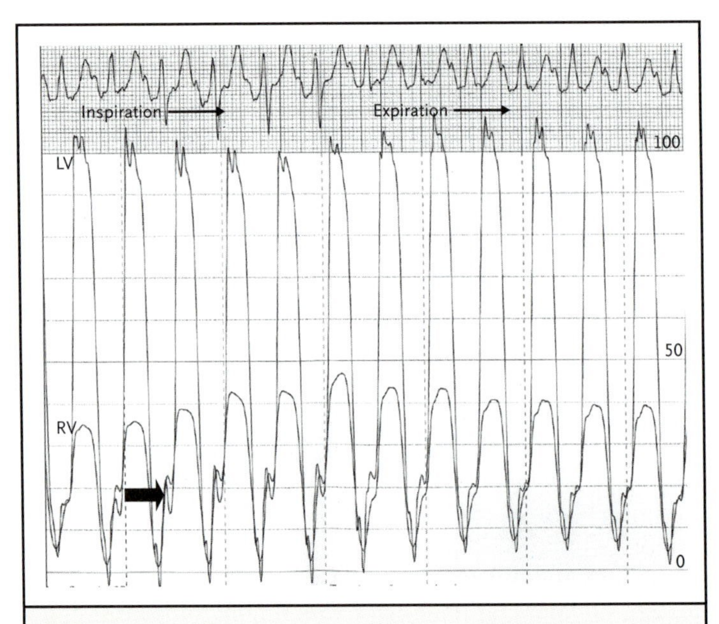

Figure 3. A Hemodynamic Tracing of Simultaneous Right Ventricular (RV) and Left Ventricular (LV) Pressures, Showing Discordant Systolic Pressures during Respiration (Thin Arrows) and Equalization of Diastolic Pressures (Thick Arrow).

during inspiration and increased intracardiac pressure during expiration. In patients with constrictive pericarditis, the heart is "shielded" from these changes in intrathoracic pressure. Increased interaction between the left and right ventricles occurs because of the decreased distensibility of the pericardium. Since ventricular filling is limited by a relatively fixed cardiac volume, increased venous return and filling of the right ventricle during inspiration impair left ventricular filling. This interdependence, evident as respiratory discordance of left and right ventricular systolic pressures, is a highly reliable hemodynamic factor for distinguishing constrictive pericarditis from other causes of heart failure.

The patient was referred to a cardiothoracic surgeon for pericardiectomy. Inspection of the pericardium revealed dense thickening of nearly 10 mm in regions. Pericardiectomy without cardiopulmonary bypass was performed with resection of the anterior pericardium between the right and left phrenic nerves and from the great arteries superiorly to the diaphragm inferiorly. During the procedure, central venous pressure decreased from 24 mm Hg after induction to 12 mm Hg at the conclusion of the procedure. Histologic

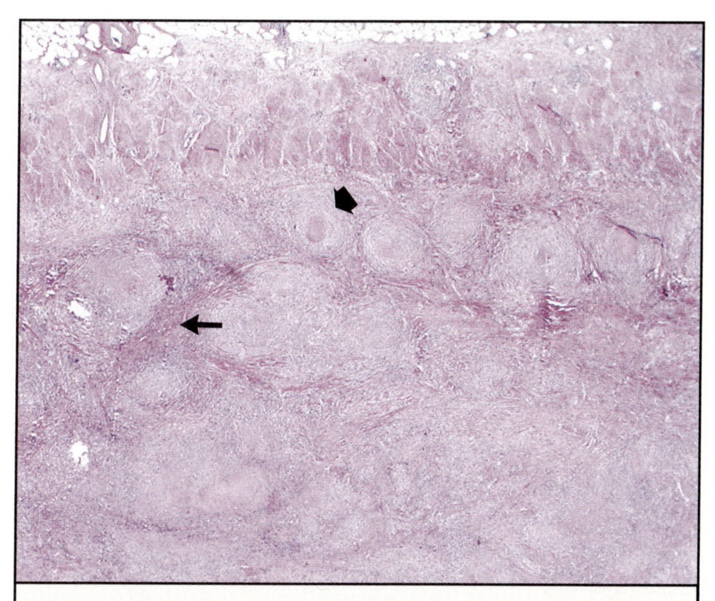

Figure 4. A Histologic Specimen of the Pericardium, Showing Fibrosis (Long Arrow) and Granulomatous Inflammation (Short Arrow) (Hematoxylin and Eosin).

examination of the pericardium revealed fibrosis with granulomatous inflammation (Figure 4). Stains and cultures for bacteria, fungi, viruses, and acid-fast bacilli were negative. The patient was discharged home five days after surgery. He has returned to a normal level of activity, with no dyspnea on exertion, and has required only low-dose oral diuretic therapy for mild edema of the bilateral lower extremities.

Although granulomatous inflammation was present in the resected pericardium, this finding is observed in several conditions, including infectious, metabolic, and rheumatologic diseases.

COMMENTARY

This case demonstrates the challenges in recognizing a slowly progressive and uncommon cause (constrictive pericarditis) of a very common clinical syndrome (heart failure). Constrictive pericarditis is defined as chronic fibrous thickening of the wall of the pericardial sac that results in abnormal diastolic filling.[1] In patients who have symptoms and signs of heart failure with preserved ventricular systolic function, the diagnosis of constrictive pericarditis as well as causes of abnormal myocardial relaxation or compliance (including myocardial hypertrophy, ischemia, restrictive cardiomyopathy, and infiltrative diseases) should be considered. Determination of the cause of left ventricular systolic dysfunction has been found to have prognostic implications for long-term survival.[2] This case illustrates that identification of the cause of diastolic heart failure, which is often overlooked, may lead to definitive therapy for the condition.

Why was there such a delay between the onset of the patient's symptoms and the diagnosis of constrictive pericarditis? The course of the disease is typically quite slow, and its symptoms and signs are not specific. As a result, in many cases symptoms are present for 12 months or longer before a diagnosis is established.[3] Prior pericarditis, cardiac surgery, and radiation therapy are the most commonly identified causes of constrictive pericarditis, accounting for approximately 50 percent of cases, but one third of cases remain idiopathic in origin.[3] This patient's medical history did not suggest a cause of constrictive pericarditis. Furthermore, the findings on physical examination may be difficult to appreciate. The jugular venous pressure and waveforms, which can offer important clues to the diagnosis, may not have been appreciated because of the patient's body habitus and the marked elevation of the venous pressure. An audible pericardial "knock," caused by the cessation of early diastolic ventricular filling (which, in turn, was caused by the constrictive pericardium),[4] is not a sensitive sign of constrictive pericarditis, particularly in the absence of pericardial calcification.[5]

Although right and left ventricular diastolic pressures are equalized in constrictive pericarditis because of limitation of diastolic filling by the pericardium, symptoms and signs of right-sided heart failure (including edema in the lower extremities and ascites) predominate. That is especially true early in the course of the disease, since the filling pressures are normally lower in the right ventricle than in the left ventricle. Consequently, the diagnosis of constrictive pericarditis should be considered in patients with evidence of right-sided heart failure that is out of proportion to the severity of pulmonary or left-sided heart disease. With progression of the disease and the associated increase in diastolic filling pressures (to levels above 15 mm Hg), symptoms and signs of left heart failure may develop.

Echocardiography is very useful for evaluating hemodynamic changes in constrictive pericarditis.[6,7] A dissociation between intrathoracic and intracardiac pressures can be detected as reciprocal changes in diastolic flow velocities across the tricuspid and mitral valves during respiration.[6,7] However, such measurements may not be routinely performed unless the diagnosis of constrictive pericarditis is suspected. As in the present case, echocardiography may be ordered to rule out common causes of heart failure, such as left ventricular systolic dysfunction or valvular disease, and signs of constrictive pericarditis are not assessed. Not infrequently, the broad, descriptive term of diastolic dysfunction is applied in the setting of symptoms or signs of heart failure with normal left ventricular systolic function.[8] Instead, a detailed examination of the diastolic filling pattern should be performed to confirm and characterize abnormal diastolic function and, potentially, to determine its specific cause.

Visualization of a thickened pericardium (3 mm or greater) by CT or magnetic resonance imaging may suggest the diagnosis of constrictive pericarditis, as it did in this patient. This finding, although a hallmark in the traditional definition of this disease,[1] has limited sensitivity,[9] and pericardial thickness may not be abnormal early in the disease process. Because of the limited sensitivity of this finding, multiple diagnostic approaches are often necessary to confirm the diagnosis of constrictive pericarditis before therapeutic intervention is undertaken.

Surgical pericardiectomy is a highly effective and potentially curative treatment for heart failure due to constrictive pericarditis. However, long-term survival is worse for patients with severe symptoms of heart failure than it is for those with milder symptoms,[3] a factor that underscores the need for early diagnosis and treatment of this frequently overlooked condition.

This article first appeared in the September 2, 2004, issue of the New England Journal of Medicine.

REFERENCES

1.
White P. Chronic constrictive pericarditis (Pick's disease): treated by pericardial resection. Lancet 1935;2:539-48, 597-603.

2.
Felker GM, Thompson RE, Hare JM, et al. Underlying causes and long-term survival in patients with initially unexplained cardiomyopathy. N Engl J Med 2000;342:1077-84.

3.
Ling LH, Oh JK, Schaff HV, et al. Constrictive pericarditis in the modern era: evolving clinical spectrum and impact on outcome after pericardiectomy. Circulation 1999;100:1380-6.

4.
Tyberg TI, Goodyer AV, Langou RA. Genesis of pericardial knock in constrictive pericarditis. Am J Cardiol 1980;46:570-5.

5.
Ling LH, Oh JK, Breen JF, et al. Calcific constrictive pericarditis: is it still with us? Ann Intern Med 2000;132:444-50. [Erratum, Ann Intern Med 2000; 133:659.]

6.
Oh JK, Hatle LK, Seward JB, et al. Diagnostic role of Doppler echocardiography in constrictive pericarditis. J Am Coll Cardiol 1994;23: 154-62.

7.
Hatle LK, Appleton CP, Popp RL. Differentiation of constrictive pericarditis and restrictive cardiomyopathy by Doppler echocardiography. Circulation 1989;79:357-70.

8.
Banerjee P, Banerjee T, Khand A, Clark AL, Cleland JG. Diastolic heart failure: neglected or misdiagnosed? J Am Coll Cardiol 2002;39:138-41.

9.
Talreja DR, Edwards WD, Danielson GK, et al. Constrictive pericarditis in 26 patients with histologically normal pericardial thickness. Circulation 2003;108: 1852-7.

Special Cure

ROBERT J. HOFFMAN, M.D., GURPREET DHALIWAL, M.D.,
DANIEL J. GILDEN, M.D., AND SANJAY SAINT, M.D., M.P.H.

A 42-year-old white man presented with a history of eight months of pain in his low back, hips, ankles, and feet. He had begun experiencing progressively severe pain during a 16-month period of incarceration. Therapy with nonsteroidal antiinflammatory medication had provided no significant improvement. The pain had become so severe that the patient had difficulty walking. He had otherwise felt well but had lost weight (from 76.2 to 67.6 kg) without a change in diet. He reported having had no fever, night sweats, diarrhea, anorexia, vomiting, abdominal distention, or dysphagia.

A number of characteristics distinguish this man's condition from that of the typical case of idiopathic low-back pain: his difficulty walking, the long duration of the condition despite conservative therapy, his weight loss, and the presence of severe pain throughout both lower extremities. These characteristics raise my concern about a neoplastic, infectious, or inflammatory disorder. His residence in prison poses certain health threats. Tuberculosis has a predilection for the thoracic and lumbar spine and can cause paralysis through vertebral destruction and compression of the spinal cord. Although tuberculosis could be manifested as an indolent monoarthritis, a symmetric bilateral polyarthritis would be decidedly uncommon. Trauma and fractures in the spine or lower extremities from altercations must also be ruled out. Another possibility is that he has an inflammatory disorder with polyarthritis. The list of possible disorders is quite long, but one of the first that comes to mind here is a seronegative spondylarthropathy, particularly reactive arthritis, which has a predilection for the lower extremities. It can be either acute and self-limited or chronic and progressive. However, weight loss is not a common feature of this disorder.

The patient had been born with gastroschisis (a congenital externalization of the bowel), which had been corrected surgically. Four years before the current evaluation, iron-deficiency anemia, hepatitis C, and hypothyroidism were diagnosed synchronously, and he was treated with oral iron and thyroxine. He had a distant history of intravenous drug use and episodic alcohol use and had a 20-pack-year history of smoking. He reported that his

mother had died of stomach cancer and had required a colostomy at the age of 27 years for an unknown condition.

I would not expect that a congenital malformation would lead to a mechanical or physiological disorder four decades after a successful repair. However, I wonder whether the genotype associated with gastroschisis could have predisposed this patient to other disorders of the gastrointestinal tract later in life. Although iron deficiency in a man is almost always explained by gastrointestinal blood loss (e.g., due to peptic ulcer disease or gastritis), it may infrequently result from failure to absorb iron due to a disorder such as celiac sprue. Hypothyroidism is usually autoimmune in origin and has been described as an extrahepatic manifestation of hepatitis C infection. The patient's history of intravenous drug use raises the possibility of infection with the human immunodeficiency virus.

The family history of stomach and colon problems and the patient's congenital malformation and iron-deficiency anemia all center around the gastrointestinal tract. Weight loss without a change in diet raises the possibility of malabsorption; other important causes of unintended weight loss with a preserved appetite are hyperthyroidism and diabetes mellitus. In trying to reconcile these possibilities with the patient's progressive symptoms in the back and lower extremities, I am still considering a seronegative spondylarthropathy, since it can occur in association with inflammatory bowel disease and other gastrointestinal conditions. One argument against this line of reasoning, however, is the absence of gastrointestinal symptoms. Another possibility is that the symptoms in his lower extremities are caused by hepatitis C–related cryoglobulinemia, with neuropathy and arthralgia. I remain uncertain of the cause of his pain at this point.

The patient's temperature was 37.1°C, his heart rate 70 beats per minute, his blood pressure 115/70 mm Hg, and his respiratory rate 20 breaths per minute. He was thin and pale but did not appear to be in distress. The examination of the heart and lungs showed no abnormalities. His abdomen had a midline scar; there was no organomegaly or tenderness. His stool was guaiac-positive. He had normal joint mobility without effusion or warmth. His muscle strength was normal without muscle tenderness. Although he had marked pain in moving any joint, the pain could not be localized to the joint itself. His reflexes were symmetric and normal throughout. He had mild clubbing of his fingers. The rest of the examination was normal.

The guaiac-positive stool points to a mucosal gastrointestinal disorder that explains the patient's iron-deficiency anemia, a finding that indicates a need for endoscopic examination. The patient does not have motor weakness; instead, his inability to walk seems to stem from pain with movement. The examination does not suggest an inflammatory arthritis, yet he cannot tolerate movement of the affected joints. Although intra-articular disease is still possible, his symptoms make me consider a pathologic process in the surrounding structures, perhaps an enthesopathy or periostitis. The fact that his fingers are clubbed would prompt me to obtain a chest radiograph in order to evaluate the possibility of lung cancer, which is very commonly associated with clubbing. Cyanotic heart disease is another major cause of clubbing and is worth mentioning, since he had another congenital malformation; however, the absence of cardiopulmonary symptoms or corrective surgery during the past four decades essentially rules out that diagnosis. Clubbing can be an extraintestinal manifestation of inflammatory bowel disease. A systemic disorder, hypertrophic osteoarthropathy may be manifested as both clubbing and periostosis, a sometimes painful condition affecting the long bones.

The hemoglobin level was 6.3 g per deciliter, the hematocrit 21.7 percent, the mean corpuscular volume 67.7 μm3, and the red-cell distribution width 20.9 percent. His white-cell count was 8300 per cubic millimeter, with a normal differential count, and the platelet count was 221,000 per cubic millimeter. The erythrocyte sedimentation rate was 70 mm per hour, and the absolute reticulocyte count was 2 percent. Other laboratory results were as follows: serum calcium, 6.9 mg per deciliter (1.7 mmol per liter); albumin, 3.2 g per deciliter; phosphorus, 1.8 mg per deciliter (0.6 mmol per liter); total protein, 6.3 g per deciliter; alanine aminotransferase, 83 U per liter; aspartate aminotransferase, 146 U per liter; alkaline phosphatase, 445 U per liter; and total bilirubin, 0.2 mg per deciliter (3.4 mmol per liter).

The patient's profound anemia is probably an important contributor to his sense of weakness. The guaiac-positive stool, the low mean corpuscular volume, and the low reticulocyte count are all consistent with iron deficiency. I wonder whether he is still taking his prescribed iron-replacement therapy. An elevated red-cell distribution width, which reflects a wide variance in the size of the red-cell population, is of limited discriminatory value. It may reflect a heterogeneous cell population due to two simultaneous effects on erythropoiesis — microcytosis from iron deficiency and macrocytosis from folate deficiency, for example — or it may reflect a nonhomogeneous population of cells due to a single disorder, such as iron deficiency.

The combination of low levels of phosphorus and calcium is characteristic of vitamin D deficiency, which is likely to be a consequence of malabsorption caused by the patient's mucosal disease. The elevated alkaline phosphatase level probably reflects the increased turnover of bone from secondary hyperparathyroidism. The aminotransferase levels can be explained by hepatitis C infection and alcoholic liver disease.

What is the nature of the patient's mucosal disease? It can be difficult to differentiate between inflammatory bowel disease, which I considered initially, and celiac sprue, another likely diagnosis. Both disorders may have extraintestinal manifestations and can cause malabsorption and iron deficiency. The family history (with colostomy), elevated sedimentation rate, and clubbing are more suggestive of inflammatory bowel disease, whereas vitamin D malabsorption and autoimmune thyroiditis are more typically associated with celiac sprue. Iron deficiency may occur in either condition, although the guaiac-positive stool is more characteristic of inflammatory bowel disease.

A plain radiograph of the patient's pelvis showed marked osteopenia (Figure 1). Dual-energy x-ray absorptiometry revealed a T score of −5.9, indicating that the patient's bone density was nearly 6 SD below the mean for normal young men. The results of laboratory tests were as follows: serum ferritin, 5 ng per milliliter (normal range, 22 to 322); free thyroxine, 0.83 ng per deciliter (10.68 pmol per liter; normal range, 0.84 to 1.51 ng per deciliter [10.81 to 19.43 pmol per liter]); and thyrotropin, 16.4 μU per milliliter (normal range, 0.35 to 5.50). The levels of vitamin B_{12} and folate were normal; HLA-B27 was not detected.

Bone densitometry reveals a severe decrease in bone density. This is probably the result of osteomalacia from vitamin D deficiency. The low level of serum ferritin confirms profound iron deficiency. The patient's hypothyroidism persists, and although it is mild, it may also be contributing to his sense of weakness. Although HLA-B27 is associated with axial arthritis (spondylitis–sacroiliitis) rather than the peripheral arthritis of spondylarthropathy, this test has limited diagnostic utility. My suspicion that the diagnosis is celiac sprue has increased substantially.

The parathyroid hormone level was extremely elevated, at 613 pg per milliliter (normal range, 15 to 65), and the 25-hydroxyvitamin D level was undetectable. The total cholesterol level was 65 mg per deciliter (1.68 mmol per liter). Endoscopy revealed a nonbleeding duodenal ulcer and a marked "scalloping" of the duodenal folds.

These values confirm hypovitaminosis D and associated secondary hyperparathyroidism. Marked hypolipidemia is seen in advanced cancer with cachexia or severe malnutrition,

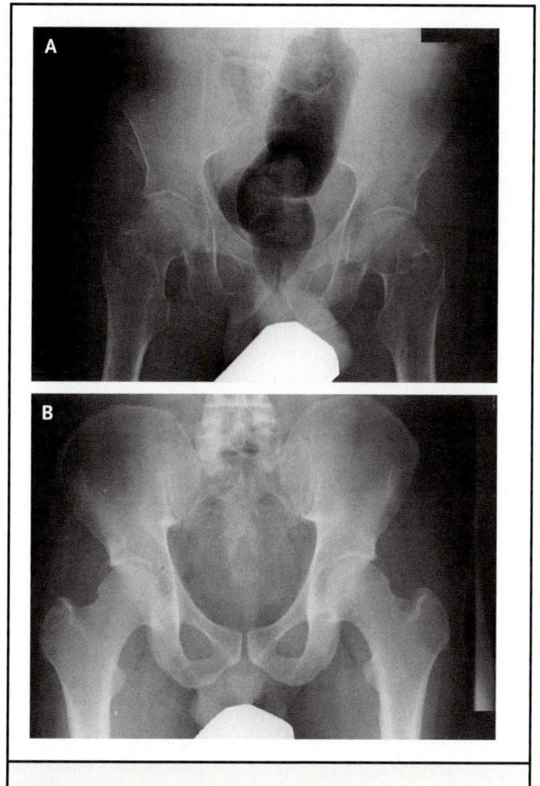

Figure 1. Radiographs of the Pelvic Area.
A plain radiograph of the patient's pelvic area shows severe osteopenia (Panel A). A radiograph of the pelvic area in a person of the same age and sex as the patient shows normal bone mineralization (Panel B).

but in this case it is explained by malabsorption. The ulcer, which I did not expect, may be explained by infection with *Helicobacter pylori* or the patient's use of nonsteroidal antiinflammatory drugs, but other causes of ulceration also merit consideration. With inflammatory bowel disease in the differential diagnosis, a biopsy would be important to rule out noncaseating granulomas, which are characteristic of Crohn's disease. Given the lymphocytic infiltration of the mucosa in celiac sprue, and the associated increase in the risk of intestinal cancer, my primary concern would be to rule out cancer, particularly lymphoma, as the cause of this ulcer.

A biopsy of the ulcer and the nonulcerated mucosa and tests for antiendomysial or antigliadin antibodies will be the definitive studies. A diffuse mucosal disease of the small intestine in the setting of severe malabsorption (with deficiencies in iron, vitamin D, and cholesterol) points to celiac sprue. Crohn's disease, which usually affects the distal small

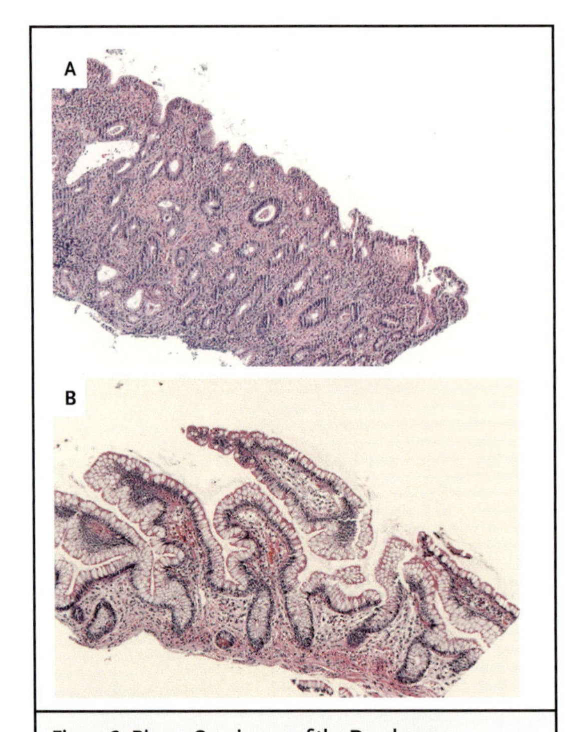

Figure 2. Biopsy Specimens of the Duodenum.

The duodenal-biopsy specimen from the patient (Panel A) reveals degeneration of surface epithelial cells with an increased number of intraepithelial lymphocytes, total villous atrophy, crypt hyperplasia, and chronic inflammation. Panel B shows normal duodenal mucosa with tall villi, normal lamina propria, and shallow crypts.

intestine, is less frequently associated with significant malabsorption. Less common enteropathies — such as tropical sprue, bacterial overgrowth, a diffuse gastrointestinal lymphoma, or Whipple's disease (even with its predilection for men and its associated arthralgia) — are unlikely.

Biopsy of the small bowel revealed marked villous atrophy (Figure 2). A test for antigliadin IgA antibodies was positive, at 209.6 enzyme-linked immunosorbent assay units, and a test for antiendomysial IgA antibodies was positive at a titer of 1:160. A diagnosis of celiac sprue was made. The patient was given a transfusion of packed red cells and intravenous iron, calcium, and vitamin D. He was discharged back to prison on a gluten-free diet.

After the patient had been on this diet (which was prepared specifically for him by the prison cafeteria staff) for four months, his pain had resolved and he had regained significant weight. His hemoglobin and calcium levels had normalized.

COMMENTARY

With a prevalence of almost 1 in 100 in the general population, celiac sprue is surprisingly common.[1-3] Unfortunately, it is a disease that also often leads to diagnostic confusion, particularly if patients do not present with chronic diarrhea and steatorrhea. This case illustrates both why the diagnosis of sprue may be challenging and how a constellation of seemingly unrelated findings led to the recognition of a pattern consistent with celiac disease.

The presenting symptom of progressive hip and leg pain with difficulty walking led the discussant to consider causes of both localized and diffuse bone pain. He initially suspected that the patient had inflammatory bowel disease complicated by a seronegative spondylarthropathy but also considered malabsorption, given the patient's history of weight loss and iron-deficiency anemia. Although both inflammatory bowel disease and celiac sprue were possibilities, the discussant settled on sprue after the discovery of vitamin D deficiency and bone loss (with osteomalacia the presumed cause of his bone pain).

A lack of awareness of the diverse clinical manifestations of celiac sprue may have led many clinicians to miss the diagnosis. In this case, the patient did not report abdominal pain or diarrhea (symptoms widely believed to be essential to the diagnosis), and the stool was guaiac-positive. However, abdominal pain or diarrhea each occurs in only about one third of patients with celiac sprue,[2] and occult blood is present in the stool in almost half of all patients with the disease.[4] In the United States, iron-deficiency anemia is the most common presentation of sprue.[5] Other common symptoms include fatigue, joint pain, diarrhea, constipation, and abdominal pain. Coexisting autoimmune diseases are common, such as hypothyroidism (in 10 percent of patients with celiac sprue), hyperthyroidism (4 percent), and type 1 diabetes mellitus (7 percent).[2,6] Gastrointestinal neoplasms and T-cell lymphomas occur in up to 11 percent of patients.[7] In patients with hepatitis C, the risk of celiac disease is increased by a factor of three,[8] but there is no recognized association between gastroschisis and sprue.

Although the diagnosis of sprue often poses challenges, the pathophysiology of the disease is well understood. Celiac sprue is a consequence of intestinal inflammation initiated in response to the wheat protein gluten. After proteolysis and activation by brush-border aminotransferases, the resultant polypeptides initiate activation of helper T cells, the release of cytokines, inflammation, and subsequent villous atrophy.[9] The diagnosis is usually made after a duodenal biopsy reveals villous atrophy with a lymphocytic infiltration in a patient with characteristic antibodies. If seen on endoscopy, scalloping of intestinal mucosa has a specificity of more than 90 percent.[10] The test for antitransglutaminase IgA antibodies has a sensitivity of 93 to 98 percent and a specificity of 94 to 100 percent[5] and is considered a test of choice for initially evaluating suspected cases and for screening high-risk patients.[5]

This clinical problem-solving exercise exemplifies the importance of efficient pattern recognition in making a correct diagnosis. Clinicians rely on a back-and-forth process of data collection and interpretation that allows for a rapid narrowing of possibilities to a few preliminary hypotheses. But the hypotheses are only as good as the templates from which they are drawn. Astute clinicians usually use a process of probabilistic reasoning (often implicit), whereby clinical findings increase or decrease the likelihood of specific disease entities.[11] The assignment of correct prior probabilities occurs only if the clinician has an accurate template of a given disease to compare with information as it is gathered. For example, most clinicians would correctly assign a very high probability to a diagnosis of hyperthyroidism in a young woman presenting with proptosis, hyperactivity, fine tremor, and diarrhea. These symptoms bring to mind the combination of signs and symptoms (i.e., the hyperthyroidism template) that is learned in medical training. In elderly patients, on the other hand, hyperthyroidism is often characterized by apathy, and this otherwise reliable template unravels, increasing the chance of missing the diagnosis.

In the present case, certain clues pointed toward the ultimate diagnosis of sprue. An expert clinician with a thorough knowledge of the signs, symptoms, associated conditions, and epidemiology of sprue might have suspected celiac disease after just the initial history — but only if armed with a correct template. The discussant's line of reasoning began with noting that a young man with iron-deficiency anemia almost certainly has a gastrointestinal lesion. In fact, up to 5 percent of cases of iron-deficiency anemia can be attributed to celiac disease.[12-14] Add in weight loss, bony pain, and a history of hypothyroidism, and one could argue that celiac sprue becomes the most likely possibility. The high prevalence of the disease provides additional support for this argument.

Skilled clinicians have a finely tuned ability to take information as it is presented and identify a pattern pointing to the ultimate diagnosis. An astute reader could have suspected the diagnosis in this case after reading the title alone. Celiac disease does indeed have a special cure: dietary modification. As an anagram for "celiac sprue," "special cure" was a hidden pattern awaiting recognition.

Supported by a Career Development Award from the Health Services Research and Development Program of the Department of Veterans Affairs and a Patient Safety Developmental Center Grant (P20-HS11540) from the Agency for Healthcare Research and Quality (both to Dr. Saint).

This article first appeared in the November 4, 2004, issue of the New England Journal of Medicine.

REFERENCES

1.
Mäki M, Mustalahti K, Kokkonen J, et al. Prevalence of celiac disease among children in Finland. N Engl J Med 2003;348:2517-24.

2.
Fasano A, Berti I, Gerarduzzi T, et al. Prevalence of celiac disease in at-risk and not-at-risk groups in the United States: a large multicenter study. Arch Intern Med 2003;163: 286-92.

3.
Hin H, Bird G, Fisher P, Mahy N, Jewell D. Coeliac disease in primary care: case finding study. BMJ 1999;318:164-7. [Erratum, BMJ 1999;318:857.]

4.
Fine KD. The prevalence of occult gastrointestinal bleeding in celiac sprue. N Engl J Med 1996;334: 1163-7.

5.
Farrell RJ, Kelly CP. Celiac sprue. N Engl J Med 2002; 346:180-8.

6.
Counsell CE, Taha A, Ruddell WS. Coeliac disease and autoimmune thyroid disease. Gut 1994;35:844-6.

7.
Green PH, Fleischauer AT, Bhagat G, Goyal R, Jabri B, Neugut AI. Risk of malignancy in patients with celiac disease. Am J Med 2003;115:191-5.

8.
Fine KD, Ogunji F, Saloum Y, Beharry S, Crippin J, Weinstein J. Celiac sprue: another autoimmune syndrome associated with hepatitis C. Am J Gastroenterol 2001;96:138-45.

9.
McManus R, Kelleher D. Celiac disease — the villain unmasked? N Engl J Med 2003;348:2573-4.

10.
Oxenteko AS, Grisolano SW, Murray JA, Burgart LJ, Dierkhising RA, Alexander JA. The insensitivity of endoscopic markers in celiac disease. Am J Gastroenterol 2002;97:933-8.

11.
Kassirer JP. Diagnostic reasoning. Ann Intern Med 1989;110:893-900.

12.
Karnam US, Felder LR, Raskin JB. Prevalence of occult celiac disease in patients with iron-deficiency anemia: a prospective study. South Med J 2004;97:30-4.

13.
McIntyre AS, Long RG. Prospective survey of investigations in outpatients referred with iron deficiency anaemia. Gut 1993;34: 1102-7.

14.
Corazza GR, Valentini RA, Andreani ML, et al. Subclinical coeliac disease is a frequent cause of iron-deficiency anaemia. Scand J Gastroenterol 1995;30: 153-6.

Why "Why" Matters

WILLIAM J. JANSSEN, M.D., GURPREET DHALIWAL, M.D., HAROLD R. COLLARD, M.D., AND SANJAY SAINT, M.D., M.P.H.

A 38-year-old woman presented to the emergency room for evaluation of shortness of breath and jaundice. The previous day, she had attended a wedding, where she felt well. Several hours after the wedding, a headache developed, she had mild dizziness, and she noticed that her urine was dark brown. The day after the wedding, she awoke with mild shortness of breath and yellow discoloration of her eyes and skin.

Jaundice is usually caused by hepatobiliary disorders or hemolysis. Biliary obstruction, acute hepatitis, or brisk intravascular hemolysis could explain the jaundice and dark urine. Wilson's disease — with hepatocellular disease and associated hemolysis — could cause jaundice and dark urine.

Dyspnea and jaundice can be related in several ways. Sepsis can cause hyperbilirubinemia and hyperventilation. Hemolysis can lead to dyspnea from anemia and to indirect hyperbilirubinemia from red-cell destruction. Some infections, such as amebiasis, can affect both the liver and the lung. In addition, in the setting of chronic liver disease with associated jaundice — which would be unlikely in this patient, since her illness was acute — dyspnea can develop as a result of the hepatopulmonary syndrome, portopulmonary hypertension, hepatic hydrothorax, or ascites.

Since the patient's illness occurred in the context of her recent attendance at a wedding, I am interested to know what she ate and drank there.

At the wedding, the patient consumed Chinese dumplings containing salt-cured meat and a glass of wine. No one else who attended the wedding became sick. The patient had no abdominal pain, nausea, vomiting, diarrhea, or fever.

I am uncertain whether the patient's illness can be attributed to events at the wedding. Acute infection with hepatitis A virus can occur with ingestion of contaminated food, but the latency period is weeks, not hours. A fatty meal might lead to cholecystitis or choledocholithiasis, but the absence of abdominal pain argues against these disorders. Enterohemorrhagic *Escherichia coli*, specifically strain O157:H7, can cause the hemolytic–uremic syndrome, although the latency period is at least 24 hours, and diarrhea and abdominal pain are typical symptoms.

In the absence of gastrointestinal symptoms, I favor the consideration of an acute hemolytic episode. A potential ingestion at the wedding, followed by hemolysis, raises the possibility of a deficiency of glucose-6-phosphate dehydrogenase (G6PD). The only food I am aware of that is associated with episodic hemolysis from G6PD deficiency is the fava bean.

The patient had a history of mild anemia. She had no history of liver disease. She took no medications or herbal supplements, had no drug allergies, and did not smoke or use illicit drugs. She drank alcohol occasionally. She was Vietnamese and had lived in the United States for seven years. She had been adopted and was unsure of her family history. She worked in a wire-manufacturing plant.

The most likely explanation for her anemia would be iron deficiency or, given her ethnic background, thalassemia. However, many of the chronic hemolytic anemias, which result from defects in the red-cell membrane, enzymes, or hemoglobin, still warrant consideration. The family history, unavailable here, is often helpful in diagnosing these disorders. Long-standing hemolytic anemia can sometimes be manifested as cholecystitis or choledocholithiasis caused by pigment gallstones. Although ingestion of a hepatotoxin might explain the patient's presentation, she reports no history of the use of potentially hepatotoxic medications or herbs and no substantial alcohol intake. Her history of having lived in Vietnam supports the consideration of hepatitis B infection as a cause of her illness.

In general, the combination of jaundice and dark urine is more likely to be a result of hepatobiliary disease than of hemolysis. However, chronic anemia, new dyspnea, and the absence of hepatotoxins, known liver disease, and gastrointestinal symptoms lead me to favor the consideration of hemolysis over an acute hepatobiliary disorder.

The patient was afebrile, with a pulse of 98 beats per minute and a blood pressure of 112/64 mm Hg. Her respiratory rate was 24 breaths per minute, and her oxygen saturation 85 percent. Her skin was jaundiced, her sclerae were icteric, and her conjunctivae were pale. An early systolic murmur was present at the right upper sternal border, and the apical impulse was hyperkinetic. Her lungs were clear on auscultation, and there was no abdominal tenderness or hepatosplenomegaly. The remainder of her physical examination was normal.

The pale conjunctivae, tachycardia, systolic murmur, and hyperkinetic apical impulse are all consistent with anemia, and the jaundice — with no evidence of hepatic or abdominal disease — suggests hemolysis as the cause. Splenomegaly may be seen in many forms of hemolysis but is not an invariable feature and can be challenging to detect by physical examination. Therefore, the absence of palpable splenomegaly is relatively uninformative.

The oxygen saturation of 85 percent is unexpected and not explained by hemolysis. Anemia is a disorder involving a decreased overall capacity to carry oxygen, but the remaining red cells should be adequately saturated in the presence of normal alveolar gas exchange. This particular oxygen saturation brings to mind methemoglobinemia, an acquired dyshemoglobinemia caused by a number of drugs or chemicals that oxidize the iron in hemoglobin, rendering it incapable of carrying oxygen. Sulfonamide antibiotics, local anesthetics such as benzocaine, and antimalarial drugs are common precipitants. Measurement of arterial blood gases with co-oximetry would provide information on the partial pressure of oxygen in arterial blood and on the fraction of the total hemoglobin that is methemoglobin. If both hemolysis and methemoglobinemia were present, I would search for an agent that could trigger both events, and I would suspect that the patient has either a G6PD deficiency or an unstable hemoglobin variant (such as hemoglobin Köln). There is no history of potential culprit drugs, such as dapsone or primaquine, but perhaps there was a component of the food or drink, such as a nitrate or sulfate, that triggered both processes.

If arterial blood analysis reveals hypoxemia without methemoglobinemia, the chest radiograph might suggest other diagnoses. Hilar lymphadenopathy might indicate lymphoma with associated autoimmune hemolysis; an infiltrate could suggest cold autoimmune hemolytic anemia with *Mycoplasma pneumoniae* infection. A normal chest radiograph would raise the possibility of a pulmonary embolism, in which case the rare disorder of paroxysmal nocturnal hemoglobinuria, characterized by hemolysis, pancytopenia, and venous thrombosis, would be worth considering.

The white-cell count was 13,600 per cubic millimeter, the hemoglobin 8.1 g per deciliter, and the platelet count 194,000 per cubic millimeter. The reticulocyte count was 1.8 percent (45,000 reticulocytes per cubic millimeter of blood [normal range, 25,000 to 75,000]). The total bilirubin level was 9.3 mg per deciliter (10.2 μmol per liter), and the lactate dehydrogenase level 2152 U per milliliter (normal range, 91 to 180). The aspartate aminotransferase and alanine aminotransferase levels were 120 U per liter (normal range, 6 to 30) and 41 units per liter (normal range, 10 to 40), respectively. The serum alkaline phosphatase, albumin, and electrolyte levels were normal. A urine dipstick test was positive for

blood; no red cells or casts were seen on microscopical examination. Viral serologic tests for hepatitis A, B, and C viruses were negative. The chest radiograph was normal. An electrocardiogram revealed sinus tachycardia.

The low hemoglobin level and elevated lactate dehydrogenase and bilirubin levels suggest ongoing hemolysis. The results of the urine studies are compatible with hemoglobinuria and indicate rapid and severe red-cell destruction; brisk hemolysis can sometimes cause elevations in aminotransferases. The initial reticulocyte count is inappropriately low, but the bone marrow can be delayed in its response to hemolysis. The normal chest radiograph increases my suspicion of methemoglobinemia.

The cause of the patient's hemolysis remains a puzzle. Given its acute onset, the preexisting anemia, the possibility of methemoglobinemia, and no clear evidence of underlying illness, I favor the hypothesis that some type of oxidant exposure at the wedding triggered a hemolytic episode in this patient, who probably has G6PD deficiency or an unstable hemoglobinopathy. Direct examination of the peripheral blood would be helpful. Disorders that render red cells susceptible to oxidant stress may result in bite cells on the peripheral smear. Heinz bodies (cellular inclusions consisting of damaged aggregated hemoglobin) may be detected with supravital staining.

Despite the administration of supplemental oxygen, the oxygen saturation remained at 85 percent. Arterial blood gas values while the patient was breathing pure oxygen by face mask were as follows: pH 7.45, partial pressure of carbon dioxide 29 mm Hg, and partial pressure of oxygen 432 mm Hg. Co-oximetry demonstrated a methemoglobin level of 8.8 percent (normal range, 0.4 to 1.5).

With the acute onset of hemolysis and methemoglobinemia, I suspect that the patient's red cells were exposed to oxidant stress and that she has either a G6PD deficiency or an unstable-hemoglobin disorder that makes her susceptible to oxidant-induced hemolysis.

How should this patient be treated? Two mechanisms — decreased red-cell mass and ineffective hemoglobin (methemoglobin) — have led to insufficient delivery of oxygen to her tissues. The first-line treatment for acquired methemoglobinemia is the administration of methylene blue, which quickly reduces methemoglobin to hemoglobin. However, G6PD deficiency is a contraindication to treatment with methylene blue because patients with this disorder are unable to metabolize methylene blue, an oxidant that can exacerbate hemolysis. With a hemoglobin level that is already quite low, this patient may not tolerate additional hemolysis.

Toxin-mediated or oxidant-mediated hemolysis is usually managed supportively after the exposure has been terminated. With G6PD deficiency, most acute episodes of hemolysis are self-limited, and only the most severe cases require transfusion. Blood transfusion would accomplish the goal of restoring a normal hemoglobin level and oxygen-carrying capacity, but it involves additional risks. I favor blood transfusion over the use of methylene blue because of the suspicion of oxidant-mediated hemolysis due to G6PD deficiency.

Intravenous methylene blue was administered. Subsequent testing demonstrated worsening anemia, with a hemoglobin value of 6.5 g per deciliter. The patient received 4 units of packed red cells, and her red-cell count was stabilized. The activity of G6PD, as measured in a blood sample obtained before transfusion, was 3.9 U per gram of hemoglobin (normal range, 4.6 to 13.5).

This measured G6PD level may actually understate the patient's degree of G6PD deficiency, since the G6PD level measured during a hemolytic episode reflects only the surviving red-cell population; these surviving red cells evade hemolysis owing to G6PD levels that are higher than average. The gene for G6PD resides on the X chromosome. In a female patient, this raises the interesting possibility that the surviving red-cell population represents cells whose precursors have selectively deactivated their deficient X chromosome.

The patient was seen in the clinic several months later and was doing well. Her hemoglobin measured 12.6 g per deciliter, and a peripheral-blood smear demonstrated only mild reticulocytosis.

COMMENTARY

A fundamental component in the care of any patient is an understanding and appreciation of the pathophysiology underlying his or her disease. Furthermore, it is essential that clinicians continue to evaluate available clinical data — even after a particular diagnosis is suspected — to ensure that there are no discordant findings. As this case illustrates, failure in these two areas can lead to inappropriate management and iatrogenic morbidity. Although the treating physicians correctly identified the patient's methemoglobinemia, the hemolytic process was not recognized as a potential contraindication to treatment. Understanding why manifestations of disease occur and incorporating this knowledge into diagnostic decision making remain important parts of the practice of medicine.

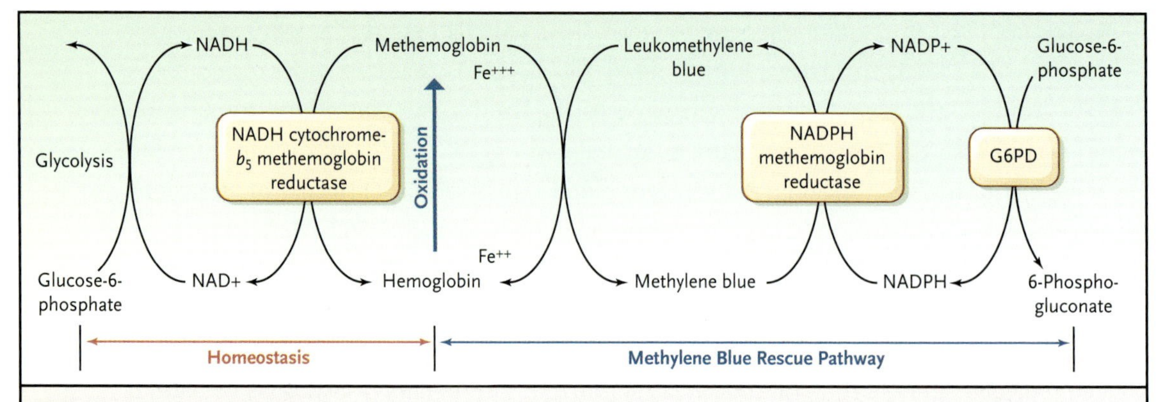

Figure 1. Reduction of Hemoglobin to Methemoglobin under Normal Circumstances and after the Administration of Methylene Blue.

Under normal circumstances, the NADH-dependent–cytochrome-b_5 methemoglobin reductase system efficiently reduces methemoglobin to hemoglobin. Methylene blue provides an alternative means by which methemoglobin can be reduced. In patients with G6PD deficiency, the production of NADPH is impaired, thereby limiting the conversion of methylene blue to its active metabolite, leukomethylene blue.

What was the pathophysiology underlying this patient's condition? Both the methemoglobinemia and the hemolytic anemia were triggered by oxidative stress. Methemoglobin (oxidized hemoglobin) is constantly produced in erythrocytes as a result of the close interaction between hemoglobin and oxygen. Under normal circumstances, methemoglobin is converted back into hemoglobin by the NADH-dependent cytochrome-b_5 methemoglobin reductase system (Figure 1), thereby maintaining an equilibrium in which less than 1 percent of hemoglobin exists as methemoglobin.[1] This balance can be upset by exposure to agents such as local anesthetics, sulfa antibiotics, and nitrite-containing compounds (including nitroglycerin and nitroprusside) that increase the levels of reactive oxygen species.[1,2]

Oxidative stress also contributes to the hemolytic anemia seen in patients with G6PD deficiency. G6PD is important for the elimination of reactive oxygen species (Figure 2). In the absence of functional G6PD, accumulated oxidant exposure leads to denaturation of hemoglobin, impaired integrity of cell membranes, and hemolysis. Common precipitants include infection, drug exposure (especially exposure to dapsone, sulfamethoxazole, and primaquine), and, in susceptible persons, ingestion of foods such as fava beans.[3,4]

Two concepts are critical for understanding how such severe hemolysis developed in this patient: inactivation of the X chromosome and activity of the G6PD enzyme. As the discussant points out, G6PD deficiency is transmitted on the X chromosome. Therefore, all men with the disease are hemizygous, and most women are heterozygous. Early in the process of female embryonic development, one X chromosome is inactivated in each

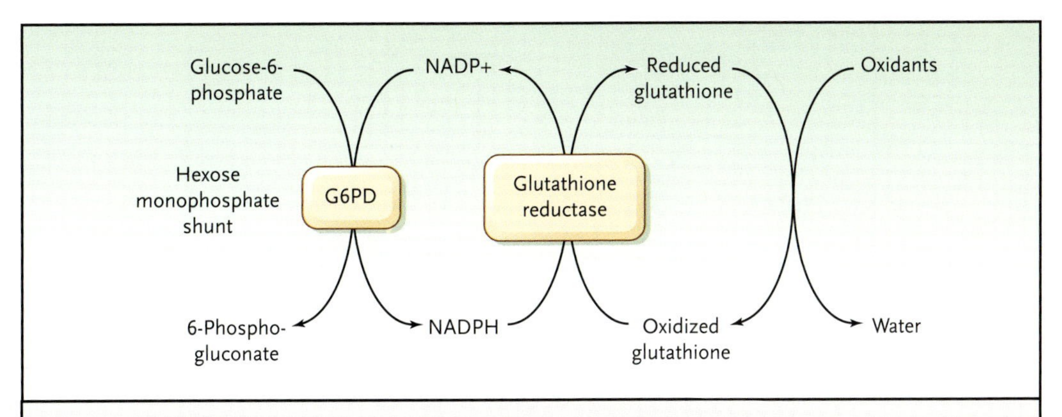

Figure 2. Role of G6PD in the Elimination of Reactive Oxygen Species in the Erythrocyte.

G6PD catalyzes the first step in the hexose monophosphate shunt by converting glucose-6-phosphate to 6-phosphogluconate. The reaction produces NADPH, which donates electrons to glutathione, thereby providing a means by which reactive oxygen species can be reduced to hydrogen peroxide and, ultimately, to water.

somatic cell, which results in two cell populations, one with normal G6PD and one with deficient G6PD (Figure 3).[4,5] The clinical phenotype is determined both by the percentage of G6PD-deficient red cells and by the degree of G6PD activity in the enzyme-deficient cells. Many of the Asian variants of G6PD deficiency are characterized by enzyme levels that are barely detectable. In persons with these variants, hemolysis can be severe and life-threatening.[6]

This case was made especially challenging by the absence of a classically recognized precipitant. Could it have been the Chinese dumplings? No localizing symptoms were present to suggest infection, which is the most common precipitant of hemolysis in patients with G6PD deficiency[3]; despite repeated review of the patient's history, no other gustatory culprit emerged. The patient specifically denied having ingested fava beans, which are uncommon in Chinese cuisine. Nitrates are converted to nitrites by intestinal bacteria, and the ingestion of foods, including dumplings, that contain high quantities of nitrates have been reported in rare cases to cause methemoglobinemia.[7-9] Sodium nitrite, a preservative commonly used to cure meats and fish, has also been implicated in outbreaks of methemoglobinemia that is related to such foods.[7,8] Nitrites can also cause brisk hemolysis in patients with G6PD deficiency.[10-12] We suspect that the dumplings were indeed the precipitating agent.

The association between methemoglobinemia and G6PD deficiency carries important implications for treatment. Although methylene blue rapidly reverses methemoglobinemia in most patients, persons with G6PD deficiency are a notable exception. Methylene

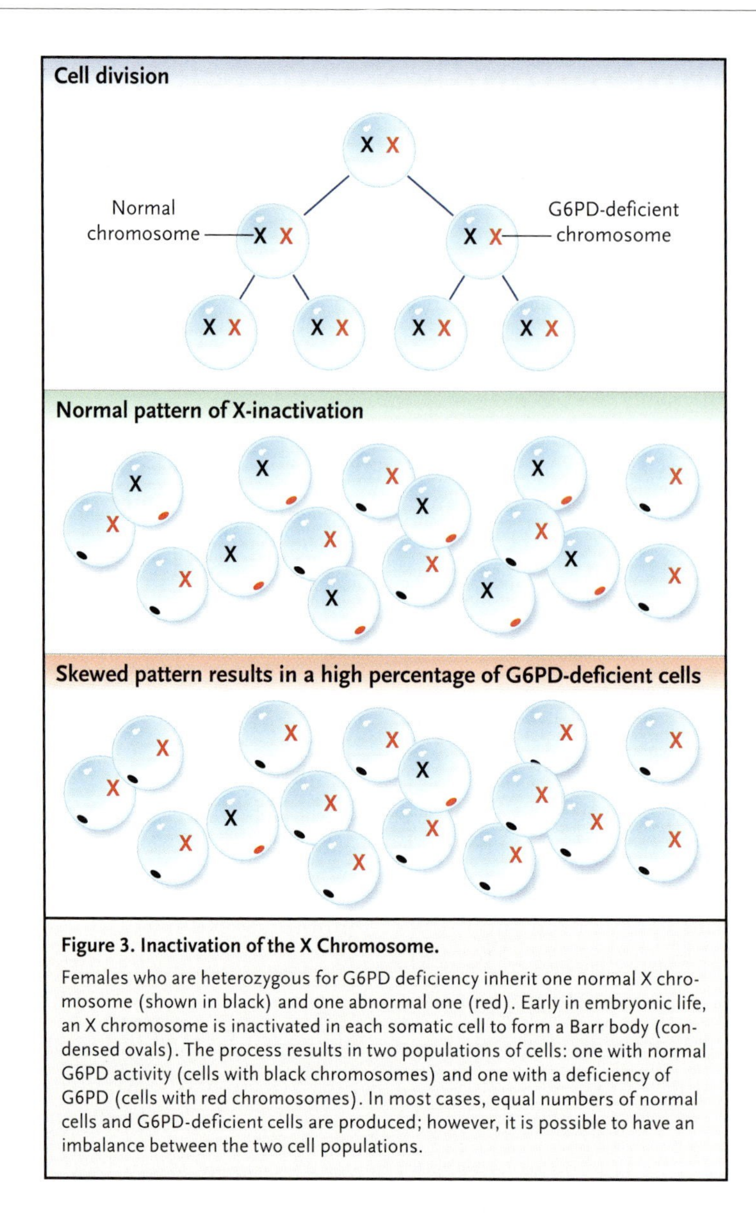

Figure 3. Inactivation of the X Chromosome.

Females who are heterozygous for G6PD deficiency inherit one normal X chromosome (shown in black) and one abnormal one (red). Early in embryonic life, an X chromosome is inactivated in each somatic cell to form a Barr body (condensed ovals). The process results in two populations of cells: one with normal G6PD activity (cells with black chromosomes) and one with a deficiency of G6PD (cells with red chromosomes). In most cases, equal numbers of normal cells and G6PD-deficient cells are produced; however, it is possible to have an imbalance between the two cell populations.

blue is largely ineffective in these patients because NADPH, which is required to reduce methylene blue to its active metabolite, leukomethylene blue, is not available (Figure 1).[13] Furthermore, methylene blue is a powerful oxidant and can precipitate or worsen hemolytic anemia associated with G6PD deficiency, as in this patient.[13,14]

The failure of the treating physicians to consider the concomitant diagnosis of G6PD deficiency in this patient and to connect the underlying pathophysiology of her hemolysis with methemoglobinemia left them at risk for making a common error in diagnostic reasoning, known as "premature closure."[15] Premature closure occurs when a diagnosis is applied to a patient's condition despite incomplete or contradictory supporting data. The danger of rendering a premature diagnosis is that diagnostic evaluation is often discontinued, and associated conditions may be overlooked or ignored. It is critical that clinicians completely analyze all available data, consider the pathophysiology of suspected diagnoses, and keep their minds open to the possibility of alternative or concomitant diagnoses. As this case illustrates, appropriate diagnosis and treatment require that clinicians understand not only what is happening but also why it is happening.

Supported by a Career Development Award from the Health Services Research and Development Program of the Department of Veterans Affairs and by a grant (P20-HS11540) from the Patient Safety Developmental Center of the Agency for Healthcare Research and Quality (both to Dr. Saint).

We are indebted to Dr. Ernest Beutler for his kind review of the manuscript.

This article first appeared in the December 2, 2004, issue of the New England Journal of Medicine.

REFERENCES

1.
Wright RO, Lewander WJ, Woolf AD. Methemoglobinemia: etiology, pharmacology, and clinical management. Ann Emerg Med 1999;34:646-56.

2.
Mansouri A, Lurie AA. Concise review: methemoglobinemia. Am J Hematol 1993;42:7-12.

3.
Beutler E. Glucose-6-phosphate dehydrogenase deficiency. N Engl J Med 1991;324:169-74.

4.
Idem. G6PD deficiency. Blood 1994;84:3613-36.

5.
Idem. The genetics of glucose-6-phosphate dehydrogenase deficiency. Semin Hematol 1990;27:137-64.

6.
Verle P, Nhan DH, Tinh TT, et al. Glucose-6-phosphate dehydrogenase deficiency in northern Vietnam. Trop Med Int Health 2000;5:203-6.

7.
Chan TY. Food-borne nitrates and nitrites as a cause of methemoglobinemia. Southeast Asian J Trop Med Public Health 1996;27:189-92.

8.
Methemoglobinemia following unintentional ingestion of sodium nitrite — New York, 2002. MMWR Morb Mortal Wkly Rep 2002;51:639-42.

9.
Walley T, Flanagan M. Nitrite-induced methaemoglobinaemia. Postgrad Med J 1987;63:643-4.

10.
Brandes JC, Bufill JA, Pisciotta AV. Amyl nitrite-induced hemolytic anemia. Am J Med 1989;86:252-4.

11.
Costello C, Pourgourides E, Youle M. Amyl nitrite induced acute haemolytic anaemia in HIV-antibody positive man. Int J STD AIDS 2000;11:334-5.

12.
Neuberger A, Fishman S, Golik A. Hemolytic anemia in a G6PD-deficient man after inhalation of amyl nitrite ("poppers"). Isr Med Assoc J 2002;4:1085-6.

13.
Rosen PJ, Johnson C, McGehee WG, Beutler E. Failure of methylene blue treatment in toxic methemoglobinemia: association with glucose-6-phosphate dehydrogenase deficiency. Ann Intern Med 1971;75:83-6.

14.
Liao YP, Hung DZ, Yang DY. Hemolytic anemia after methylene blue therapy for aniline-induced methemoglobinemia. Vet Hum Toxicol 2002;44:19-21.

15.
Voytovich AE, Rippey RM, Suffredini A. Premature conclusions in diagnostic reasoning. J Med Educ 1985;60:302-7.

Unfashionably Late

MICHAEL LUKELA, M.D., DAVID DEGUZMAN, M.D.,
STEVEN WEINBERGER, M.D., AND SANJAY SAINT, M.D., M.P.H.

An 18-year-old man presented with shortness of breath, a cough that was productive of clear sputum, and a two-week history of pleuritic chest pain. He also reported night sweats, fever, and fatigue, but no hemoptysis, weight loss, recent travel, or new environmental exposures.

The combination of progressive shortness of breath and pleuritic chest pain suggests either of two pathogenetic sequences. In one scenario, the primary process could have originated at the pleural surface and produced either a pleural effusion or a pneumothorax large enough to cause dyspnea. Alternatively, the process could have originated in the pulmonary parenchyma (causing dyspnea) and extended to the pleural surface (causing pleuritic chest pain). In either case, the presence of night sweats, fever, and fatigue suggests an underlying infection or a noninfectious inflammatory process, although a neoplasm (such as lymphoma) or even recurrent pulmonary embolism is also possible.

The patient had had two episodes of community-acquired pneumonia as a teenager; the last episode occurred two years before the current illness. Other than having a cyst removed from his neck as a child, he reported no serious illnesses or operations. He was taking no medications. There was no family history of cystic fibrosis, lung disease, or immune deficiencies. His immunizations were current. He was a recent high-school graduate who lived with his parents in suburban Michigan. He said that he did not use alcohol, tobacco, or illicit drugs, and he had no pets.

The patient's history of previous episodes of community-acquired pneumonia raises the question of an underlying susceptibility to bacterial or other infections, either because of a systemic problem associated with impaired pulmonary defense mechanisms (such as an immune deficiency, ciliary dysfunction, or cystic fibrosis) or because of focal endobronchial disease predisposing him to postobstructive infection (especially if the earlier bouts of pneumonia were in the same anatomic location). Although what he described as a neck cyst was probably unrelated to the current symptoms, the possibility of an underlying anatomic problem or complication following excision or that the cyst had been an infected lymph node (as in cases of tuberculous lymphadenitis), rather than a sterile cyst, should also be considered.

The patient was a thin white man in no acute distress. His temperature was 36.6°C, the heart rate 88 beats per minute, the respiratory rate 18 breaths per minute, the blood pressure 106/56 mm Hg, and the oxygen saturation 98 percent while he was breathing ambient air. His height was 163 cm, and his weight 55 kg. He had no cervical lymphadenopathy. He had bronchial breath sounds at both lung bases and egophony in his right mid-chest area. His back and both thighs were noted to have small acneiform lesions; he had no clubbing. The remainder of his physical examination was normal.

The white-cell count was 7.0 per cubic millimeter, with 74 percent neutrophils, 16 percent lymphocytes, and 10 percent monocytes. The hematocrit was 40 percent, and the platelet count 344,000 per cubic millimeter. The levels of aspartate and alanine aminotransferase were normal at 30 and 22 units per liter, respectively. The serum level of lactate dehydrogenase was 325 units per liter (normal range, 60 to 200). The results of an electrolyte panel and urinalysis were normal, as was the level of creatinine. A chest radiograph showed air-space opacities in the right middle lobe, lingula, and both lower lobes (Figure 1).

The extensive air-space opacities and the consolidation suggest that the process causing pleuritic chest pain started in the pulmonary parenchyma and extended to the pleural surface. In addition, the multifocal nature of the opacities on the chest radiographs is inconsistent with a focal endobronchial obstruction leading to recurrent postobstructive pneumonia. My primary diagnostic considerations remain infection and noninfectious inflammatory disease, specifically bronchiolitis obliterans with organizing pneumonia or hypersensitivity pneumonitis, since both can have patchy airspace opacities that mimic bacterial pneumonia. The subacute clinical presentation, which took place over a number of weeks, combined with constitutional symptoms is particularly suggestive of bronchiolitis obliterans with organizing pneumonia, whereas the history of what was reported as two previous episodes of community-acquired pneumonia raises the possibility of recurrent episodes of hypersensitivity pneumonitis misdiagnosed as pneumonia.

The patient was admitted to the hospital and was given ceftriaxone and azithromycin. A test for the human immunodeficiency virus was negative, as were the results of tuberculin skin testing. Quantitative levels of immunoglobulins and of complement were normal. Tests for the presence of antinuclear antibody and antineutrophil cytoplasmic antibody

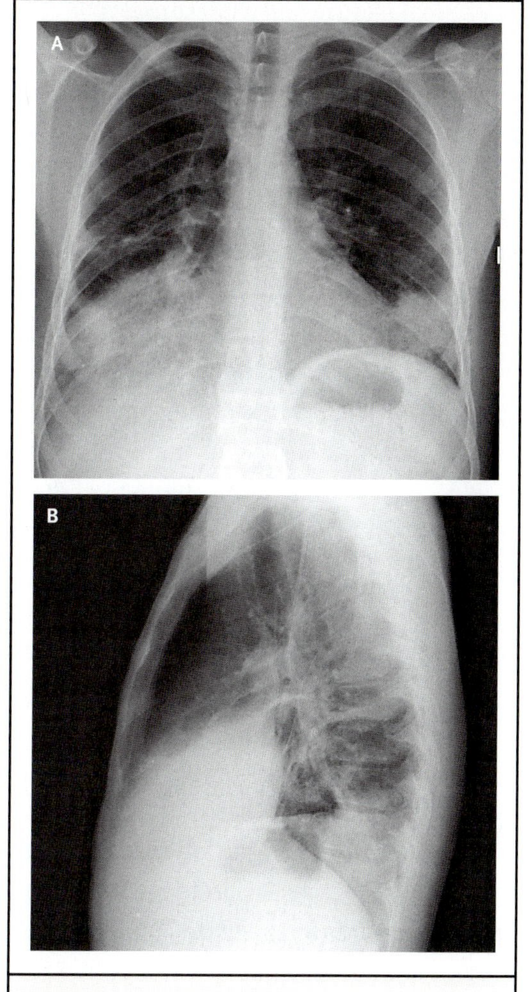

Figure 1. Chest Radiographs.

A posteroanterior view (Panel A) and a lateral view (Panel B) show bilateral air-space opacities in the right middle lobe, lingula, and both lower lobes.

were both negative; the Westergren erythrocyte sedimentation rate was 57 mm per hour. Several blood and sputum cultures obtained during febrile periods revealed no growth. Serologic tests for the presence of cytomegalovirus, Epstein–Barr virus, herpes simplex virus, and parvovirus B19 were negative. Immunodiffusion studies for histoplasmosis, coccidioidomycosis, and blastomycosis were nonreactive. A transthoracic echocardiogram showed no abnormalities.

Although patients with a clinical picture and a chest radiograph such as this patient had are typically given a diagnosis of bacterial pneumonia and started empirically on antibiotic treatment, the normal leukocyte count and the subacute presentation argue against this diagnosis. Consequently, my preference would have been to withhold empirical antibiotic therapy, unless the patient appeared particularly ill. One nonbacterial infection I would consider is blastomycosis, and the negative results on the immunodiffusion study do not dissuade me from this possibility, given the relatively poor diagnostic sensitivity of the test. The chest radiograph in a patient with pulmonary blastomycosis often shows one or more areas of consolidation that may mimic the appearance of a bacterial pneumonia — similar to the abnormalities seen in this patient.

Furthermore, if the acneiform lesions noted on the physical examination appear to be quite new, they could represent an early cutaneous manifestation of *Blastomyces dermatitidis*, whose name reminds us of the potential for involvement of the skin. However, I remain concerned about bronchiolitis obliterans with organizing pneumonia. As with blastomycosis, the areas of consolidation on the chest radiograph mimic the signs of pneumonia, but the clinical onset of bronchiolitis obliterans with organizing pneumonia is typically more gradual than the onset of bacterial pneumonia. The absence of a response to antibiotic treatment is often a clue to the diagnosis of bronchiolitis obliterans with organizing pneumonia.

High-resolution computed tomographic (CT) scans of the chest (Figure 2) revealed extensive air-space opacification involving the right lower lobe, accompanied by additional patchy and confluent areas of air-space opacification in the right middle lobe, lingula, and left lower lobe. There was also mild bronchiectasis. No lymphadenopathy was present. Examination by bronchoscopy showed normal airways; bronchoalveolar-lavage fluid was negative for acid-fast bacilli, as determined by staining, and for *Pneumocystis carinii*, as determined by polymerase-chain-reaction (PCR) assay. A transbronchial biopsy revealed nonspecific plasma-cell and lymphocytic infiltrates. The patient's fever abated and his dyspnea improved while he was receiving ceftriaxone and azithromycin. He was discharged to his home without antibiotics, having completed a 10-day course of treatment as an inpatient.

Although the dense areas of consolidation in both lungs, as seen on the CT scans, are consistent with a diagnosis of bacterial pneumonia, they are also consistent with either blastomycosis or bronchiolitis obliterans with organizing pneumonia. In particular, the peripheral nature of some of the areas of consolidation may be indicative of bronchiolitis

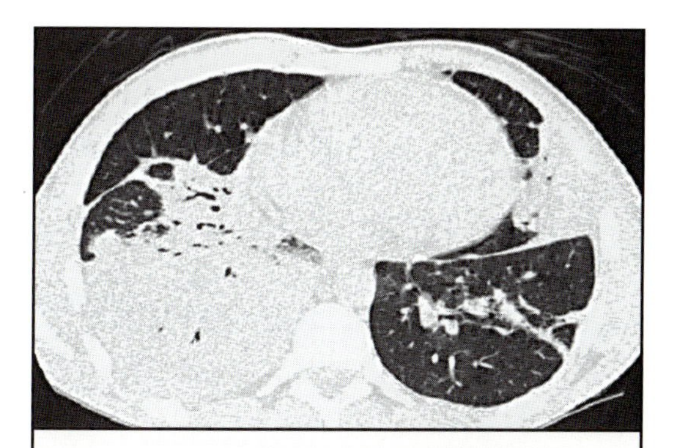

Figure 2. High-Resolution CT Scan of the Chest.

A representative CT image shows extensive air-space opacification involving the right lower lobe, accompanied by additional patchy and confluent areas of opacification in the lingula and the left lower lobe and by mild bronchiectasis. An area of opacification was also present in the right middle lobe (not shown).

obliterans with organizing pneumonia. The presence of plasma-cell and lymphocytic infiltrates in the absence of neutrophils argues against a diagnosis of bacterial pneumonia, and the absence of eosinophils makes a diagnosis of either acute or chronic eosinophilic pneumonia improbable.

Although the patient is reported to have improved while receiving antibiotic agents, it is unclear whether the improvement was spontaneous and coincidental with institution of this treatment or was actually due to antibiotic action. At the moment, my leading diagnosis would be bronchiolitis obliterans with organizing pneumonia, but respiratory infections can be the precipitant for an inflammatory response with the pattern of bronchiolitis obliterans with organizing pneumonia, so that the diagnoses of infection and bronchiolitis obliterans with organizing pneumonia are not mutually exclusive.

During the two weeks after discharge, the patient became febrile, with a temperature as high as 40°C. He was readmitted to the hospital and given treatment with cefepime, clindamycin, and azithromycin. He showed little improvement after five days of hospitalization. Since the previous transbronchial biopsy had been nondiagnostic, open-lung biopsy with mediastinoscopy was performed and revealed necrotizing granulomas with atypical lymphocytic infiltration. Immunophenotyping showed no evidence of lymphoma. Staining for organisms was also negative. Initial cultures of the tissue specimen obtained during the lung biopsy showed no growth.

Despite the presumed improvement associated with the first regimen of antibiotic agents, it is clear that the clinical problem was far from resolved, and the biopsy to obtain tissue was appropriate. The finding of necrotizing granulomas with atypical lymphocytic infiltration on histopathological examination is not diagnostic, but it makes some earlier diagnostic considerations less probable and at the same time raises new possibilities. Mycobacterial or fungal infections, especially blastomycosis, remain a concern, despite the negative tuberculin skin test and the negative serologic studies for fungus. The histopathological features were not suggestive of bronchiolitis obliterans with organizing pneumonia, so among the noninfectious inflammatory (or even neoplastic) disorders, I would now be more concerned about those entities with prominent atypical lymphocytic or necrotizing granulomatous inflammation, such as lymphomatoid granulomatosis. The patient's history of persistent cough, dyspnea, and fever is consistent with this disorder, although imaging studies typically show nodules or masses, rather than air-space opacification. Nevertheless, at this point, my leading diagnosis would be either lymphomatoid granulomatosis or an infectious process, either fungal (especially blastomycosis) or mycobacterial.

In light of the pathological findings on lung biopsy, the patient was given a preliminary diagnosis of either bronchiolitis obliterans with organizing pneumonia or a lymphoproliferative disorder of unclear cause; he was started on oral prednisone (60 mg daily). He noted moderate improvement in his dyspnea and cough. He was discharged to his home, still taking corticosteroids, and with close outpatient follow-up included in his treatment plan.

I am concerned about the empirical use of corticosteroids in this setting, without a definite diagnosis. Through the nonspecific suppression of the inflammatory response, corticosteroids can result in initial symptomatic improvement in many clinical conditions, but the ultimate control or cure of the underlying problem requires additional or alternative treatment. The early improvement in the patient's dyspnea and cough after the institution of corticosteroids does not assure me that the presumed diagnosis of either bronchiolitis obliterans with organizing pneumonia or a lymphoproliferative disorder is correct. The possibility of an unrecognized infection remains, and the use of corticosteroids in the absence of appropriate antimicrobial coverage carries a risk, since these drugs will suppress his cellular immune response.

The patient continued with the oral prednisone at 60 mg daily. He was seen in the clinic three weeks after his discharge, and while he was there, the return of his dyspnea, fevers

as high as 39.4°C, and cough with pleuritic chest pain were noted. He was admitted again to the hospital, and a review of the culture from the lung-biopsy specimen obtained three weeks earlier revealed growth of *Burkholderia cepacia*. He was started on intravenous ceftazidime and levofloxacin. A repeated high-resolution CT scan of the chest showed consolidation in both lower lobes and the right middle lobe, findings that were unchanged from the previous examination.

We now have an organism growing in culture from a lung-biopsy specimen, and the results are surprising. *B. cepacia* can be an environmental contaminant, a colonizer, or a true cause of disease; in this particular case, I would worry that it is a real pathogen. However, it typically occurs in the setting of certain disorders characterized by impaired pulmonary defense mechanisms, specifically in patients with cystic fibrosis or chronic granulomatous disease. Although both of these diseases are usually diagnosed during childhood, they can sometimes be found in late adolescence or early adulthood. Recurrent pneumonia and mild bronchiectasis could be sequelae of cystic fibrosis, and the necrotizing granulomas found on biopsy could indicate coexistent infection with nontuberculous mycobacteria, a well-recognized complication of cystic fibrosis. Alternatively, recurrent *B. cepacia* pneumonia associated with chronic granulomatous disease is also possible, in which case the granulomatous inflammation found on biopsy is a characteristic of the underlying disease.

Careful review of this patient's family history again revealed no relatives with cystic fibrosis or immune deficiencies. The sweat chloride test was normal, with a sweat weight of 22 g and a sweat chloride level of 24 mEq per liter (normal range, 1 to 39). A PCR assay for an abnormal cystic fibrosis transmembrane regulator (*CFTR*) gene was negative for a standard panel of 25 genes. The patient remained febrile while receiving intravenous antibiotics; the results of a repeated bronchoscopy showed normal airways. Bronchoalveolar lavage was performed, and the fluid was negative for bacteria and viruses on culture, for acid-fast bacilli on staining, and for *Pneumocystis carinii* on PCR assay.

Although a normal result from a chloride sweat test and negative test results for the standard panel of abnormal *CFTR* genes, taken alone, can each miss a small percentage of cases of cystic fibrosis, the fact that both of these tests were negative makes a diagnosis of cystic fibrosis extremely unlikely. Therefore, I believe that the unexpected growth of *B. cepacia*, in the setting of a negative workup for cystic fibrosis, leads us to chronic granu-

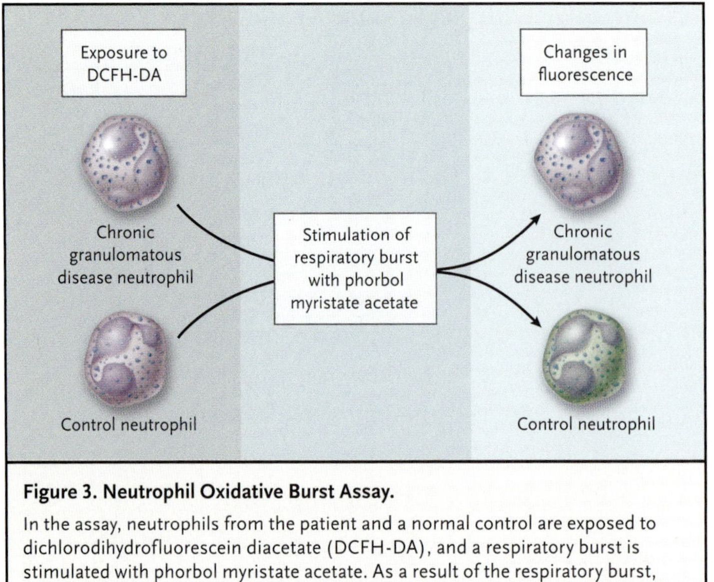

Figure 3. Neutrophil Oxidative Burst Assay.

In the assay, neutrophils from the patient and a normal control are exposed to dichlorodihydrofluorescein diacetate (DCFH-DA), and a respiratory burst is stimulated with phorbol myristate acetate. As a result of the respiratory burst, DCFH-DA is oxidized to the green fluorescent compound dichlorodihydrofluorescein. Changes in fluorescence are then measured by a fluorescence reader and quantified as a change in the relative fluorescence units. In patients with chronic granulomatous disease, no oxidative burst is seen in response to stimulation with phorbol myristate acetate, and therefore there is little or no change in the relative fluorescence.

lomatous disease as the most likely disorder responsible for this patient's clinical presentation, course, and histologic findings. Whereas we often consider an unusual presentation of a common disease to be more likely than a typical presentation of an uncommon disease, I think we may be dealing here with an even less likely scenario: an unusual presentation of an uncommon disease.

A neutrophil oxidative burst assay was performed. The patient's neutrophils showed no evidence of an oxidative burst in response to stimulation, whereas an assay performed concurrently in a normal person as a control showed a normal oxidative burst pattern (Figure 3). The results in the patient were considered diagnostic of chronic granulomatous disease. Another review of his history showed no evidence of recurrent infections or lymphadenopathy as a child, stomatitis, or enteritis. Genetic screening was offered to the patient's family.

COMMENTARY

Physicians are often confronted with the question of whether a premature disorder is the cause of a patient's symptoms; coronary artery disease as the cause of chest pain in a 36-year-old patient is one such example. The opposite phenomenon — considering illnesses that should have presented years earlier — is a less familiar scenario. In this case, perhaps if the patient's physicians had further considered disorders with delayed presentation earlier, the patient's condition might have been diagnosed sooner.

As the discussant points out, recurrent pneumonia in an otherwise healthy adolescent patient merits further investigation. Even though this young man had had two previous episodes of pneumonia, the reappearance of extensive lung disease and the subacute presentation should have raised the possibility of an underlying inherited disease at an earlier stage of his evaluation.

The clinical team, however, can hardly be faulted for not quickly recognizing an atypical presentation of chronic granulomatous disease. The disease was first described in 1957 as a "fatal granulomatosus of childhood."[1,2] It soon became clear that neutrophils from affected patients, although capable of phagocytosis, were unable to generate active microbicidal oxygen species necessary to eradicate infection.[3,4] The most common defect present in the X-linked recessive condition affects $gp91^{phox}$, an integral membrane protein of NADPH oxidase.[5] Three additional forms of the disease are due to autosomal recessive defects in other major components of the oxidase, $p22^{phox}$, $p47^{phox}$, and $p67^{phox}$.[5,6]

It has been estimated that chronic granulomatous disease has an incidence of 1 per 200,000 births in the United States.[5] Of 368 patients enrolled in a national registry of patients with chronic granulomatous disease, 70 percent had the X-linked recessive form and 22 percent had an autosomal recessive form; the genetic basis of the disease could not be determined in the remaining 8 percent.[5] Eighty-five percent of the patients in these cases were male; 83 percent were white, 11 percent were black, 2 percent were Asian, less than 1 percent were Native American, 1 percent were of mixed ancestry, and 3 percent were of unknown race or ethnic group, on the basis of demographic information obtained from the physicians who enrolled patients in the registry. The mean age at diagnosis was three years in patients with the X-linked recessive form and eight years in those with autosomal recessive disease.[5,7]

Infection represents the most common clinical finding in patients with chronic granulomatous disease. The leading infections are pneumonia, abscess formation, suppurative adenitis, and osteomyelitis.[5,7] Noninfectious complications related to granuloma formation have also been described and include colitis, gastric-outlet obstruction, and skin ulceration.[6,8]

The diagnosis of chronic granulomatous disease has historically been confirmed by the nitroblue tetrazolium test. Functioning neutrophils reduce the nitroblue tetrazolium dye from a clear yellow, water-soluble compound to a dark blue precipitant (formazan) in the presence of oxygen species produced during the respiratory burst.[6,9] More sensitive tests are now available that involve probes whose fluorescent or chemiluminescent properties are altered by their reaction with reactive oxidants, such as the dihydrorhodamine-123 fluorescence test.[6,10] After confirmation of the diagnosis with functional assays, the genotype can be determined by immunoblotting or direct sequencing.

The outcome for patients has improved substantially as compared with outcomes in earlier cohorts, in which only 70 percent of children with chronic granulomatous disease survived beyond the age of eight years.[11,12] Currently, median survival is into the second decade of life.[5] This improvement in survival is attributed primarily to widespread antimicrobial prophylaxis with trimethoprim–sulfamethoxazole.[11,12] Adjunctive use of itraconazole has been effective as prophylaxis against fungal pathogens.[12] Whereas treatment with interferon gamma reduces the frequency and severity of infections, when used alone or in conjunction with antimicrobial prophylaxis, its cost and side effects have limited its use.[13] Newer methods, such as gene therapy and bone marrow transplantation, may one day represent curative options.[14]

Chronic granulomatous disease is only one example of a genetic disorder that may present later than usually described; other genetic disorders — for example, Tay–Sachs disease and cystic fibrosis — may do the same. This case reminds us to keep in mind conditions that show up earlier or later than expected, however unfashionable their arrival may seem.

Dr. Saint is the recipient of a Career Development Award from the Health Services Research and Development Program of the Department of Veterans Affairs and a Patient Safety Developmental Center Grant from the Agency for Healthcare Research and Quality (P20-HS11540).

This article first appeared in the January 6, 2005, issue of the New England Journal of Medicine.

REFERENCES

1.
Berendes H, Bridges RA, Good RA. A fatal granulomatosus of childhood: the clinical study of a new syndrome. Minn Med 1957;40:309-12.

2.
Bridges RA, Berendes H, Good RA. A fatal granulomatous disease of childhood: the clinical, pathological, and laboratory features of a new syndrome. AMA J Dis Child 1959;97:387-408.

3.
Baehner RL, Nathan DG. Leukocyte oxidase: defective activity in chronic granulomatous disease. Science 1967;155:835-6.

4.
Quie PG, White JG, Holmes PG, Good RA. In vitro bactericidal capacity of human polymorphonuclear leukocytes: diminished activity in chronic granulomatous disease of childhood. J Clin Invest 1967;46:668-79.

5.
Winkelstein JA, Marino MC, Johnston RB Jr, et al. Chronic granulomatous disease: report on a national registry of 368 patients. Medicine (Baltimore) 2000;79:155-69.

6.
Segal BH, Leto TL, Gallin JI, Malech HL, Holland SM. Genetic, biochemical, and clinical features of chronic granulomatous disease. Medicine (Baltimore) 2000;79:170-200.

7.
Johnston RB Jr. Clinical aspects of chronic granulomatous disease. Curr Opin Hematol 2001;8:17-22.

8.
Barton LL, Moussa SL, Villar RG, Hulett RL. Gastrointestinal complications of chronic granulomatous disease: case report and literature review. Clin Pediatr (Phila) 1998;37:231-6.

9.
Baehner RL, Boxer LA, Davis J. The biochemical basis of nitroblue tetrazolium reduction in normal human and chronic granulomatous disease polymorphonuclear leukocytes. Blood 1976;48:309-13.

10.
Jirapongsananuruk O, Malech HL, Kuhns DB, et al. Diagnostic paradigm for evaluation of male patients with chronic granulomatous disease, based on the dihydrorhodamine 123 assay. J Allergy Clin Immunol 2003;111:374-9.

11.
Cale CM, Jones AM, Goldblatt D. Follow up of patients with chronic granulomatous disease diagnosed since 1990. Clin Exp Immunol 2000;120:351-5.

12.
Mouy R, Fischer A, Vilmer E, Seger R, Griscelli C. Incidence, severity, and prevention of infections in chronic granulomatous disease. J Pediatr 1989;114:555-60.

13.
Gallin JI, Malech HL, Weening RS, et al. A controlled trial of interferon gamma to prevent infection in chronic granulomatous disease. N Engl J Med 1991;324:509-16.

14.
Malech HL. Progress in gene therapy for chronic granulomatous disease. J Infect Dis 1999;179:Suppl 2:S318-S325.

The Unturned Stone

CHRISTOPHER J. GOULET, M.D., RICHARD H. MOSELEY, M.D., CLAUDE TONNERRE, M.D., IQBAL S. SANDHU, M.D., AND SANJAY SAINT, M.D., M.P.H.

A 20-year-old man was transferred to an academic medical center in Salt Lake City for further evaluation of diarrhea, abdominal pain, and fever. Two months before admission, he presented to a community hospital with dull, intermittent pain in the right lower quadrant. A colonoscopy performed at that time showed patchy erythema, edema, and ulcerations from the transverse colon to the cecum. The terminal ileum also appeared inflamed and had linear ulcerations. Pathological examination of specimens revealed nonspecific chronic inflammation.

The patient's symptoms have been present for two months, defining this as a case of chronic diarrhea. Acute diarrhea, most often caused by infectious agents, resolves within four weeks. Among the four major categories of chronic diarrhea — osmotic, secretory, fatty, and inflammatory — the fever and endoscopic and pathological findings point to an inflammatory process. Disorders to consider include Crohn's disease, Behçet's disease, and chronic infections such as gastrointestinal tuberculosis, histoplasmosis, and amebiasis. Ulcerating viral infections (such as cytomegalovirus and herpes simplex infection) would be important concerns in an immunocompromised patient.

While at the community hospital, the patient tested positive for *Clostridium difficile* toxin, but did not improve despite treatment with oral metronidazole and, subsequently, oral vancomycin. He was also treated aggressively for presumed Crohn's disease with mesalamine, corticosteroids (prednisone, 60 mg daily), and two infusions of infliximab — with no improvement. Because of increasing pain and abdominal distention, the patient was placed on total parenteral nutrition and transferred to the academic medical center for further management of his condition.

Risk factors for *C. difficile* infection include advanced age, hospitalization, and antibiotic exposure. Even without prior antibiotic use, the patient may have become colonized during a hospitalization. Most infections with *C. difficile* respond to vancomycin or metronidazole, and the lack of a response warrants a search for an alternative diagnosis. Furthermore, although rectal sparing has been described, the endoscopic findings are inconsistent with the diagnosis of *C. difficile* colitis. A flare-up of Crohn's disease is possible; an association between *C. difficile* infection and exacerbations of inflammatory bowel disease is well recognized. Although most patients with moderate-to-severe Crohn's disease respond to prednisone or infliximab (a chimeric tumor necrosis factor monoclonal antibody), the absence of a response does not rule out the diagnosis. Treatment with corticosteroids and infliximab for presumptive Crohn's disease without convincing histopathological evidence is potentially hazardous, given that chronic infections are well known to mimic Crohn's disease.

The patient was born in Guatemala and adopted at birth. He moved to the western United States at nine years of age with his adoptive family. He said that he had not traveled recently. He had had lifelong diarrhea, with several watery stools daily. The stools were small to moderate in volume, occasionally tinged with blood, but not greasy or notably foul smelling. He had undergone multiple evaluations and lower endoscopies and had been given a diagnosis of nonspecific colitis. Treatment with aminosalicylates and corticosteroids led to minimal improvement. At 12 years of age, he was diagnosed with colonic malacoplakia (yellowish, soft papules or nodules) at another academic medical center after colonic biopsy revealed histiocytes with intracytoplasmic inclusion bodies and intracellular bacilli. Extensive evaluation at that time showed no evidence of inflammatory bowel disease. Bacterial cultures and examination of stool samples for signs of ova and parasites were negative. In addition, acid-fast staining and cultures, including fungal cultures, of colonic-biopsy specimens were negative. He was treated with trimethoprim–sulfamethoxazole with moderate but temporary improvement, and diarrhea soon recurred. Further details of the medical history included a positive tuberculin skin test but a normal chest radiograph; he subsequently received oral isoniazid for six months. The patient reported no use of alcohol, tobacco, or illicit drugs, and he was not sexually active. He had received a blood transfusion during infancy for unknown reasons.

The patient's history of immigration from Central America suggests the possibility of tropical sprue, a syndrome that can occur in persons residing in certain tropical locations, which is presumed to be caused by small-bowel bacterial overgrowth and characterized by chronic diarrhea and malabsorption. However, tropical sprue is rare in Guatemala, and the characteristic pathological findings are limited to the small intestine, rather than the colon. Predisposing conditions for colonic malacoplakia include chronic infections by coliform bacteria and granulomatous processes, such as sarcoidosis and tuberculosis. Colonic tuberculosis usually causes ulcers with associated nodularity, a finding not observed in this patient. The diagnosis is established by culture or histologic examination, both of which were negative. Nonetheless, the yield from cultures and biopsy material may be low, and diagnosing intestinal tuberculosis may be particularly challenging in the absence of extraintestinal manifestations. The history of a blood transfusion during infancy raises the possibility of an underlying infection with the human immunodeficiency virus (HIV).

The patient appeared to be underdeveloped and chronically ill, with diminutive stature and decreased muscle mass. On physical examination, his height was 160 cm and his weight 47.5 kg. His temperature was 39.2°C, his blood pressure 98/40 mm Hg, his heart rate 94 beats per minute, and his respiratory rate 20 breaths per minute. His lungs were clear, and his cardiac examination showed no abnormalities. His abdomen was soft, with mild distention, normal bowel sounds, and no organomegaly. There was diffuse tenderness to palpation that was worse in the right lower quadrant, but without rebound tenderness. A rectal examination revealed no masses; a small amount of brown stool was obtained, which tested positive for occult blood. An examination of the skin revealed no lesions, and a neurologic examination showed no abnormalities.

The patient clearly has chronic diarrhea and resulting nutrient malabsorption, as reflected in his habitus. A complete blood count and measurements of prothrombin time and serum levels of electrolytes, albumin, calcium, phosphate, magnesium, iron, folate, and vitamin B_{12} should be obtained to screen for malabsorption; blood cultures should also be obtained. Abdominal computed tomography (CT) should be performed, with special attention to the ileocecal region for signs of mural and omental thickening, lymphadenopathy, ascites, or abscess. Fever, right-lower-quadrant pain, and an ileocecal distribution of inflammation may be clues to the presence of Crohn's disease, but they may also suggest a neoplasm or an infection that might include tuberculosis, histoplasmosis, amebiasis, *Mycobacterium avium* complex, and *Yersinia enterocolitica*.

The white-cell count was 5500 per cubic millimeter, with 10 percent band forms. The hematocrit was 36 percent, with a mean corpuscular volume of 81 μm^3, and the platelet count was 146,000 per cubic millimeter. Other laboratory values were as follows: sodium, 138 mmol per liter; chloride, 101 mmol per liter; potassium, 4.6 mmol per liter; bicarbonate, 33 mmol per liter; blood urea nitrogen, 11 mg per deciliter (3.93 mmol per liter); cre-

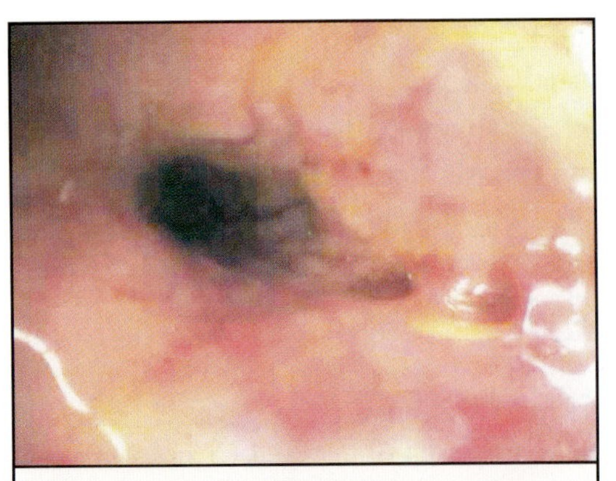

Figure 1. Stricture at the Hepatic Flexure on Endoscopy with Edema, Erythema, and Linear Ulcerations.

atinine, 0.9 mg per deciliter (79.6 mmol per liter); and lipase, 20 U per liter (normal range, 30 to 190). The calcium level was normal. The serum albumin level was 2.9 g per deciliter. The aspartate aminotransferase level was 95 U per liter (normal range, 15 to 59); the alanine aminotransferase level was normal. The prothrombin time was prolonged at 17.8 seconds (international normalized ratio, 1.4) with a normal partial thromboplastin time of 31 seconds. Chest radiography revealed no abnormalities. CT of the abdomen and pelvis showed a thickened cecum and terminal ileum, without signs of fistula, abscess, or free air.

The patient has mild anemia, probably the result of iron deficiency due to either malabsorption or chronic blood loss. Alternatively, an ongoing infection or inflammatory process could result in anemia of chronic disease. His prolonged prothrombin time is likely to reflect a deficiency of vitamin K resulting from malabsorption of fat-soluble vitamins, in which case I would expect it to be corrected with parenteral supplementation. Celiac sprue has been associated with elevated levels of serum aminotransferase that become normal when the patient adopts a gluten-free diet. A high prevalence of amebiasis is seen in the general population in Central America. Although the manifestation of intestinal amebiasis is typically subacute, it may be associated on rare occasions with a chronic nondysenteric infection accompanied by diarrhea, abdominal pain, and weight loss that may be present for years. The diagnosis rests on microscopical evidence of cysts or trophozoites in stool or endoscopic biopsy samples, both of which were negative in this patient. Tuberculosis is also a major health problem in Central America, particularly infection with drug-resistant strains. Exacerbations of intestinal tuberculosis mimicking Crohn's

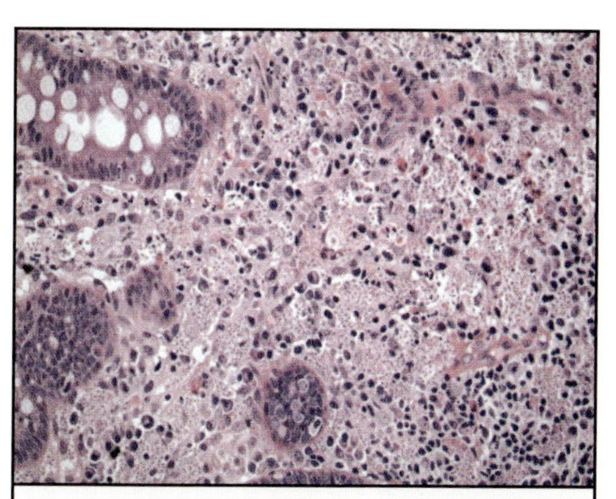

Figure 2. Colonic Mucosa with Chronic Inflammatory Infiltrate and Numerous *H. capsulatum* in Macrophages (Hematoxylin and Eosin).

disease have been reported after infliximab treatment similar to that received by this patient. I remain concerned about an undiagnosed intestinal infection.

The patient received intravenous fluids and total parenteral nutrition. His treatment with mesalamine was continued, and the dosage of prednisone was increased to 80 mg daily. Testing for HIV was negative. A repeated colonoscopy revealed normal-appearing mucosa from the distal colon to the proximal transverse colon, where patchy erythema, edema, and linear ulcerations were seen. A narrow stricture was encountered at the hepatic flexure, preventing safe advancement of the endoscope (Figure 1). Multiple biopsy samples were obtained, including tissue for viral and fungal cultures. A biopsy specimen was obtained from a single 4-mm nodule at the rectosigmoid junction. The clinical findings were thought to be consistent with Crohn's disease, and plans were made for surgery.

In reviewing all the data, including the poor response to therapy, I remain skeptical of the diagnosis of Crohn's disease. I am still concerned about a chronic infection; this should be ruled out before proceeding to surgery. Gastrointestinal tuberculosis, histoplasmosis, amebiasis, and actinomycosis have all been reported to mimic Crohn's disease. Aeromonas and yersinia, although typically self-limited infections, may last several weeks and would be considerations were this illness the patient's initial presentation. The patient's stool samples should be examined again for *Entamoeba histolytica* cysts and trophozoites. The cultures and histologic sections obtained from the endoscopic-biopsy specimens should be carefully evaluated for evidence of any of these pathogens.

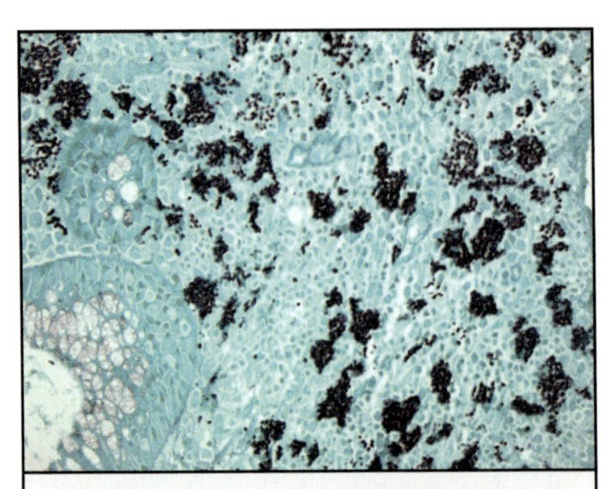

Figure 3. Sheets of *H. capsulatum* Staining Black with Gomori–Methenamine–Silver Stain.

Before surgery, the biopsy specimens were reviewed. Both the samples from the right-sided biopsies and the sample from the rectosigmoid nodule included numerous macrophages containing organisms compatible with *Histoplasma capsulatum* (Figure 2 and Figure 3). This was confirmed with Gomori–methenamine silver staining. There was no distortion in colonic crypts to suggest inflammatory bowel disease. A review of the peripheral-blood smear revealed previously undetected organisms in leukocytes, a finding that is consistent with histoplasmosis (Figure 4). The serum was strongly positive for histoplasma antigen, at 30 enzyme immunoassay units.

The patient has disseminated histoplasmosis, which involves the gastrointestinal tract in up to 70 percent of patients. The usual treatment is itraconazole, although amphotericin B is used in severely immunocompromised patients. This patient tested negative for HIV, but prolonged courses of corticosteroids and a potential underlying immunodeficiency that might have predisposed him to disseminated histoplasmosis support the use of amphotericin B until a clinical response, which may be slow, is observed.

The patient was started on therapy with amphotericin B, and the corticosteroids were slowly decreased. Three days after the new drug was introduced, hypotension and a rigid abdomen developed. Exploratory laparotomy revealed extensive bowel necrosis; a right hemicolectomy and distal ileal resection with ileostomy were performed. Blood cultures grew *Streptococcus mitis*. The resected bowel showed extensive histoplasmosis. The patient's hospital course was complicated by nosocomial pneumonia and the abdominal compartment syndrome, which required prolonged open decompression of the abdomen. He

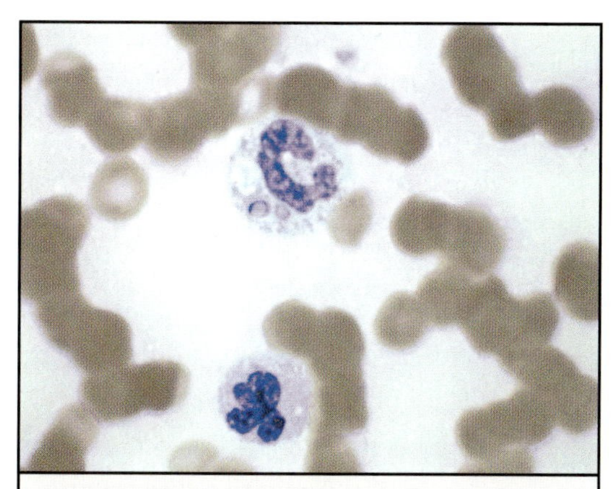

Figure 4. Peripheral-Blood Smear Showing Intracellular Organisms.

eventually underwent partial surgical closure of his abdomen with mesh placement. Superficial layers healed subsequently by secondary intention. He was discharged to his home with treatment with oral itraconazole to continue for six months. Sixteen months after hospital discharge, he reported feeling well and had gained 25 kg.

Abdominal perforation is a recognized complication of gastrointestinal histoplasmosis — a complication that might have been avoided with an earlier diagnosis and medical treatment. Despite his complicated course, his improved general health and weight gain at follow-up indicate successful treatment of his infection.

COMMENTARY

A challenge that clinicians face on a daily basis is deciding when they have sufficient information to make a diagnosis. Clinical medicine is filled with scenarios in which ruling out a condition that mimics another disorder is important. One example is the necessity to rule out pulmonary tuberculosis or an anaerobic infection in an elderly patient with a history of smoking who presents with a cavitary lung mass. The current case provides another example: the need to consider infections that may mimic inflammatory bowel disease.

Unfortunately, no single test is perfectly sensitive and specific for Crohn's disease. The diagnosis relies on a consistent historical, endoscopic, radiographic, and histopathological pattern. As was seen with the patient in this case, management with early, aggressive immunosuppression without a definitive diagnosis can lead to catastrophic consequences when a chronic infection goes undiagnosed.

Histoplasmosis, which primarily affects the lungs, is caused by a dimorphic fungus endemic to river valleys in the midwestern and southeastern United States, as well as Central America and South America. The organism is transmitted by inhalation of spores from soil contaminated by bat or bird droppings. Histoplasmosis is not an easy diagnosis to make. Indeed, Goodwin and colleagues noted two decades ago that "the diagnosis of histoplasmosis begins with thinking of it."[1]

More than 90 percent of infected persons remain asymptomatic and are identified only as a result of abnormal chest radiographs or positive skin testing.[2] Fewer than 10 percent of all recognized cases represent disseminated disease. Disseminated disease is uncommon in immunocompetent patients, but it is common when infection occurs in immunocompromised patients.[3] Gastrointestinal involvement occurs in 70 to 90 percent of patients with disseminated disease and has been reported primarily in immunocompromised patients.[3-6]

Clinical manifestations of gastrointestinal histoplasmosis range from none, in asymptomatic infection, to nausea, vomiting, diarrhea, bleeding, abdominal pain, weight loss, obstruction, and perforation. The most frequently involved sites are the terminal ileum and cecum.[4] Endoscopic findings include plaques, small polyps, mucosal edema, ulcerations, strictures, and masses.[3,6] Definitive diagnosis is made by histologic examination or culture growth, with subsequent identification of *H. capsulatum*. Histoplasmosis antigen in serum or urine is specific and sensitive, and organisms may occasionally be detected on a peripheral-blood smear. Serologic testing for antibodies is less reliable, since immunocompromised patients may be anergic.[4] Treatment options include intravenous amphotericin B or oral itraconazole; early treatment usually results in good outcomes.

Certainly, this patient's diarrhea, right-lower-quadrant pain, and endoscopic findings of ileocecal inflammation and stricture could have been consistent with Crohn's disease. Several clues, however, raised the suspicion of a chronic infection that mimicked Crohn's disease, including the patient's childhood in Central America and the substantial mononuclear cell inflammation on colonic-biopsy specimens, in the absence of the distortion of crypt architecture or granulomas typical of Crohn's disease.

An important additional clue that the diagnosis was incorrect was the poor clinical response to aggressive treatment for Crohn's disease. Corticosteroid therapy typically results in short-term response rates of 80 to 90 percent among patients with moderate-to-severe Crohn's disease.[7] Patients with Crohn's disease that is refractory to aminosalicylates and corticosteroids have short-term responses to infliximab 50 to 80 percent of the time.[8] Rather than improving while receiving these agents, this patient's condition worsened. In retrospect, the infliximab may have led to his decompensation.

Infliximab, along with etanercept, exerts biologic effects through antagonism of tumor necrosis factor α. Several reports have documented disseminated histoplasmosis in patients treated with infliximab or etanercept for rheumatoid arthritis or Crohn's disease.[9-11] Cell cultures infected with *H. capsulatum* and treated with infliximab show proliferation of the organism and decreased lymphocyte proliferation.[9] Tuberculosis has also been reported in patients treated with infliximab, and tuberculin skin testing is routinely performed before the initiation of infliximab therapy.[12] Although routine testing for histoplasmosis is not recommended before infliximab therapy is initiated, a test for histoplasmosis antigen in urine or serum could have been helpful in this case, especially since the diagnosis was uncertain.

The lack of a pathognomonic test for Crohn's disease makes this condition one that is frequently misdiagnosed.[13] The identification of chronic infections may be particularly challenging, since their diagnosis may require multiple biopsies, large amounts of sample tissue, special culture media, and prolonged culture times. This case demonstrates that infections precipitated by antagonists to tumor necrosis factor α may mimic Crohn's disease. Diligence — leaving no stone unturned — will facilitate the appropriate diagnosis and treatment of these challenging conditions.

Dr. Saint is the recipient of a Career Development Award from the Health Services Research and Development Program of the Department of Veterans Affairs; his work is supported by a Patient Safety Developmental Center Grant (P20-HS11540) from the Agency for Healthcare Research and Quality.

Dr. Moseley reports having received consulting fees from Pfizer for serving as an expert witness.

This article first appeared in the February 3, 2005, issue of the New England Journal of Medicine.

Figures 2 and 3 have been revised in this version to correct an error in the original publication. A correction notice was published in the April 21, 2005, issue.

REFERENCES

1. Goodwin RA, Loyd JE, Des Prez RM. Histoplasmosis in normal hosts. Medicine (Baltimore) 1981;60:231-66.

2. Deepe GS Jr. *Histoplasmosis capsulatum*. In: Mandell GL, Bennett JE, Dolin R, eds. Mandell, Douglas, and Bennett's principles and practice of infectious disease. 5th ed. Philadelphia: Churchill Livingstone, 2000: 2718-33.

3. Lamps LW, Molina CP, West AB, Haggitt RC, Scott MA. The pathologic spectrum of gastrointestinal and hepatic histoplasmosis. Am J Clin Pathol 2000;113: 64-72.

4. Cappell MS, Mandell W, Grimes MM, Neu HC. Gastrointestinal histoplasmosis. Dig Dis Sci 1988;33:353-60.

5. Mullick SS, Mody DR, Schwartz MR. Cytology of gastrointestinal histoplasmosis: a report of two cases with differential diagnosis and diagnostic pitfalls. Acta Cytol 1996;40:989-94.

6. Hertan H, Nair S, Arguello P. Progressive gastrointestinal histoplasmosis leading to colonic obstruction two years after initial presentation. Am J Gastroenterol 2001;96:221-2.

7. Sands B. Crohn's disease. In: Feldman M, Friedman LS, Sleisenger MH, eds. Sleisenger and Fordtran's gastrointestinal and liver disease. 7th ed. Philadelphia: Saunders, 2002:2005-38.

8. Targan SR, Hanauer SB, van Deventer SJ, et al. A short-term study of chimeric monoclonal antibody cA2 to tumor necrosis factor α for Crohn's disease. N Engl J Med 1997;337: 1029-35.

9. Wood KL, Hage CA, Knox KS, et al. Histoplasmosis after treatment with anti-tumor necrosis factor-α therapy. Am J Respir Crit Care Med 2003;167:1279-82.

10. Lee JH, Slifman NR, Gershon SK, et al. Life-threatening histoplasmosis complicating immunotherapy with tumor necrosis factor α antagonists infliximab and etanercept. Arthritis Rheum 2002;46: 2565-70.

11. Colombel JF, Loftus EV Jr, Tremaine WJ, et al. The safety profile of infliximab in patients with Crohn's disease: the Mayo Clinic experience in 500 patients. Gastroenterology 2004;126: 19-31.

12. Keane J, Gershon S, Wise RP, et al. Tuberculosis associated with infliximab, a tumor necrosis factor α–neutralizing agent. N Engl J Med 2001;345:1098-104.

13. Lavy A, Militianu D, Eidelman S. Diseases of the intestine mimicking Crohn's disease. J Clin Gastroenterol 1992;15: 17-23.

On the Threshold — A Diagnosis of Exclusion

PETER CLARKE, M.D., SUSAN GLICK, M.D.,
AND BRENDAN M. REILLY, M.D.

A 48-year-old airline mechanic from Belize presented to the emergency department with fever and altered mental status.

Two weeks earlier, fever, myalgias, and dry cough had developed. His maximal daily temperature reached as high as 41.1°C, and one week before coming to the emergency department, the patient awakened unable to speak. At a hospital in Belize, he was febrile and aphasic without other focal neurologic findings. The results of computed tomography (CT) of the brain were normal. Examination of the cerebrospinal fluid revealed a protein level of 157 mg per deciliter and a glucose level of 44 mg per deciliter (2.4 mmol per liter) but no cells or microorganisms. The patient received treatment with chloroquine and acyclovir for the next five days but did not improve and was flown to Chicago for further care.

On examination, the patient was agitated and unable to speak or follow verbal commands. The blood pressure was 132/74 mm Hg, the pulse 82 beats per minute, and the respiratory rate 20 breaths per minute. The temperature was 39.5°C. The results of the general examination were normal, without meningismus. A neurologic examination revealed global aphasia but was otherwise normal except for an equivocal extensor plantar response on the right. The optic fundi appeared normal.

Fever with aphasia and an absence of other neurologic abnormalities suggest an inflammatory process involving a discrete area of the dominant cerebral cortex in the temporoparietal or frontal region, or both. The apparently sudden onset of aphasia suggests a vascular process, such as a septic embolism, vasculitis, or hemorrhage into an abscess or neoplasm. In a patient from Central America, neurocysticercosis must also be considered. Has the patient had seizures? Other primary infections that might occur in an immunocompetent patient include viral encephalitis (especially due to herpes simplex virus), acute disseminated encephalomyelitis, and tuberculosis — but the reported absence of cells in the spinal fluid argues against these diagnoses. Because the patient's immune status is unknown, I would also be concerned about fungal disease, toxoplasmosis, and other opportunistic infections.

I would reexamine the patient, looking particularly for signs of infective endocarditis (such as Roth's spots or splinter hemorrhages). I would also obtain additional images of the brain, preferably with magnetic resonance imaging (MRI), obtain blood cultures and malaria smears, and test for the human immunodeficiency virus (HIV).

The white-cell count was 10,300 per cubic millimeter, with 80 percent polymorphonuclear leukocytes. The hematocrit, platelet count, electrolyte levels, levels of urea nitrogen and creatinine, liver-enzyme levels, smears for malaria, and results of the urinalysis, toxicologic screen, chest radiography, and the test for HIV were normal. Blood cultures were obtained. The findings on contrast-enhanced CT of the brain were normal.

Examination of cerebrospinal fluid revealed 15 red cells and 30 white cells per cubic millimeter (21 lymphocytes and 9 neutrophils); the protein level was 140 mg per deciliter, the glucose level 33 mg per deciliter (1.8 mmol per liter), and the serum glucose level 100 mg per deciliter (5.5 mmol per liter). But the results of Gram's staining, a smear for acid-fast bacilli, India-ink preparation, and a test for cryptococcal antigen were negative.

The patient was hospitalized, and treatment was begun with intravenous ceftriaxone, vancomycin, and acyclovir.

The normal results of the patient's imaging studies are perplexing. A cortical infarct, abscess, or mass should be visible by now, one week after the onset of aphasia. Is it certain that the patient is aphasic? Mutism associated with cerebellar or brain-stem disease (for which CT may be a less reliable method of diagnosis) can be confused with aphasia.

Lymphocytic pleocytosis with hypoglycorrhachia suggests tuberculous, fungal, or carcinomatous meningitis, any of which can cause stroke due to contiguous vascular involvement. Has the patient lost weight or had prior systemic symptoms?

I would immediately perform MRI of the brain and a tuberculin skin test. In addition to bacterial, fungal, and mycobacterial cultures, I would test the cerebrospinal fluid with the polymerase chain reaction (PCR) for herpes simplex virus and *Mycobacterium tuberculosis*. Pending the results of these studies, broad-spectrum antibiotics, including acyclovir, should be continued.

A neurology consultant agreed that the patient was globally aphasic, with no other focal neurologic findings. MRI of the brain revealed increased signal intensity along the left sylvian fissure and the adjacent left frontal lobe, with localized leptomeningeal enhancement (Figure 1). The neuroradiologist's impression was that the focus of the differential diagnosis should be "meningoencephalitis versus vasculitis."

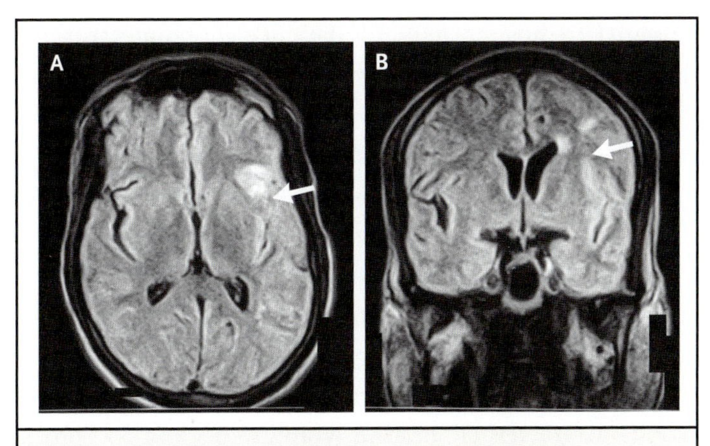

Figure 1. Axial (Panel A) and Coronal (Panel B) Magnetic Resonance Images of Left Frontotemporal Parietal Abnormality (Arrows).

Additional information was obtained. Three months before the current illness, the patient had been aphasic for several days without other symptoms. At that time, he was flown to Houston, where MRI abnormalities in the left frontal cortex were reported as "consistent with possible vasculitis." He was treated with phenytoin prophylactically. His aphasia subsequently resolved, and he stopped taking phenytoin one month later. In the ensuing six weeks before his current presentation, he was reportedly well.

His history was otherwise remarkable only for infrequent migraine headaches that occurred over a period of 20 years, without associated neurologic symptoms, and recurrent oral ulcers. He did not use tobacco, alcohol, or drugs. He had not lost weight.

A relapsing course of symptoms such as the patient had over three months argues against most of the infectious disorders initially considered. Noninfectious inflammatory processes, such as sarcoidosis or vasculitis, are possible. The history of oral ulcers is intriguing, but no other clinical findings suggest systemic lupus erythematosus or Behçet's disease. Giant-cell arteritis is very improbable in a patient of this age. Primary central nervous system (CNS) angiitis, a granulomatous vasculitis limited to the nervous system that may cause either focal or diffuse neurologic impairment (and lymphocytic pleocytosis), is rare but must be considered.

I would perform tests for antinuclear and antineutrophil cytoplasmic antibodies and also try to obtain further information about the patient's previous evaluations in Houston and Belize. If initial cultures are negative, I would repeat the lumbar puncture.

On the second through fifth hospital days, the patient had a temperature as high as 40.0°C. The results of a neurologic examination showed no change.

Blood and cerebrospinal fluid cultures revealed no growth after 72 hours. Transesophageal echocardiography showed no abnormalities. Tests of serum and cerebrospinal fluid for syphilis and a tuberculin skin test were negative. Assays for toxoplasma IgG and *Borrelia burgdorferi* antibodies were negative. An electroencephalogram showed nonspecific diffuse slowing. The results of tests for antinuclear and antineutrophil cytoplasmic antibodies, protein electropheresis, and evaluation of complement levels were normal. The sedimentation rate was 69 mm per hour.

On the sixth hospital day, a repeated lumbar puncture showed 130 red cells and 510 white cells per cubic millimeter (61 percent lymphocytes and 39 percent neutrophils), with negative results on Gram's staining, an acid-fast smear, an India-ink preparation, and cytologic evaluation. Protein and glucose levels in the cerebrospinal fluid were not measured; oligoclonal bands were absent. Ceftriaxone and vancomycin were discontinued. A treatment regimen of isoniazid, rifampin, pyrazinamide, ethambutol, and pyridoxine was begun.

Considering the diagnostic importance of hypoglycorrhachia in a febrile patient with lymphocytic pleocytosis, the level of glucose in the spinal fluid should be measured again. Fungal meningitis is very improbable in an immunocompetent patient. A prolonged, relapsing clinical course is unusual in tuberculous or carcinomatous meningitis, but I agree with the recommendation of empirical antituberculosis treatment, and I would search for a primary cancer.

CT of the neck, chest, abdomen, and pelvis revealed no abnormalities. The serum level of angiotensin-converting enzyme (ACE) was normal.

Cerebrospinal fluid PCR tests were negative for *M. tuberculosis*, cytomegalovirus, the Epstein–Barr virus, herpes simplex virus, herpes zoster virus, and enteroviruses. Tests of serum for antibodies to the California, eastern equine, western equine, and St. Louis encephalitis viruses were negative. Acyclovir was discontinued.

On the sixth through ninth hospital days, the patient's condition remained unchanged. His temperature was as high as 40°C daily, and he remained unable to communicate. Treatment with doxycycline was begun, pending the results of serologic studies for rickettsia and brucella.

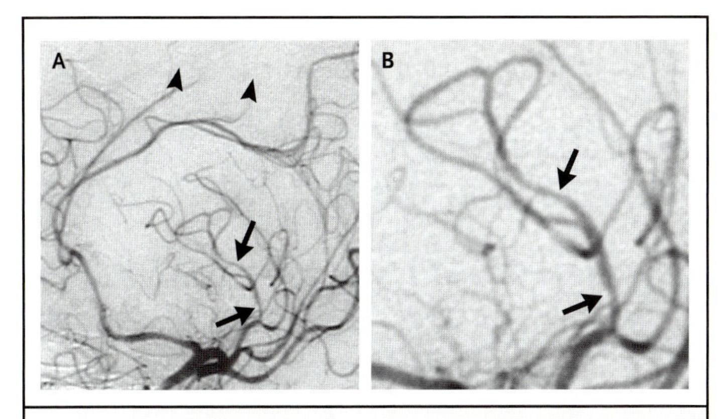

Figure 2. Cerebral Angiogram.

Panel A shows irregular narrowing of the middle cerebral artery (arrows) and decreased parenchymal blush in the distribution of the middle and anterior cerebral arteries (arrowheads). Panel B is a magnification of the same area.

The normal results on CT imaging of the body reaffirm the probability that the disease is limited to the brain. A normal serum level of ACE does not rule out the diagnosis of sarcoidosis, but isolated CNS sarcoid is very rare. Coverage with doxycycline is appropriate because the patient's clinical findings and cerebrospinal fluid findings are consistent with brucellosis. Rickettsial diseases seem highly improbable, with the possible exception of Q fever (caused by *Coxiella burnetii*).

Unless the patient has a dramatic response to the current antibiotic therapy, I would push for brain biopsy. I doubt that cerebral angiography would be definitive.

On the 10th hospital day, cerebral arteriography revealed marked attenuation, narrowing, and irregularities of the left middle and anterior cerebral arteries, with decreased parenchymal blush (small-vessel perfusion) in those regions (Figure 2). The neuroradiologist's impression of the findings was "focal asymmetric cerebral angiitis, primary versus secondary to meningoencephalitis." Treatment with felodipine was begun.

The angiographic findings correlate with the patient's clinical findings, but the underlying cause of the vascular abnormalities remains unclear. We must consider systemic vasculitides, drug-induced vasculitis (e.g., due to amphetamines), and neoplasms (including lymphoma), but none of these diagnoses seem likely. The patient's high fever — not a common finding in primary CNS angiitis — mandates that we rule out infection with vasculotropic organisms such as herpesviruses, fungi, and other organisms, including *M. tuberculosis*, that are known to cause secondary CNS angiitis.

On hospital days 10 through 17, the patient's temperature spiked to 40°C daily despite antituberculosis therapy and treatment with doxycycline, phenytoin, and felodipine. He remained aphasic. All cultures were negative.

On hospital day 18, intravenous methylprednisolone therapy was begun for probable primary CNS angiitis, on the advice of a consulting rheumatologist. The neurology consultant recommended brain biopsy.

The patient has shown no signs of improvement after almost two weeks of broad-spectrum antibiotic therapy, and the diagnosis remains unclear. As I have already noted, I agree with the recommendation for brain biopsy.

On hospital day 19, an open left-frontal brain biopsy was performed. Grossly, the dura was thickened and adherent to the arachnoid and the pia. The adjacent cerebral cortex was noted to feel rubbery. Biopsy specimens were obtained from the cortex and leptomeninges.

During the next 48 hours, low-grade fever (38.3°C) persisted, but the patient's condition appeared improved, and he began to speak haltingly. Serum titers of antibodies to rickettsia and brucella were negative. Doxycycline was stopped.

Microscopical examination of biopsy specimens revealed noncaseating granulomas and an intense lymphocytic infiltrate involving small blood vessels, the leptomeninges, and the adjacent cerebral cortex (Figure 3). Tissue and cerebrospinal fluid smears for bacteria, acid-fast bacilli, parasites, fungi, and malignant cells were negative. PCR testing was negative for *M. tuberculosis*, cytomegalovirus, herpes simplex virus, varicella–zoster virus, human herpesvirus 6, and JC and BK viruses.

We have now done all we can to make a diagnosis. The granulomatous histologic findings are nonspecific. However, I believe we can rule out viral, fungal, and rickettsial causes with confidence. Given the patient's relapsing clinical course; the negative tuberculin test, acid-fast smears, and DNA tests on multiple spinal-fluid and brain-tissue specimens; and the lack of clinical improvement after two weeks of antituberculosis therapy, the diagnosis of tuberculosis seems so unlikely that I believe that empirical antituberculosis therapy can be discontinued. There is no evidence of neoplasm or systemic vasculitis. By a process of exclusion, primary CNS angiitis is the most likely diagnosis.

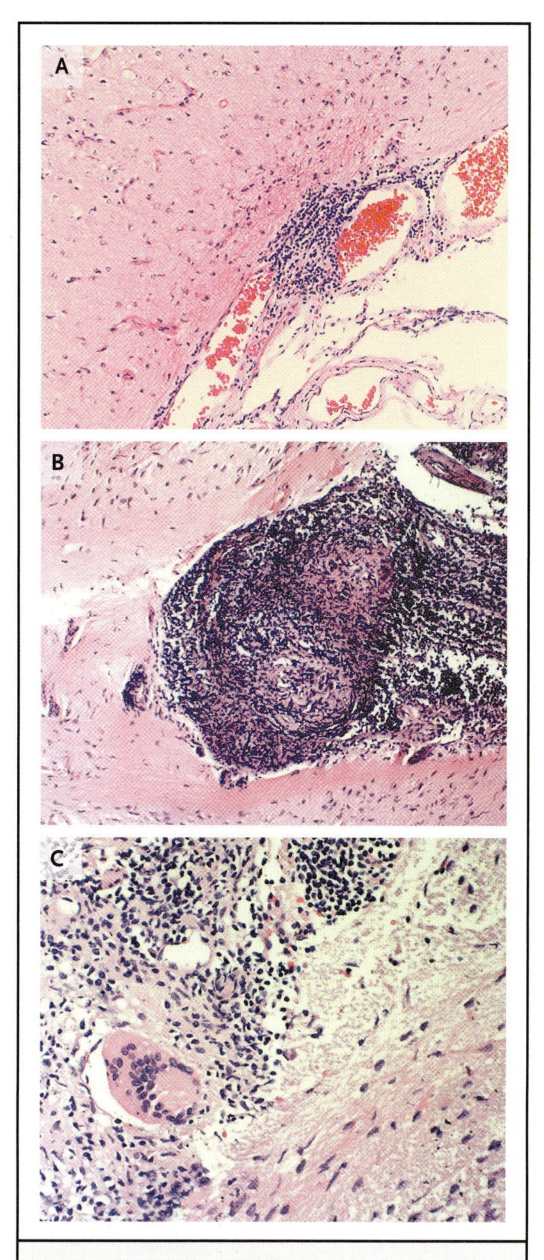

Figure 3. Brain-Biopsy Specimen (Hematoxylin and Eosin).

Panel A shows a lymphocytic infiltrate involving the leptomeninges, adjacent cerebral cortex, and small blood vessels with noncaseating granulomas. Panels B and C show higher-power magnifications of the granulomas.

I would treat the patient with corticosteroids and follow his response clinically and with MRI.

During the following week, the patient's fever resolved, and he became more interactive verbally, but he remained markedly dysphasic (with poor comprehension, repetition, and naming facilities). Treatment with prednisone (60 mg daily) and the antituberculosis therapy were continued. The results of bronchoscopic biopsy and transbronchial biopsies were normal. In light of the patient's persistent severe verbal disability, the rheumatology consultant recommended the addition of high-dose cyclophosphamide therapy for primary CNS angiitis. The consultants in neurology and infectious diseases agreed but also recommended full antituberculosis treatment for 12 months.

An intravenous infusion of 1300 mg of cyclophosphamide was given.

The evidence to support the addition of cyclophosphamide as first-line therapy for primary CNS angiitis is not strong. In this case, the patient's condition is already improving, and we must consider the potential toxicity of cyclophosphamide. My recommendation would be to treat with corticosteroids alone and follow the patient carefully.

All cultures remained negative. On hospital day 35, the patient was discharged to his home in Belize while receiving daily prednisone and antituberculosis therapy, with plans for a second infusion of high-dose cyclophosphamide in the next month. At the time of discharge, he appeared greatly improved but remained dysphasic.

Three weeks later, the laboratory reported positive cerebrospinal fluid cultures for isoniazid-sensitive *M. tuberculosis.* Cultures of brain and lung tissue were sterile. Cyclophosphamide was stopped. Antituberculosis therapy was continued, and prednisone therapy was tapered gradually.

One year later, the patient is doing well.

Hats off to those who insisted on treatment for tuberculosis despite the patient's unusual clinical presentation and multiple negative tests. That decision may well have been lifesaving.

COMMENTARY

During the primary infection, *M. tuberculosis* disseminates widely before cell-mediated immune mechanisms either kill or contain the organisms.[1] In the latter event, caseous tubercles containing live bacilli (so-called Rich foci) can be found in the CNS many years after the primary infection.[2] If one of these foci ruptures, typically when host immunity wanes, tuberculous meningitis (rupture into the ventricle or subarachnoid space) or tuberculoma (rupture into the brain or spinal cord) will develop. We speculate that our patient's initial aphasia resulted from rupture of a caseous tubercle into his frontotemporal cortex. After improving temporarily, he worsened as the infection and local inflammatory response spread to involve the adjacent blood vessels and meninges.

This clinical syndrome — tuberculous meningoencephalitis with granulomatous vasculitis — is rarely seen today in immunocompetent adults native to North America. However, it remains an important concern in people living in or emigrating from countries with a high prevalence of tuberculosis.[3] The prevalence of tuberculosis in Belize, for example, is about 10 times that in the United States.

The diagnosis of CNS tuberculosis is notoriously difficult to make.[1] Half of afflicted patients show no clinical signs of pulmonary (or other extraneural) involvement. Typical symptoms (e.g., headache and low-grade fever) are nonspecific. Progressive worsening is the rule, but relapsing clinical courses, as in this patient, have been reported.[4] Abnormal neurologic findings may be absent (in stage 1 disease) or striking (stupor, coma, or dense hemiplegia in stage 3 disease), but most patients present with stage 2 disease, accompanied by signs (confusion, cranial-nerve palsies, or hemiparesis) that mimic many other disorders.[5,6] Abnormalities on CT and MRI scanning are common (in 70 to 80 percent of patients) but nonspecific; hydrocephalus, meningeal or parenchymal enhancement, mass lesions, or infarction may be seen.[7,8] Cerebrospinal fluid may be normal on examination early in the clinical course, and 25 percent of patients never have what would be considered the classic cerebrospinal fluid profile (lymphocytic pleocytosis, elevated protein levels, and low glucose levels). Smears for acid-fast bacilli in cerebrospinal fluid are positive in only 20 percent of cases,[1] and the sensitivity of PCR testing (30 to 80 percent) has been disappointing.[9,10] The gold standard test — spinal-fluid culture for *M. tuberculosis* — requires several weeks to complete and is negative in as many as half of all patients who improve clinically with antituberculosis treatment. Thus, the diagnosis requires both a high index of suspicion and the knowledge that, as Zuger and Lowy have stated, "All premortem means of diagnosing [CNS tuberculosis] must be assumed to be fallible."[1]

As the discussant noted, primary CNS angiitis is very rare; there were only 108 cases reported in the English-language literature over a 40-year period.[11,12] Such so-called zebra diagnoses should always prompt skepticism, because a common presentation of a rare disease is less likely than a rare presentation of a common disease. This rule of thumb is especially germane to our case, because primary CNS angiitis is a diagnosis of exclusion: it cannot be made until all other secondary causes are disproved, especially infectious diseases, such as tuberculosis, that may worsen if treated mistakenly with corticosteroids alone. Fortunately for our patient, his physicians knew this. Untreated CNS tuberculosis is invariably fatal. With treatment, 70 to 85 percent of patients survive, half of them with no residual neurologic disability.[5]

Even if primary CNS angiitis were considered the more probable diagnosis, a "threshold approach" to clinical problem-solving could have avoided the discussant's (potentially disastrous) treatment error in this case.[13] Under conditions of diagnostic uncertainty, empirical treatment is indicated for all diagnoses whose probability exceeds their treatment threshold. (This term refers to the probability of disease at which there is no clear advantage for either empirical treatment or no treatment.) For CNS tuberculosis, this threshold probability is very low because the potential harm of antituberculosis drugs is very small (risk of fatal hepatitis, approximately 0.1 percent)[14] and their potential benefit very great.[5] In other words, empiric antituberculosis treatment should be given even if the probability of CNS tuberculosis is very low and another diagnosis seems more plausible. Once this critical decision is made to "cover" the patient for tuberculosis, the decision also to begin corticosteroid treatment is an easy one. Corticosteroids are not only the mainstay of treatment for primary CNS angiitis[12]; they are also recommended (as adjunctive treatment) for CNS tuberculosis.[15]

This article first appeared in the March 3, 2005, issue of the New England Journal of Medicine.

REFERENCES

1.
Zuger A, Lowy FD. Tuberculosis. In: Scheld WM, Whitley RJ, Durack DT, eds. Infections of the central nervous system. 2nd ed. Philadelphia: Lippincott-Raven, 1997:417-43.

2.
Rich AR, McCordock HA. The pathogenesis of tuberculous meningitis. Bull Johns Hopkins Hosp 1933;52:5-37.

3.
Dye C, Scheele S, Dolin P, Pathania V, Raviglione MC. Consensus statement: global burden of tuberculosis: estimated incidence, prevalence, and mortality by country. JAMA 1999;282:677-86.

4.
Kasik J. Central nervous system tuberculosis. In: Schlossberg D, ed. Tuberculosis and nontuberculous mycobacterial infections. 4th ed. Philadelphia: W.B. Saunders, 1999:175-85.

5.
Humphries M. The management of tuberculous meningitis. Thorax 1992;47:577-81.

6.
Kennedy DH, Fallon RJ. Tuberculous meningitis. JAMA 1979;241:264-8.

7.
Ozates M, Kemaloglu S, Gurkan F, Ozkan U, Hosoglu S, Simsek MM. CT of the brain in tuberculous meningitis: a review of 289 patients. Acta Radiol 2000;41:13-7.

8.
Offenbacher H, Fazekas F, Schmidt R, et al. MRI in tuberculous meningoencephalitis: report of four cases and review of the neuroimaging literature. J Neurol 1991;238:340-4.

9.
Nguyen LN, Kox LFF, Pham LD, Kuijper S, Kolk AHJ. The potential contribution of the polymerase chain reaction to the diagnosis of tuberculosis meningitis. Arch Neurol 1996;53:771-6.

10.
Sarmiento OL, Weigle KA, Alexander J, Weber DJ, Miller WC. Assessment by meta-analysis of PCR for diagnosis of smear-negative pulmonary tuberculosis. J Clin Microbiol 2003;41:3233-40.

11.
Calabrese LH, Mallek JA. Primary angiitis of the central nervous system: report of 8 new cases, review of the literature, and proposal for diagnostic criteria. Medicine (Baltimore) 1987;67:20-39.

12.
Calabrese LH, Furlan AJ, Gragg LA, Ropos TJ. Primary angiitis of the central nervous system: diagnostic criteria and clinical approach. Cleve Clin J Med 1992;59:293-306.

13.
Pauker SG, Kassirer JP. The threshold approach to clinical decision making. N Engl J Med 1980;302:1109-17.

14.
Chitturi S, Farrell GC. Drug-induced liver disease. In: Schiff ER, Sorrell MF, Maddrey WC, eds. Schiff's diseases of the liver. 9th ed. Philadelphia: Lippincott Williams & Wilkins, 2003:1059-127.

15.
American Thoracic Society/Centers for Disease Control and Prevention/Infectious Diseases Society of America: treatment of tuberculosis. Am J Respir Crit Care Med 2003;167:603-62.

INDEX

Page numbers followed by italic f or t denote figures or tables, respectively.

C

D